Schizophrenia in children and adolescents

The earlier in life schizophrenia manifests itself, the poorer the long-term prognosis, and although it is very difficult to diagnose in the young, early treatment is now thought to improve outcome. Recent research also suggests that early onset schizophrenia has developmental precursors, making it difficult to distinguish from a number of other developmental disorders. In this timely book, an international team of psychiatrists, psychotherapists and psychologists give an up-to-date review of the latest findings in the diagnosis and treatment of schizophrenia in children and adolescents to give a comprehensive account of the current state of knowledge and the therapeutic options available to clinicians. They examine the disorder from developmental and clinical perspectives, with a focus on diagnosis, etiology, therapy, and rehabilitation. This book is essen~ young people with schizophrenia

Helmut Rem rtment of Child and Adolescent Ps videly in the field of child and adolescent psychiatry, with p developmental psychopathology, schizophrenia research, psychiatric genetics, valuation research.

Cambridge Child and Adolescent Psychiatry

Child and adolescent psychiatry is an important and growing area of clinical psychiatry. The last decade has seen a rapid expansion of scientific knowledge in this field and has provided a new understanding of the underlying pathology of mental disorders in these age groups. This series is aimed at practitioners and researchers both in child and adolescent mental health services and developmental and clinical neuroscience. Focusing on psychopathology, it highlights those topics where the growth of knowledge has had the greatest impact on clinical practice and on the treatment and understanding of mental illness. Individual volumes benefit both from the international expertise of their contributors and a coherence generated through a uniform style and structure for the series. Each volume provides firstly an historical overview and a clear descriptive account of the psychopathology of a specific disorder or group of related disorders. These features then form the basis for a thorough critical review of the etiology, natural history, management, prevention and impact on later adult adjustment. Whilst each volume is therefore complete in its own right, volumes also relate to each other to create a flexible and collectable series that should appeal to students as well as experienced scientists and practitioners.

Editorial board

Already published in this series:

Schizophrenia in children and adolescents

Edited by

Helmut Remschmidt

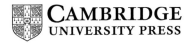

CAMBRIDGE
UNIVERSITY PRESS

PUBLISHED BY THE PRESS SYNDICATE OF THE UNIVERSITY OF CAMBRIDGE

The Pitt Building, Trumpington Street, Cambridge, United Kingdom

CAMBRIDGE UNIVERSITY PRESS

The Edinburgh Building, Cambridge CB2 2RU, UK

40 West 20th Street, New York, NY 10011-4211, USA

10 Stamford Road, Oakleigh, VIC 3166, Australia

Ruiz do Alarcón 13, 28014 Madrid, Spain

Dock House, The Waterfront, Cape Town 8001, South Africa

http://www,cambridge.org

First published 2001

Printed in the United Kingdom at the University Press, Cambridge

Typeset in Dante MT 11/14pt [VN]

A catalogue record for this book is available from the British Library

Library of Congress Cataloguing in Publication data

ISBN 0 521 79428 5 paperback

Every effort has been made in preparing this book to provide accurate and up-to-date information which is in accord with accepted standards and practice at the time of publication. Nevertheless, the authors, editors and publisher can make no warranties that the information contained herein is totally free from error, not least because clinical standards are constantly changing through research and regulation. The authors, editors and publisher therefore disclaim all liability for direct or consequential damages resulting from the use of material contained in this book. Readers are strongly advised to pay careful attention to information provided by the manufacturer of any drugs or equipment that they plan to use.

This book is dedicated to the memory of
William Ll. Parry-Jones and Michael Goldstein.

Contents

Contributors

Joan R. Asarnow
UCLA Neuropsychiatric Institute and
Hospital
Division of Child and Adolescent Psychiatry
760 Westwood Plaza
Los Angeles, CA 90024-1759,
USA

Robert F. Asarnow
UCLA Neuropsychiatric Institute and
Hospital
Division of Child and Adolescent Psychiatry
760 Westwood Plaza
Los Angeles, CA 90024-1759,
USA

Christopher Gillberg
Section of Child and Adolescent Psychiatry
Annedals Clinics
S-41345 Göteborg
Sweden

Michael J. Goldstein (deceased)
UCLA Neuropsychiatric Institute and
Hospital
Division of Child and Adolescent Psychiatry
760 Westwood Plaza
Los Angeles, CA 90024-1759,
USA

Klaus Hennighausen
Abt. für Psychiatrie und Psychotherapie
im Kindes- und Jungendalter
Albert Ludwigs Universität
Hauptstr. 8
D-79104 Freiburg
Germany

Chris Hollis
Department of Child and Adolescent
Psychiatry
University of Nottingham
Queen's Medical Centre
Clifton Boulevard
Nottingham NG7 2UH
UK

Canan Karatekin
UCLA Neuropsychiatric Institute and
Hospital
Division of Child and Adolescent Psychiatry
76 Westwood Plaza
Los Angeles, CA 90024-1759
USA

Matthias Martin
Klinik für Psychiatrie und Psychotherapie
des Kindes- und Jugendalters der
Philipps-Universität
Hans-Sachs-Str.6
D-35033 Marburg
Germany

Peter McGuffin
Institute of Psychiatry
Denmark Hill
London SE 58 AF
UK

Sally N. Merry
School of Medicine, University of Auckland
Department of Psychiatry and Behavioural
Science
32 Glendowie Road, Auckland
New Zealand

William Ll. Parry-Jones (deceased)
Dept. of Child and Adolescent Psychiatry
Royal Hospital for Sick Children
Glasgow G3 8SJ,
UK

Helmut Remschmidt
Klinik für Psychiatrie und Psychotherapie
des Kindes- und Jugendalters der
Philipps-Universität
Hans-Sachs-Str. 6
D-35033 Marburg
Germany

Eberhard Schulz
Abt. für Psychiatrie und Psychotherapie
im Kindes- und Jugendalter
Albert Ludwigs Universität
Hauptstr. 8
D-79104 Freiburg
Germany

Jane Scourfield
University of Wales College of Medicine
Division of Psychological Medicine
Heath Park
Cardiff CF4 4XN,
UK

Martha C. Tompson
Boston University
Department of Psychology
64 Cummington Street
Boston, MA 02215,
USA

Fred R. Volkmar
Child Study Center
Yale University
PO Box 207900
New Haven, CT 06520,
USA

John Scott Werry
School of Medicine, University of Auckland
Department of Psychiatry and Behavioural
Science
32 Glendowie Road
Glendowie, Auckland
New Zealand

Preface

Schizophrenic psychoses in childhood are important but rare disorders within the spectrum of psychoses. They become increasingly common during adolescence and the symptomatology with age becomes increasingly similar to the adult disorder. After Kraepelin (1893) first described dementia praecox and Bleuler (1911) introduced the term "schizophrenia," Homburger (1926) asserted the existence of childhood schizophrenia in his classic textbook and described some characteristic features of the disorder including those today known as "negative symptoms."

Kanner (1943) and Asperger (1944) differentiated the meanwhile well-known autistic syndromes (early infantile autism and autistic personality disorder) from the pool of the childhood psychoses. Finally, Leonhard's work is worthy of note (1986). He emphasized that schizophrenic psychoses comprise a very heterogeneous group of disorders, and that it was an illusion to think that one could find a unique etiology in schizophrenia. Unlike many other authors, he subdivided the schizophrenic disorders into unsystematic and systematic schizophrenias. According to this classification, unsystematic schizophrenias are characterized by primarily affective symptoms (e.g., extreme anxiety states, delusions, hallucinations, ideas of reference) with an acute, sometimes periodic course and periods of good remission. They have more in common with affective psychoses than with the group of systematic schizophrenias. Systematic schizophrenias show predominantly cognitive disturbances and disturbances of voluntary functions. Their course is generally chronic without recovery to former cognitive levels and the prognosis is poor. As a special form of childhood schizophrenia, Leonhard distinguishes early infantile catatonia, which is characterized by motor symptoms, absent or poor language development, circumscribed intellectual impairments, negativism, a periodic course, and dominance amongst males. So far, to our knowledge, there is no study that has replicated Karl Leonhard's results on early infantile catatonia. However, such studies are necessary to validate the modern classification criteria of

ICD-10 and DSM-IV, which it is suggested do not cover the whole range of schizophrenic disorders, at least at a very young age.

Studies in recent years have very much focused on the neurobiological and neurodevelopmental approaches, including genetics, and have produced interesting results which have not yet been integrated into a conclusive and convincing theory of schizophrenia. The results of this work can be condensed along the following lines (Remschmidt, 1993; Remschmidt et al., 1994):

– Schizophrenia in childhood and adolescence is not a sudden event befalling patients out of the blue.

– Schizophrenic psychoses have a long history within the individual patient and there are many precursors in the shape of developmental, cognitive and emotional symptoms or retardation. It is difficult to ascertain which precursors are specific for schizophrenia and which are uncharacteristic features that may increase the risk of schizophrenia, but possibly also of other disorders. However, it is striking how many children and adolescents with this disorder seem to be multidimensionally impaired. One consequence of these results is that the dimensional model may be more appropriate to our understanding of schizophrenia than a categorial one.

– In spite of the fact that childhood and adolescent schizophrenia lie on a continuum with schizophrenia in adults, there are special difficulties in applying the "adult criteria" to younger children with suspected schizophrenia. Symptoms at an early age are less specific and show remarkable overlap with a number of developmental disorders. This leads to a greater uncertainty regarding diagnosis especially in younger children.

– This uncertainty can lead to the desire to confirm the diagnosis over a period of time which in turn can result in the loss of valuable time for early treatment. Recent research suggests that early treatment seems to improve the outcome especially with the new atypical neuroleptics.

– Recently, the question of primary prevention has been discussed; the prescribing of medication to subjects at high risk of schizophrenia. As far as children and adolescents are concerned, our knowledge is not yet sufficient to justify this as "preschizophrenic states" cannot be reliably diagnosed.

These and other issues are discussed in the ten chapters of this volume, written by experienced clinicians and researchers from Europe, the United States and New Zealand.

The intention of this book is to give a comprehensive overview of the current state of knowledge and therapeutic options. It also clearly states which aspects of the disorder are not yet well understood and the research questions for the future.

I would like to thank the authors for their valuable contributions, Dr Philip Heiser and Dr Peter M. Wehmeier for their considerable editorial work, Johanna Schneider and Elisabeth Le Guillarme for help in preparing the manuscript and the editorial staff of Cambridge University Press for their excellent co-operation during the preparation of this book.

The book is devoted to the memory of two colleagues and friends who contributed to this volume and who died during the preparation of this book: Michael Goldstein (Los Angeles) and William Parry-Jones (Glasgow).

Helmut Remschmidt

Marburg, August 1999

REFERENCES

Asperger, H. (1944). Die "autistischen Psychopathen" im Kindesalter. *Archiv für Psychiatrie und Nervenkrankheiten*, **117**, 76–136.

Bleuler, E. (1911). *Dementia praecox oder die Gruppe der Schizophrenien*. Leipzig: Deuticke.

Homburger, A. (1926). *Vorlesungen über Psychopathologie des Kindesalters*. Berlin: Springer.

Kanner, L. (1943). Autistic disturbances of affective contact. *The Nervous Child*, **2**, 217–50.

Kraepelin, E. (1893). *Ein kurzes Lehrbuch für Studierende und Ärzte*, 4th edn. Leipzig: Abel.

Leonhard, K. (1986). *Aufteilung der endogenen Psychosen und ihre differenzierte Ätiologie*, 6th edn. Berlin: Akademie Verlag.

Remschmidt, H. (1993). Childhood and adolescent schizophrenia. *Current Opinion in Psychiatry*, **6**, 470–9.

Remschmidt, H., Schulz, E., Martin, M., Warnke, A., & Trott, G-E. (1994). Childhood-onset schizophrenia: history of the concept and recent studies. *Schizophrenia Bulletin*, **20**, 722–45.

Childhood psychosis and schizophrenia: a historical review

The late William Ll. Parry-Jones

Introduction

For over 100 years, the onset of schizophrenia during adolescence has been accepted, but its onset in childhood, the question of its equivalence with the adult disorder, and the possibility of childhood antecedents of the adult form have been controversial clinical and research issues. Until 20 to 30 years ago, child psychiatrists were reluctant to acknowledge or diagnose psychoses in children and adolescents, and various euphemistic terms tended to be used. Even at present, there may be a disinclination to do so because of fears about the potentially adverse consequences of diagnostic labeling. Many factors have contributed to this, principally infrequency of presentation and uncertainty about diagnosis and classification, since formerly, the term schizophrenia has been used to refer to a remarkable range of severe, chronic disorders arising in children, with little or no differentiation. Furthermore, there has been a lack of research-based therapeutic guidelines. Recent years, however, have witnessed a rebirth of interest in schizophrenia in children, especially in identifying continuities and discontinuities with the condition presenting in adolescents and adults. In this context, the general aim of this chapter is to review the literature relating to schizophrenia in children and adolescents up to the 1970s, setting in historical perspective some of the issues presented and discussed in subsequent chapters, particularly in relation to diagnosis and classification.

Historiography of schizophrenia

Historical consideration of the concept of schizophrenia in children has to be located in the wider context of historical research on the functional psychoses as a whole, particularly schizophrenia (Howells, 1991; Berrios & Porter, 1995, pp. 261–430). The historiography of a subject of such complexity is fraught with methodological difficulties, including wide variation in the content and quality of sources, especially manuscript material; uncertainty and imprecision about which symptoms or morbid processes constitute schizophrenia, even at the present day; and all the hazards associated with retrospective diagnosis and interpretation of both theoretical constructs and clinical practice.

Limited historical research has been undertaken on the history of schizophrenia in children using primary printed or manuscript sources. However, the historical background has been the subject of a number of reviews, including those by Bradley (1942), Lurie and Lurie (1950), Eisenberg (1957), Goldfarb (1970), Rutter (1972), Fish and Ritvo (1979), Cantor (1988), Bender (1991), Werry (1992) and Remschmidt et al. (1994). An annotated bibliography by Goldfarb and Dorsen (1956) reviewed the relevant literature up to 1954, and further coverage to 1969 was provided by Tilton et al. (1966) and Bryson and Hintgen (1971).

Before 1900: pre-nineteenth century

There has been considerable controversy whether schizophrenia has always existed or if it is of relatively recent origin (Klaf & Hamilton, 1961; Hare, 1988). The search for evidence of schizophrenia in the past is complicated by frequent terminological and nosological changes and overlaps. For example, since it was not viewed as a discrete entity until the end of the nineteenth century, it might have been perceived as a form of delirium, mania, melancholia, dementia, imbecility or idiocy. In general, the historical evidence lends support for its enduring nature, albeit associated with changing manifestations (Jeste et al., 1985; Howells, 1991). Up to the medieval period, the evidence is highly equivocal, but subsequently, to the end of the nineteenth century, the case for the existence of schizophrenia strengthens. In the absence of precisely defined diagnostic entities, it is difficult to reconstruct a picture of psychosis in juveniles or to estimate its prevalence in pre-nineteenth century accounts of insane children and young people. Instead, the focus has to be on common denominators, such as evidence of a qualitative difference in mental state and behavior in the absence of overt organic brain disease, such as odd, bizarre, incongruous, unintelligible thinking and behavior, and the presence of delusions and hallucinations. A diverse range of literature requires scrutiny including, for example, accounts of alleged demonic possession in juveniles (e.g., Baddeley, 1622), since seventeenth century perceptions of madness were intertwined with beliefs in witchcraft. Childhood disorders featured only sporadically in eighteenth-century lunacy texts (e.g., Perfect, 1791).

Nineteenth century

During the first half of the century, increasing publication of unusual cases and references to young lunatics indicated mounting medical interest. Haslam's detailed account, in 1809, of a disorder occurring in young persons associated with "hopeless and degrading change" is widely quoted as an early, if not the first, description of schizophrenia (Haslam, 1809, p. 64). The prevailing view was that madness rarely occurred before puberty, although a small number of cases of insane children were described (e.g., Cox, 1804; Rush, 1812; Burrows, 1828; Morison, 1828). Esquirol (1845), whose account of mania strongly suggests schizophrenia, described cases of mania in children, one child being reported as having hallucinations of taste and vision, but no link was established with a progressive dementing process. This emerged when Morel (1860) drew attention, ahead of Kraepelin, to premature dementia (*démence précose*) in a 14-year-old boy.

From the 1860s onwards, childhood insanity featured regularly in psychiatric publications, with references to conditions comparable to psychosis. It was accepted that all forms of mental disease that occurred in adults could present in children (e.g., Crichton-Browne, 1860; Maudsley, 1867). The relationship between the occurrence and form of insanity and the developmental stage was recognized. For example, Griesinger (1867) observed that monomania was "uncommonly rare" in children, because "no persistent ego is as yet formed in which there could occur a lasting radical change." It was noted also that hallucinations and "fixed delirious ideas" were rarer than in adults (Griesinger, 1867, p. 143). However, mental diseases were regarded as more frequent after the age of 16 (Griesinger, 1867, p. 145). Similarly, Ireland described the changing manifestations of insanity in children according to age and development (Ireland, 1898, pp. 271–302). These could include hallucinations, especially in older children, but again, "fixed ideas and delusions" were not common, "even when derangement is very decided, there is a want of persistence in the mental delusions of children." Down (1887) reported that cases had come to his attention with "well-marked delusions of suspicion" (Down, 1887, p. 92) and another example was provided by the ten cases of childhood psychoses described by Schöntal (1892).

Towards the end of the century, monographs on childhood insanity appeared, including innovative works by Emminghaus (1887) in Germany and Moreau de Tours (1888) and Manheimer (1899) in France. In addition, adolescent disorders became a new focus of interest, with puberty recognized increasingly as a physiological cause of mental disturbance. "Developmental," "pubescent" or "adolescent" insanity was described frequently (e.g., Clouston,

1892). Adolescence was perceived as an important period for the emergence of "ancestral influences" and atavisms and for its predisposition to dementia praecox and manic-depressive insanity.

In addition to Morel's description of *démence précose*, other psychotic syndromes were delineated in the late-nineteenth century. Hebephrenia was reported by Hecker (1871), and Kahlbaum (1874) described catatonia in adolescents, culminating in terminal deterioration. In his seminal work, publicized in 1898, Kraepelin (1919) grouped together such syndromes within the diagnostic entity of dementia praecox, which in his view, was based on organic brain pathology and progressed inevitably towards mental deterioration. The subtypes were catatonic, hebephrenic, paranoid and simple. He made brief reference to the possibility of early onset during adolescence. Dementia praecox could commence in childhood and, in at least 3.5% of his 1054 cases, onset was before the age of 10 years, with another 2.7% of cases beginning between 10 and 15 years.

Twentieth century

The literature on psychoses in the early twentieth century was influenced strongly by Kraepelinian ideas, including the concept of dementia praecox as a discrete disease entity. These were reflected in the growing consideration of psychosis in children. Increasingly, individual case reports of juvenile psychosis, especially those occurring in the prepubertal period appeared, and the diagnosis tended to become inclusive, comprising many types of pubertal and adolescent insanity. It was accepted that all known psychoses could present during this period, the only form occurring exclusively at this time being hebephrenia. The latter was characterized by "a change of superficial emotional conditions, beginning with mental depression, followed by odd, fantastic delusions, eccentric, silly behavior, and intense motor activity, and resulting often in a rapid or gradual passage into chronic dementia or into the condition of catatonia" (Noyes, 1901).

In 1906, de Sanctis described *dementia praecocissimia*, in cases occurring in very early life, presenting with mannerisms, negativism and catatonic symptoms, which he thought resembled demmentia praecox (de Sanctis, 1906, 1925). Later, it was shown to comprise a collection of heterogeneous diseases, including the sequelae of encephalitis. In 1908, Heller described cases of a condition that he termed *dementia infantilis* (previously used by Weygandt), in which, like dementia praecocissima, there was rapid and profound speech disturbance, extreme restlessness and dementia, beginning in the third or fourth years, in previously normal children (Heller, 1908; Hulse, 1954). Other authors (e.g., Zappert, 1921) described similar conditions (Lay, 1938), but differentiated from schizophrenia, and by the mid-1930s, Kanner felt able to assert that Heller's syndrome was "an illness *sui generis* and should not be identified with schizophrenia" (Kanner, 1935, p. 493). Nevertheless, the concept of a disintegrative psychosis continued to feature in the differential diagnosis of childhood schizophrenia.

Introduction of the term "schizophrenia"

In his 1911 monograph, Bleuler (1950) introduced the term schizophrenia for dementia praecox. Although he was thinking of "the group of schizophrenias," in practice, the two disorders came to be viewed as synonymous. There was, however, a widening of Kraepelin's diagnostic construct, making schizophrenia progressively less readily definable. Bleuler estimated that 0.5 to 1% of schizophrenia cases had onset before the age of 10, 4% beginning before 15 years. He stated that "schizophrenia is not a puberty psychosis in the strict sense of the word, although in the majority of patients the sickness becomes manifest soon after puberty." Further, he noted that "we know of no differences between the infantile and other forms of the disease. If we observe patients during childhood, they present the same symptoms as those seen in adults. We did note, however, that the analyses of such youthful patients are more difficult. In contrast to adults, children are not less clear in their desires and wishes, but the content is less clearly defined. The difficulty may also be due to our inadequate experience with the technique of handling youthful psychotics. The prognosis of those cases in which the onset of the illness occurs before puberty does not appear to be poorer for the next few years" (Bleuler, 1950, pp. 240–1). Unlike Kraepelin, Bleuler did not believe that schizophrenia led inevitably to deterioration and emphasized intrapsychic and psychosocial aspects, encouraging a more positive and optimistic therapeutic attitude. In this respect, his views resembled those of Meyer (1906), who first raised the issue of the patient's previous personality and proposed a unique psychobiological basis for disorder, whereby schizophrenia could be regarded as the consequence of defective life accommodation. Such approaches were found more applicable to children than the more restrictive, pessimistic Kraepelinian views.

Increasing recognition of schizophrenia in childhood: the 1930s and 1940s

Up to the 1930s, dementia praecox or schizophrenia was described and diagnosed in small numbers of children using the same criteria as applied to adult patients (see Lay, 1938 for early twentieth century reflection, e.g., to the contributions of Vogt, Aubry, Voigt, and Weber). Initially, the literature on childhood psychoses was limited compared with that about psychoses in adolescents and adults (e.g., Lutz, 1937; Bellak, 1948) and many psychiatrists disputed the existence of childhood schizophrenia. Subsequently, this concept became increasingly accepted, with wider and more encompassing criteria, and attention shifted from the study of a disease entity to the personal and developmental characteristics and family environment of psychotic children. This encouraged the polarization of the concepts of child and adult schizophrenia, with emphasis on the differences in causation, diagnosis and treatment, particularly on the developmental aspects. In this context, concurrent developments in child and adolescent psychiatry were relevant. During the late 1920s and 1930s, a recognizably separate discipline of child psychiatry emerged, accompanied by the rapid widening of the number and range of disturbed children presenting to child guidance clinics and to the early hospital-based outpatient departments (Parry-Jones, 1993). Further, new psychological and psychiatric methods of investigation came into use for the objective study of the child. The developing speciality directed attention away from the impersonal disease model, organ pathology, heredity, syndromal description and physical treatment, towards psychosocial and psychodynamic theories. In the process, it distanced itself from asylum psychiatry and from the most severely disturbed subjects, particularly adolescents with psychotic disorders.

Interest in schizophrenia in children and its diverse connotations expanded rapidly (e.g., Kasanin & Kaufman, 1929) and from the 1930s, there was a striking increase in related literature (Goldfarb & Dorsen, 1956), including sections in child psychiatry textbooks (e.g., Homberger, 1926; Kanner, 1935). The crucial questions were whether childhood schizophrenia was the same as adult dementia praecox, and what constituted the adult outcome of the childhood disorder. In a widely reported paper, Potter (1933) described six cases of childhood schizophrenia, which, typically, could occur before pubescence, including paranoid delusions, bizarre fantasies, auditory hallucinations and thought disorder. His diagnostic criteria were broad and he recognized the importance of developmental stage, since children "do not possess the facility to fully verbalise their feelings, nor are they capable of complicated abstractions," their "delusional formations" are relatively simple and "symbolisation is particularly naive." In the first edition of his influential textbook, Kanner (1935, pp. 484–507), discussed the major psychoses or "parergastic reaction forms" (characterized by odd, archaic types of behavior), using Meyerian concepts, to distinguish them from "thymergastic reaction forms" or affective disorders. He included three case illustrations, in which he emphasized antecedent factors, and observed that "schizophrenic difficulties did not come upon the patients out of a clear sky as a result of some cellular destruction or abscessed teeth or endocrine disorder or whatnot" (Kanner, 1935, p. 500). Even though there was little to be done once "dilapidation" had set in, Kanner supported the notion of prophylaxis with children displaying "daydreaming preoccupations, seclusive trends, oversensitiveness, and peculiar behavior" (Kanner, 1935, pp. 501–2). Individual case reports and discussions proliferated, especially those relating to early onset psychosis (e.g., Lutz, 1937) and one of the first comprehensive reviews was published by Bradley (1942), in which he emphasized the primary significance of seclusiveness, bizarre behavior and regression. Based on work at the New York State Psychiatric Institute, from 1930 to 1937, Despert (1938) defined schizophrenia as a "disease process in which the loss of affective contact with reality is coincident with or determined by the appearance of autistic thinking and accompanied by specific phenomena of regression and dissociation." Attention was given to onset history in clarifying life course and treatment response. The therapeutic task was to establish affective contact and to break into the child's autistic world. Although the ideas of Kraepelin and Bleuler continued to be influential, the Freudian psychoanalytic system (Freud, 1924) and Meyerian views were having an increasing effect. In the 1920s, for example, Klein started to use psychoanalytic treatment with young schizophrenic children, and later developed her techniques in conjunction with A. Freud.

Difficulties in the differentiation of childhood schizophrenia from mental deficiency and from deafness with mutism began to be reported. It was recognized that schizophrenia could be diagnosed as mental deficiency, and that schizophrenic children could be sent erroneously to institutions for the mentally deficient. Alternatively, schizophrenia could be superimposed on underlying feeble-mindedness to create the condition known as *pfropfhebephrenia* (Kasanin & Kaufman, 1929) or *pfropfschizophrenia* (Bromberg, 1934; Bergman et al., 1951), and Earl (1934) described a condition in low-grade mental defectives as "primative catatonic psychosis of idiocy," characterized by signs of deterioration, catatonia and emotional dissociation. Ambiguities persisted and O'Gorman (1954) for example, considered schizophrenia as a possible cause, rather than a sequel, of mental deficiency.

The greatest problems in differential diagnosis arose, however, following Kanner's introduction of the term *early infantile autism* (Kanner, 1943), to classify certain conditions regarded as psychoses that occurred as early as in the first 2 years of life, characterized by extreme aloneness, impaired communication, obsessive insistence on sameness and fascination for objects. This was followed by application of the term to a wider group of disturbed children and confusion about its relationship to schizophrenia. For example, Kanner (1949) noted that "the basic nature of its manifestations is so intimately related to the basic nature of childhood schizophrenia as to be indistinguishable from it, especially from cases with insidious onset." Although there were claims that autistic children became schizophrenic, findings were controversial and uncorroborated (Bender, 1953) and, finally, Kanner changed his view (Kanner, 1971). The description of "hyperkinetic disease" in children in the early 1930s, and its classification as a form of childhood psychosis, further complicated the diagnostic picture (Lay, 1938). In general, psychoses caused by organic brain disease, whether due to trauma, neoplasms, infection, toxic agents, metabolic aberrations or degenerative diseases, were categorized separately. Isolated accounts of mania and hypomania, similar to the adult picture appeared more frequently among adolescents than prepubertal children (Parry-Jones, 1995). With regard to the manifestations of psychosis in children, there was particular controversy about the frequency and form of hallucinations and delusions (Lurie & Lurie, 1950).

Towards a unitary view of childhood psychosis: 1950s to 1970s

During the 1950s and 1960s, American and European concepts of schizophrenia diverged increasingly. In the USA, it had broadened and become much less precisely defined, while in Europe, the somatic Kraepelinian model tended to be retained and popularized by Schneider's publication of the first- and second-rank symptoms of schizophrenia, as defined in German psychiatry (Schneider, 1939). During the 1970s, the introduction of research-based diagnostic criteria was to change the situation, attaining increasing consensus (e.g., Feighner et al., 1972).

The amorphous nature of the symptoms of schizophrenia spawned many studies in the 1950s and 1960s, which reviewed and revised the diagnostic criteria of childhood psychoses, drawing on highly diversified clinical descriptions and causative theories. By this stage, an essentially unitary view of chidhood psychosis had emerged. As well as having specific meanings, the labels of childhood psychosis, or childhood schizophrenia, were employed to cover the whole range of psychotic conditions of childhood, as well as many different types of disturbance which might incorporate mental deficiency, severe emotional and behavioral disorders, and the effects of severe deprivation. Harms (1952) asserted that, "If anyone were to take the trouble to summarize the descriptions of childhood schizophrenia by various authors in the past fifteen years, they would find every symptom ever occurring in abnormal psychology." This amalgamation was to be reflected formally in

DSM-II (American Psychiatric Association, 1968) and ICD-8 (World Health Organization, 1967), which used a single generic category of "childhood schizophrenia." Many authors, however, were critical of the lack of clarity in diagnostic criteria (e.g., Harms, 1952) and were concerned especially about the differential diagnosis between disorders with, and without, evidence of brain damage. Kestenberg (1952) discussed differentiation from a specific type of severe neurosis, which she termed *pseudo-schizophrenia*. Other groups of workers continued to dispute whether schizophrenia occurred at all in children and Rank (1949), for example, preferred to apply the term "atypical" to children displaying "arrested emotional development" and "fragmented scattered personality." Although there was greater acceptance of the occurrence of schizophrenia in adolescents, there was uncertainty about its nature, its relationship to adolescent maturation and "whether or not an individual who becomes schizophrenic in adolescence is manifesting a disease that had been lurking within the personality since childhood, or earlier" (Neubauer & Steinert, 1952).

Long-term work, commencing in the 1940s, of Bender and colleagues at Bellevue Hospital, New York, who observed more than 100 preadolescent children suffering from schizophrenia, was especially influential. It emphasized positive diagnostic criteria, rather than diagnosis by exclusion, in that "the child must not be mentally defective, must not be post-encephalitic, the disturbance must not be understandable in mechanistic terms like a deeply inhibited or discouraged neurosis, and the child must not be a psychopathic personality" (Bender, 1941). Bender (1958) viewed childhood schizophrenia as a "total psychobiologic disorder" and distinguished between the early onset "pseudo-defective group," resembling infantile autistic children with onset in the first 2 years, the "pseudo-neurotic," aged between 3 and 5 years, who displayed anxiety, and the "pseudo-psychopathic or antisocial," aged 10 or 11 years. The same child, therefore, might pass through all these reactions, thereby blurring the definition between autism and schizophrenia. Her theories centered around the concept that schizophrenia was the consequence of a developmental lag of the biological processes from which behavior developed by maturation at an embryological level, characterized by embryonic plasticity, resulting in anxiety and neurotic defence mechanisms. Precipitation could be by physiological crisis in the perinatal period, leading to brain damage or personality deterioration, and the pattern of psychosis would be determined by psychological and environmental factors (Bender, 1966, 1991). Regarding outcome, she concluded that most schizophrenic children continued to be diagnosed as schizophrenic in adolescence and adulthood (Bender, 1953).

The psychoanalytic perspective was well established, based on the view that schizophrenia was determined psychodynamically, like a neurosis. In this context, Mahler, a child analyst of the ego psychology school, played an important part in developing the concept of symbiotic psychosis in children who were deeply dependent on an overanxious mother, becoming disorganized and regressed at the prospect of psychological separation (Mahler, 1952). This condition was distinguished from autistic psychosis, which arose if the infant failed to grow beyond the earlier, normal autistic phase. Similarly, Szurek (1956) and his colleagues were strong protagonists of the psychogenic basis of psychotic disorder, viewing it as the consequence of emotional conflict. With regard to adolescence, the general psychoanalytic view of adolescent "storm and stress" leading to a variety of clinical pictures (Freud, A., 1958), even to "normal psychosis," created a heritage of diagnostic and therapeutic uncertainty for clinicians.

In the early 1960s, deliberations by a British Working Party, led by Creak (1961, 1964), proposed "nine points" as diagnostic criteria for the "schizophrenic syndrome in childhood," without specifying age of onset. These comprised: (1) "Gross and sustained impairment of emotional relationships with people;" (2) "Apparent unawareness of his own personal identity to a degree inappropriate to his age;" (3) "Pathological preoccupation with particular objects or certain characteristics of them, without regard to their accepted functions;" (4) "Sustained resistance to change in the environment and a striving to maintain or restore sameness;" (5) "Abnormal perceptual experience (in the absence of discernible organic abnormality) implied by excessive, diminished or unpredictable response to sensory stimuli;" (6) "Acute, excessive, and seemingly illogical anxiety;" (7) "Speech may have been lost, or never acquired, or may have failed to develop beyond a level appropriate to an earlier stage;" (8) "Distortion in motility patterns;" (9) "A background of serious retardation in which islets of normal, near normal or exceptional intellectual function or skill may appear." According to Goldfarb (1970, pp. 780–1), a review of 52 published reports of schizophrenia indicated that all behavioral symptoms were comprised in the nine points. The emergent model, therefore, based on the nine points, was that differing pathological processes might all result in a similar clinical picture.

Resolution of terminological and diagnostic chaos

By the early 1970s, dilution of the concept of childhood schizophrenia had resulted in a chaotic diagnostic situation and the term was misused widely. According to Rutter (1972), childhood schizophrenia had been used "as a generic term to include an astonishingly heterogeneous mixture of disorders with little in common other than their severity, chronicity and occurrence in childhood . . . A host of different syndromes have been included . . . infantile autism, the atypical child, symbiotic psychosis, dementia praecosissima, dementia infantilis, schizophrenic syndrome of childhood, pseudo-psychopathic schizophrenia, and latent schizophrenia to name but a few." To this list, organic psychosis and borderline psychosis (Ekstein & Wallerstein, 1957) might have been added. It was in this context that studies by Anthony (1958), Rutter, Greenfield and Lockyer (1967) and Kolvin et al. (1971) made a major contribution to a changed approach towards the diagnosis and classification of psychotic syndromes in children and adolescents. It was demonstrated that symptoms, including delusions, hallucinations and thought disorder, similar to those in adults, occurred in children. This enabled a clear distinction to be drawn between early-onset autism of the Kanner type, adult-form schizophrenia with late-childhood onset, and other psychoses with no clear relation to schizophrenia. The child and adult forms could be regarded as qualitatively similar and continuous, while allowing for developmental variation. A wide range of psychological tests had been used from the 1940s (Mehr, 1952; Goldfarb, 1970, p. 781). Later, in conjunction with the new diagnostic and nosological developments, there were major advances in the assessment techniques in schizophrenia, using interview schedules, rating scales, and measures of thought disorder.

The revised, differentiated view and subclassification of childhood psychosis was incorporated in ICD-9 (World Health Organization, 1978) and DSM-III (American Psychiatric Association, 1980), which advocated the application of the same diagnostic criteria as for adult-type disorders, with some allowance for different manifestations. Nevertheless, some ambiguity remained in ICD-9. For example, there continued to be a category for "psychoses with origin specific to childhood," including early infantile autism, disintegrative psychosis and other atypical and unspecified conditions, such as "schizophrenic syndrome of childhood NOS." The same general principles were incorporated in ICD-10 (World Health Organization, 1992) and DSM-IV (American Psychiatric Association, 1994), using symptoms derived, essentially, from the original work of Kraepelin, Bleuler and Schneider.

Psychotic juveniles in asylums

Throughout the nineteenth century, there is conclusive evidence that children and young people were admitted alongside adult patients to private and public asylums (Parry-Jones, 1993). This practice continued into the twentieth century, until separate facilities were provided for juveniles, predominantly after the Second World War. The clearest profile of presenting clinical problems is derivable from asylum records, but medical labeling and precise diagnostic statements were rare, permitting only speculative retrospective diagnosis.

Very few studies of juveniles in asylums have been undertaken. In one such investigation of a series of patients aged up to 16, admitted to asylums in Oxfordshire, England, from 1846 to 1866 (Parry-Jones, 1990), only two children were hallucinated and, of four with delusional ideas, two were paranoid. Some excited states suggested mania, and one girl aged 16 was restless, talked incessantly and unconnectedly and uttered profanities. Acutely disturbed, noisy and destructive behavior was characteristic, as well as in other contemporaneous case reports. In a major study of 1069 juvenile admissions to Bethlem Royal Hospital, England, from 1815 to 1899, Wilkins (1987, 1993) investigated patterns of hallucinations and delusions and their possible relevance to the incidence of schizophrenia.

Premorbid characteristics and borderline disorder

From the 1920s, there was growing interest in the premorbid characteristics of childhood schizophrenia and the childhood antecedents of adult-onset schizophrenia. A few authors described children displaying symptoms resembling those characteristic of the early stages of schizophrenia. Childers (1931) applied the term "schizoid" to problem children on the basis of "(i) the nature and extent of the child's social incapacity; (ii) his habitual reaction to the situations and requirements of reality by withdrawal rather than by attack or conforming; (iii) the nature, extent, and purpose of his phantasies; (iv) the occurrence in a given child of such definite mental symptoms as are usually observed in adult schizophrenics." Speculation has continued about the nature and inter-relationship of a group of poorly defined conditions, including schizoid personality type and schizotypical borderline configuration. Wolff and Chick (1980) used the term schizoid personality of childhood to refer to children with distinctive personality characteristics, but differentiation from Asperger's Syndrome has remained controversial (Asperger, 1944).

Epidemiology

In the nineteenth century, madness in children, in a form comparable to psychosis, was regarded as rare, although its occurrence increased steadily after puberty. During this period, overall admissions to asylums increased rapidly and Hare (1983) has put forward the interesting theory that this may have been due to cases of dementia praecox, possibly produced by a "slow epidemic" of viral origin. Subsequently, until recent years (e.g., Remschmidt et al., 1994), limited epidemiological data continued to be available, complicated by the lack of a uniform system of diagnostic classification and variation in population sampling. No comprehensive reviews on the historical aspects of the epidemiology of childhood psychosis and schizophrenia have been published, although Lay (1938) summarized briefly a number of studies. In the early twentieth century, schizophrenia in children was regarded as extremely uncommon, but by the 1930s this view began to be revised (Potter, 1933; Despert, 1938; Bradley, 1942). Three representative studies are referred to briefly. At the Boston Psychopathic Hospital, during the period 1923–5, there were 160 children under 16 years among the 6000 admissions and only 65 cases were diagnosed as psychotic (Kasanin & Kaufman, 1929). A survey of 1000 randomly selected problem children in a child guidance home by Lurie et al. (1936) showed that 1.3% were diagnosed as dementia praecox. A study by Tizard (1966), using the "nine points" of the British Working Party, indicated a prevalence of psychosis of 4 per 10 000. Higher ratios of boys to girls have been reported in the literature on childhood psychosis, but, in general, sex ratios have varied with the populations studied.

Theories of causation

Multiple factors and morbid processes have been implicated in the causation of dementia praecox, schizophrenia and childhood psychosis, over the last century, and of analogous abnormal states in previous centuries. In general, disagreement has centered around the question whether the disorder was determined by an inherent biological defect or by psychological factors. Although consistently viewed as conditions characterized by psychological disturbance, causation has been attributed frequently to primary vulnerability generated by anatomical, biochemical and endocrine factors, toxins and infections, autointoxication, brain damage or disease, and to generic aberrations. With regard to the latter, Canavan and Clark (1923) followed up the children of dementia praecox patients and found five out of 381 with dementia praecox. Several studies, from the 1950s onwards, suggested that schizophrenia in children was associated with a high level of familial aggregation, e.g., a study by Kallman & Roth, (1956) of 52 sets of twins and 50 singletons. These confirmed the views of many other researchers, including some psychoanalysts, that there was a hereditary or constitutional basis. Bender (1958), for example, concluded that the primary cause, namely, a form of encephalopathy-related maturational lag at the embryonic level, was genetically determined, and emphasized the significance of "soft neurological signs" (Bender, 1947). From the 1960s, increasing research attention was being given to the role of cognitive development, perception, speech, linguistic processes, neurobiological correlates, including biochemical and EEG studies, and the effects of pregnancy and birth complications.

Numerous hypotheses have implicated the psychosocial environment and interpersonal experiences. In particular, attention was paid to the parent–child relationship and the home atmosphere. In the 1930s, Potter (1933) listed various psychological factors, especially a dominant, overprotective mother, an unassertive father, and dependence on mother. Similar conclusions were reached by many other authors (e.g., Kasanin et al., 1934; Kanner, 1943; Rank, 1949) and the "pernicious" role of maternal overprotection–rejection became popular as an alleged precipitant of both early infantile autism and schizophrenia in children. The concept of the rejecting "schizophrenogenic mother" was introduced (Fromm-Reichmann, 1948) and the "parental perplexity" hypothesis was developed by Meyers and Goldfarb (1961). Parental attitudes, family characteristics and the family environment attracted increasing interest, as precipitating factors (e.g., Lidz & Lidz, 1949). These theories were not without their detractors, especially because of the variance in clinical observations and Rutter (1965) challenged the attribution of childhood psychosis to abnormal parental attitudes. Such views survived, however, for example, in the parental communication theories of Singer and Wynne (1963).

From an early stage, psychodynamic interpretations of the causation of schizophrenia were introduced, theories being dependent on various schools of thought (Stone, 1991). Brill (1926), one of the foremost early analytic theorists, concluded confidently that "the nucleus of all these psychoses just as of the neuroses is a psycho-sexual maladjustment in childhood." The important contributions of Mahler (1952) and Szurek (1956) have been referred to previously. Szurek's theoretical position, in which psychotic symptoms were viewed as the consequence of self-destructive postnatal conflict, and its resolution, provided a particularly constructive basis for psychotherapy.

Treatment and outcome

Despite the extensive literature on schizophrenia in children and adolescents, there was relatively little discussion of treatment and outcome until the 1950s.

Treatment approaches have been remarkably diverse, often associated with evanescent, idiosyncratic etiological hypotheses and, generally, lacking evaluative research and controlled studies.

Pharmacological treatments of all descriptions have been utilized to alleviate symptoms and improve the psychotic child's accessibility, each generation producing its innovations, e.g., ephedrine, caffeine, tri-iodothyronine, sodium amytal and LSD-25, culminating in modern neuroleptics. Similarly, physical treatments have followed fashionable theories, so that, for example, shock therapy using insulin, metrazol or electric shock (Cottington, 1941; Bender, 1947) and prefrontal leukotomy (Freeman & Watts, 1950) have been utilized for juveniles with schizophrenia. Despite the disproportionately high mortality rates associated with leukotomy in children, Angus (1949) considered the risk "legitimate in view of the long hospitalization and unfavorable outlook of cases selected as these are on the basis of a hopeless prognosis from other methods of treatment."

From the early twentieth century, various forms of individual psychotherapy were practiced, with children with schizophrenia. Escalona (1948) categorized these methods as both "expressive" and "suppressive." Despite enduring criticism that psychotherapeutic approaches were not possible because of "the lack of an essential emotional rapport" (Potter, 1933), some authors claimed it was the most successful treatment method (Lourie et al., 1943). Specific psychoanalytic treatment was advocated by many authors, e.g., Klein (1949). During the 1960s, the role of behavior modification to improve language and social behavior was explored actively (Leff, 1968). An important aspect of management was work with parents, concerned principally to develop a positive and realistic attitude towards the child's illness (e.g., Kaufman et al., 1957).

In general, it has been recognized consistently that children with schizophrenia required a broad, multidimensional approach, including institutional treatment, to promote socialization and rehabilitation, thus creating the setting for milieu therapy. Bender's views, in the mid-1950s (Bender, 1958), based on her "maturational lag" theory, illustrate the range of treatment goals and therapeutic programs thought to be required. These were "(i) to stimulate maturation and patterning in all of the lagging and embryonically plastic biological and psychological processes; (ii) to relieve anxiety; (iii) to protect, correct or help the formation of adequate defense mechanisms; (iv) to place a high value on the time factor in children by promoting maturation at the earliest and most favorable period in order to avoid or shorten isolation experiences ...; (v) to help the child learn to tolerate and live with his schizophrenic illness, and similarly to help the parents, the schools and the community." To achieve these goals, the lifelong treatment program required "milieu or environmental therapy," "specific psychotherapy," "specific remedial procedures . . . such as remedial tutoring . . .," "physiological therapies, especially electric convulsive treatment," "pharmacological therapies with antihistamines, amphetamines, mephenesins, anticonvulsants, growth vitamins, etc.," and "organizations and discussion groups for parents." Despite recognition of their often long-term institutional needs, special inpatient facilities for juveniles with psychoses did not develop, to any significant extent, until the 1940s and 1950s, and children and adolescents shared the same regime as adults.

A very variable historical picture emerges of the prospects of recovery and actual outcome, complicated, inevitably, by widely different diagnostic criteria, variation in the selection procedures in the different treatment settings, the length of follow-up, and the number and age of the subjects (Eggers, 1978). In general, while stopping short of therapeutic nihilism, most reports have indicated a uniformly poor prognosis (e.g., Bradley, 1942). At Bellevue Hospital, New York, however, Cottington (1941) felt that there was scope for progress using socialization, psychotherapy and shock therapy. The most satisfactory responses were reported following psychodynamic treatments (e.g., Klein, 1949; Kaufman et al., 1963). However, in a follow-up of 100 children diagnosed as suffering from schizophrenia, from 1935 to 1952, Bender (1970) showed that the disorder "is an early onset of a life course of schizophrenia of every possible type," although the criteria used in adulthood have been questioned. Carter (1942) provided a brief, useful review of the prognostic factors in adolescent psychoses.

Conclusions

The historical study of schizophrenia highlights the remarkable degree of fluidity that has characterized its definition and diagnostic criteria and the special problems in relation to the existence and features of the disorder in children. The findings incorporated in this chapter broadly endorse the key historical trends identified by Goldfarb (1970, pp. 776–7), which may be summarized as follows: (i) "Profound alterations in biological development, either in the form of regressions or of arrests, are noted by all observers;" (ii) "All workers refer to the very global and total integrative failure demonstrated by schizophrenic children. The total personality is disordered;" (iii) "Observers frequently refer to the highly variable and changing nature of the symptomatic expressions of schizophrenic children;" (iv) "All observers note a serious disturbance of emotional organization;" (v) "A major advance in rationalizing the disorders subsumed by the diagnosis of childhood schizophrenia, or any of the other labels for childhood psychosis, is represented in the concept of ego aberration;" (vi) "If there has been a "break through" in the study of etiology, it consists of the implementation of the concept of a multiplicity of factors, centred in the child and in the environment, to explain the adaptive accommodation of the child, which is then classified as psychosis."

Since the 1970s, nosological anomalies and confusion in relation to the disorders subsumed in the category of childhood psychosis have been largely resolved, with the application of the same core criteria for schizophrenia across all developmental periods and the recognition of very similar clinical features and comparable responses to pharmacological treatment. A universally accepted definition of schizophrenia, however, has remained elusive and evidence of causation is fragmentary. In historical terms, the present stage simply sets the scene for further fundamental clinical and research questions concerning the origins of schizophrenia, the significance of early onset, developmental variation in the expression of the disorder, the status of atypical symptomatic presentations that lie outside the current narrow ICD-10 and DSM-IV criteria, and the significance of comorbidity. Schizophrenia at all ages continues to be a perplexing and challenging disorder, in both clinical and research terms. Consequently, historical research has more relevance than its purely antiquarian interest, since it both elucidates the condition and establishes future research directions by highlighting enduring ambiguities. Finally, the historical dimension provides a corrective warning to each generation about the potential fallibility of received wisdom.

REFERENCES

American Psychiatric Association (1968). *DSM-II. Diagnostic and Statistical Manual of Mental Disorders*, 2nd edn. Washington, DC: APA.

American Psychiatric Association (1980). *DSM-III. Diagnostic and Statistical Manual of Mental Disorders*, 3rd edn. Washington, DC: APA.

American Psychiatric Association (1994). *DSM-IV. Diagnostic and Statistical Manual of Mental Disorders*, 4th edn. Washington, DC: APA.

Angus, L.R. (1949). Prefrontal lobotomy as a method of therapy in a special school. *American Journal of Mental Deficiency*, **53**, 470–6.

Anthony, E.J. (1958). An experimental approach to the psychopathology of childhood autism. *British Journal of Medical Psychology*, **31**, 211–25.

Asperger, H. (1944). Die "austistischen Psychopathien" im Kindesalter. *Archiv für Psychiatrie und Nervenkrankheiten*, **117**, 76–136.

Baddeley, R. (1622). *The boy of Bilson: or a true discovery of the late notorious impostures of certaine Romish priests in their pretended exorcisme, or expulsion of the devill out of a young boy.* London: F.K. for W. Barret.

Bellak, L. (1948). *Dementia Praecox.* New York: Grune & Stratton.

Bender, L. (1941). Childhood schizophrenia. *Nervous Child*, **1**, 138–40.

Bender, L. (1947). One hundred cases of childhood schizophrenia treated with electric shock. *Transactions of the American Neurological Association*, **72**, 165–9.

Bender, L. (1953). Childhood schizophrenia. *Psychiatric Quarterly*, **27**, 663–81.

Bender, L. (1958). Psychiatric problems of childhood. *Medical Clinics of North America*, **42**, 755–67.

Bender, L. (1966). The concept of plasticity in childhood schizophrenia. In *Psychopathology of Schizophrenia*, ed. P.H. Hoch & J. Zubin. New York: Grune & Stratton.

Bender, L. (1970). The life course of schizophrenic children. *Biological Psychiatry*, **2**, 165–72.

Bender, L. (1991). The historical background of the concept of childhood schizophrenia. In *The Concept of Schizophrenia: Historical Perspectives*, ed. J.G. Howells, pp. 109–24. Washington DC: American Psychiatric Press.

Bergman, M., Waller, H., & Marchand, J. (1951). Schizophrenic reactions during childhood in mental defectives. *Psychiatric Quarterly*, **25**, 294–333.

Berrios, G. & Porter, R. (1995). *A History of Clinical Psychiatry. The Origin and History of Psychiatric Disorders.* London: Athlone.

Bleuler, E. (1950). *Dementia Praecox or the Group of Schizophrenias* (trans. by J. Zinkin). New York: International Universities Press.

Bradley, C. (1942). *Schizophrenia in Childhood.* New York: Macmillan.

Brill, A.A. (1926). Psychotic children: treatment and prophylaxis. *American Journal of Psychiatry*, **5**, 357–64.

Bromberg, W. (1934). Schizophrenic-like psychoses in the defective child. *Proceedings of the American Association for Mental Deficiency*, **58**, 226–57.

Bryson, C.Q. & Hintgen, J.N. (1971). *Early Childhood Psychosis: Infantile Autism, Childhood Schizophrenia and Related Disorders. An annotated bibliography 1964 to 1969.* Rockville, MD: Institute of Mental Health.

Burrows, G.M. (1828). *Commentaries on the Causes, Forms, Symptoms, and Treatment, Moral and Medical of Insanity.* London: Underwood.

Canavan, M.M. & Clark, R. (1923). The mental health of 463 children from dementia-praecox stock. *Mental Hygiene*, **7**, 137–48.

Cantor, S. (1988). *Childhood Schizophrenia.* New York: Guilford Press.

Carter, A.B. (1942). The prognostic factors of adolescent psychoses. *Journal of Mental Science*, **88**, 31–81.

Childers, A.T. (1931). A study of some schizoid children. *Mental Hygiene*, **15**, 106–34.

Clouston, T.S. (1892). Developmental insanities and psychoses. In *A Dictionary of Psychological Medicine*, ed. D.H. Tuke, vol. 1, pp. 357–71. London: Churchill.

Cottington, F. (1941). Treatment of childhood schizophrenia by metrazol shock modified by beta-erythroidine. *American Journal of Psychiatry*, **98**, 397–400.

Cox, J.M. (1804). *Practical Observations on Insanity*. London: C. & R. Baldwin.

Creak, M. (1961). Schizophrenic syndrome in childhood. Progress Report (April, 1961) of a working party. *British Medical Journal*, **2**, 889–90.

Creak, M. (1964). Schizophrenic syndrome in childhood. Further progress report of a working party (April, 1964). *Developmental Medicine and Child Neurology*, **4**, 530–5.

Crichton-Browne, J. (1860). Psychological diseases of early life. *Journal of Mental Science*, **6**, 284–320.

De Sanctis, S. (1906). Sopra alcuna varieta della demenza precoce. *Rivista Sperimentale di Freniatria e Medicina Legale delle Alienazioni Mentale*, 141–65.

De Sanctis, S. (1925). *Neuropsichiatria Infantile. Patologia e Diagnostica*. Turin: S. Lattes & Co.

Despert, J.L. (1938). Schizophrenia in children. *Psychiatric Quarterly*, **12**, 366–71.

Down, J.L. (1887). *On Some of the Mental Affections of Childhood and Youth: Being the Lettsomian Lectures Delivered before the Medical Society of London in 1887 Together with Other Papers*. London: J. & A. Churchill.

Earl, C.J.C. (1934). The primative catatonic psychosis of idiocy. *British Journal of Medicine Psychology*, **14**, 230–53.

Eggers, C. (1978). Course and prognosis of childhood schizophrenia. *Journal of Autism and Childhood Schizophrenia*, **8**, 21–36.

Eisenberg, L. (1957). The course of childhood schizophrenia. *A.M.A. Archives of Neurology and Psychiatry*, **78**, 69–83.

Ekstein, R. & Wallerstein, J. (1957). Choice of interpretation in the treatment of borderline and psychotic children. *Bulletin of the Menninger Clinic*, **21**, 199–207.

Emminghaus, H. (1887). *Die psychischen Störungen des Kindesalters*. Tübingen: Laupp.

Escalona, S. (1948). Some considerations regarding psychotherapy with psychotic children. *Bulletin of the Menninger Clinic*, **12**, 126–34.

Esquirol, E. (1845). *Mental Maladies. A Treatise on Insanity* (trans. by E.K. Hurt). Philadelphia: Lea & Blanchard.

Feighner, J.P., Robins, E., Guze, S.B. Woodruff, R.A. jr, Winokur, G. & Munoz, R. (1972). Diagnostic criteria for use in psychiatric research. *Archives of General Psychiatry*, **26**, 57–63.

Fish, B. & Ritvo, E.R. (1979). Psychoses of childhood. In *Basic Handbook of Child Psychiatry*, vol. 2, ed. J.D. Noshpitz, pp. 249–304. New York: Basic Books.

Freeman, W. & Watts, J.W. (1950). *Psychosurgery*, 2nd edn. Springfield: Thomas.

Freud, A. (1958). Adolescence. *Psychoanalytic Study of the Child*, **13**, 255–78.

Freud, S. (1924). The loss of reality in neurosis and psychosis. *Collected Papers*, II. London: Hogarth Press.

Fromm-Reichmann, F. (1948). Notes on the treatment of schizophrenia by psychoanalytic psychotherapy. *Psychiatry*, **11**, 263–??.

Goldfarb, W. (1970). Childhood psychosis. In *Carmichael's Manual of Child Psychology*, 3rd edn, ed. P.H. Mussen, pp. 765–830. New York: John Wiley.

Goldfarb, W. & Dorsen, M.M. (1956). *Annotated Bibliography of Childhood Schizophrenia and Related Disorders*. New York: Basic Books.

Griesinger, W. (1867). *Mental pathology and therapeutics* (trans. C.L. Robertson & J. Rutherford). London: New Sydenharm Society.

Hare, E. (1983). Was insanity on the increase? *British Journal of Psychiatry*, **142**, 439–55.

Hare, E. (1988). Schizophrenia as a recent disease. *British Journal of Psychiatry*, **153**, 521–31.

Harms, E. (1952). Essential problems regarding our present knowledge of childhood schizophrenia. *Nervous Child*, **10**, 7–8.

Haslam, J. (1809). *Observations on Madness and Melancholy*. London: G. Hayden.

Hecker, E. (1871). Die Hebephrenie. *Archiv für pathologische Anatomie und Physiologie und linische Medizin*, **52**, 394–429.

Heller, Th. (1908). Über Dementia Infantilis. *Zeitschrift zur Erforschung und Behandlung des jugendlichen Schwachsinns*, **2**, 17.

Homberger, A. (1926). *Vorlesungen über Psychopathologie des Kindesalters*. Berlin: Springer.

Howells, J. (ed.) (1991). *The Concept of Schizophrenia: Historical Perspectives*. Washington, DC: American Psychiatric Press.

Hulse, W.C. (1954). Dementia infantilis. *Journal of Nervous and Mental Disease*, **119**, 471–77.

Ireland, W.W. (1898). *The Mental Affections of Children, Idiocy, Imbecility and Insanity*. London: J. & A. Churchill.

Jeste, D.V., Del Carmen, R., Lohr, J.B. et al. (1985). Did schizophrenia occur before the 18th century? *Comprehensive Psychiatry*, **26**, 493–503.

Kahlbaum, K.L. (1874). *Die Katatonie oder das Spaltungsirresein*. Berlin: Hirschwald.

Kallmann, F.J. & Roth, B. (1956). Genetic aspects of pre-adolescent schizophrenia. *American Journal of Psychiatry*, **112**, 599–606.

Kanner, L. (1935). *Child Psychiatry*, pp. 484–507. London: Baillière, Tindall & Cox.

Kanner, L. (1943). Autistic disturbances of affective contact. *Nervous Child*, **2**, 217–50.

Kanner, L. (1949). Problems of nosology and psychodynamics of early infantile autism. *American Journal of Orthopsychiatry*, **19**, 416–26.

Kanner, L. (1971). Follow-up study of eleven autistic children originally reported in 1943. *Journal of Autism and Childhood Schizophrenia*, **1**, 119–45.

Kasanin, J. & Kaufman, M.R. (1929). A study of the functional psychoses in childhood. *American Journal of Psychiatry*, **9**, 307–84.

Kasanin, J., Knight, E., & Sage, P. (1934). The parent–child relationship in schizophrenia. I. Overprotection–rejection. *Journal of Nervous and Mental Disease*, **79**, 249–63.

Kaufman, I., Rosenblum, E., Heims, L., & Willer, L. (1957). Childhood schizophrenia: treatment of children and parents. *American Journal of Orthopsychiatry*, **27**, 683–90.

Kaufman, I., Frank, T., Friend, J.G., Heims, L.W., & Weiss, R. (1963). Adaptation of treatment techniques to a new classification of schizophrenic children. *Journal of the American Academy of Child Psychiatry*, **2**, 460–83.

Kestenberg, J.S. (1952). Pseudo-schizophrenia in childhood and adolescence. *Nervous Child*, **10**, 146–62.

Klaf, F.S. & Hamilton, J.G. (1961). Schizophrenia – a hundred years ago and today. *Journal of Mental Science*, **107**, 819–27.

Klein, M. (1949). *The Psycho-analysis of Children* (trans. A. Strachey). London: Hogarth.

Kolvin, I., Ounsted, C., Humphrey, M., & McNay, A. (1971). The phenomenology of childhood psychoses. *British Journal of Psychiatry*, **118**, 385–95.

Kraepelin, E. (1919). *Dementia Praecox and Paraphrenia* (trans. R.M. Barclay of the eighth German edition of the *Textbook of Psychiatry*, vol. iii, part ii). Edinburgh: E. & S. Livingstone.

Lay, R.A.Q. (1938). Schizophrenia-like psychoses in young children. *Journal of Mental Science*, **84**, 105–33.

Leff, R. (1968). Behavior modification and the psychoses of childhood: a review. *Psychological Bulletin*, **69**, 396–409.

Lidz, R.W. & Lidz, T. (1949). The family environment of schizophrenic patients. *American Journal of Psychiatry*, **106**, 332–45.

Lourie, R.S., Pacella, B.L., & Piotrowski, Z.A. (1943). Studies on the prognosis in schizophrenic-like psychoses in children. *American Journal of Psychiatry*, **99**, 542–??.

Lurie, L.A. & Lurie, M.L. (1950). Psychoses in children – a review. *Journal of Pediatrics*, **36**, 801–9.

Lurie, L.A., Tietz, E.B., & Hertzman, J. (1936). Functional psychoses in children. An analysis of the findings in twenty cases of psychotic children studied at the child guidance home. *American Journal of Psychiatry*, **92**, 1169–83.

Lutz, J. (1937). Über die Schizophrenie im Kindesalter. *Schweizer Archiv für Neurologie, Neurochirurgie und Psychiatrie*, **39**, 335–72.

Mahler, M.S. (1952). On child psychosis and schizophrenia. *Psychoanalytic Study of the Child*, **7**, 286–305.

Manheimer, M. (1899). *Les Troubles Mentaux de l'Enfance: Précis de Psychiatrie Infantile*. Paris: Société d'Éditions Scientifiques.

Maudsley, H. (1867). *The Physiology and Pathology of the Mind*. London: Macmillan.

Mehr, H.M. (1952). The application of psychological tests and methods to schizophrenia in children. *Nervous Child*, **10**, 63–93.

Meyer, A. (1906). Fundamental conceptions of dementia praecox. *British Medical Journal*, **2**, 757–60.

Meyers, D.I. & Goldfarb, W. (1961). Studies of complexity in mothers of schizophrenic children. *American Journal of Orthopsychiatry*, **31**, 551–64.

Moreau de Tours, P. (1888). *La Folie chez les Enfants*. Paris: Baillière.

Morel, B.A. (1860). *Traité des Maladies Mentales*. Paris: V. Masson.

Morison, A. (1828). *Cases of Mental Disease, with Practical Observations on the Medical Treatment*. London: Longman / S. Highley.

Neubauer, P.B. & Steinert, J. (1952). Schizophrenia in adolescence. *Nervous Child*, **10**, 129–34.

Noyes, W.B. (1901). The mental diseases of childhood. *New York Medical Journal*, **73**, 1132–6.

O'Gorman, G. (1954). Psychosis as a cause of mental defect. *Journal of Mental Science*, **100**, 934–43.

Parry-Jones, W.Ll. (1990). Juveniles in 19th-century Oxfordshire asylums. *British Journal of Clinical and Social Psychiatry*, **7**, 51–8.

Parry-Jones, W.Ll. (1993). History of child and adolescent psychiatry. In *Child and Adolescent Psychiatry, Modern Approaches*, 3rd edn, ed. M. Rutter, L. Hersov & E. Taylor, pp. 794–812. Oxford: Blackwell Scientific.

Parry-Jones, W.Ll. (1995). Historical aspects of mood and its disorders in young people. In *The*

Depressed Child and Adolescent: Developmental and Clinical Perspectives, ed. I.M. Goodyer, pp. 1–25. Cambridge: Cambridge University Press.

Perfect, W. (1791). *A Remarkable Case of Madness, with the Diet and Medicines used in the Cure.* Rochester, Great Britain: W. Perfect.

Potter, H.W. (1933). Schizophrenia in children. *American Journal of Psychiatry*, **12**, 1253–70.

Rank, B. (1949). Adaptation of the psychoanalytic technique for the treatment of young children with atypical development. *American Journal of Orthopsychiatry*, **19**, 130–9.

Remschmidt, H.E., Schulz, E., Martin, M., Warnke, A. & Trott, G-E. (1994). Childhood-onset schizophrenia: history of the concept and recent studies. *Schizophrenia Bulletin*, **20**, 727–45.

Rush, B. (1812). *Medical Inquiries and Observations upon the Dreams of the Mind.* Philadelphia: Kimber & Richardson.

Rutter, M. (1965). The influence of organic and emotional factors on the origins, nature and outcome of childhood psychosis. *Developmental Medicine and Child Neurology*, **7**, 518–28.

Rutter, M. (1972). Childhood schizophrenia reconsidered. *Journal of Autism and Childhood Schizophrenia*, **2**, 315–37.

Rutter, M., Greenfield, D., & Lockyer, L. (1967). A five to fifteen year study of infantile psychosis. II. Social behavioural outcome. *British Journal of Psychiatry*, **113**, 1183–99.

Schneider, K. (1939). *Psychischer Befund und psychiatrische Diagnose.* Leipzig: Thieme.

Schönthal, Dr. (1892). Beiträge zur Kenntnis der im frühen Lebensalter auftretenden Psychosen. *Archiv für Psychiatrie*, **23**, 799–837.

Singer, M. & Wynne, L.C. (1963). Differentiating characteristics of the parents of childhood schizophrenics, childhood neurotics, and young adult schizophrenics. *American Journal of Psychiatry*, **120**, 234–43.

Stone, M. (1991). The psychodynamics of schizophrenia. I: Introduction and Psychoanalysis. In *The Concept of Schizophrenia: Historical Perspectives*, ed. J.G. Howells, pp. 125–51. Washington, DC: American Psychiatric Press.

Szurek, S. (1956). Psychotic episodes and psychotic maldevelopment. *American Journal of Orthopsychiatry*, **26**, 519–43.

Tilton, J., De Myer, M., & Loew, L. (1966). *Annotated Bibliography on Childhood Schizophrenia: 1955–1964.* New York: Grune & Stratton.

Tizard, J. (1966). Mental subnormality and child psychiatry. *Journal of Child Psychology and Psychiatry*, **7**, 1–15.

Werry, J.S. (1992). Child and adolescent (early-onset) schizophrenia: a review in light of DSM-III-R. *Journal of Autism and Developmental Disorders*, **22**, 601–24.

Wilkins, R. (1987). Hallucinations in children and teenagers admitted to Bethlem Royal Hospital in the 19th century and the possible relevance to the incidence of schizophrenia. *Journal of Child Psychology and Psychiatry*, **28**, 569–80.

Wilkins, R. (1993). Delusions in children and teenagers admitted to Bethlem Royal Hospital in the 19th century. *British Journal of Psychiatry*, **162**, 487–92.

Wolff, S. & Chick, J. (1980). Schizoid personality in childhood: a controlled follow-up study. *Psychological Medicine*, **10**, 85–100.

World Health Organization (1967). *International Classification of Diseases.* Eighth revision. Geneva: WHO.

World Health Organization (1978). *Mental Disorders: Glossary and Guide to their Classification in Accordance with the Ninth Revision of the International Classification of Diseases.* Geneva: WHO.

World Health Organization (1992). *The ICD-10 Classification of Mental and Behavioural Disorders.* Geneva: WHO.

Zappert, J. (1921). Dementia infantilis (Heller). *Wiener med. Wochensch,* **20**(30), 1328.

2

Definition and classification

Helmut Remschmidt

Introduction

Schizophrenic psychoses in childhood are important but rare disorders within the spectrum of psychoses. They were delineated as specific psychotic disorders only in the late 1930s (Lutz, 1937/38). By the 1950s and 1960s, it was evident that age and developmental stage were important criteria for the classification of childhood psychoses (Group for the Advancement of Psychiatry, 1966; Stutte, 1969). Their importance was demonstrated by several empirical studies (Rutter & Lockyer, 1967; Rutter et al., 1967; Kolvin, 1971; Kolvin et al., 1971a,b,c,d,e). Finally, these studies confirmed the notion of Kanner (1943, 1957), who subdivided childhood psychoses into three groups: early infantile autism, childhood schizophrenia, and disintegrative psychoses of childhood. Disintegrative psychoses comprise disorders such as dementia infantilis (Heller, 1908) and psychoses related to different kinds of brain damage. These subdivisions have also influenced the multiaxial classification systems of the International Classification of Diseases on the basis of ICD-9 and ICD-10 (WHO, 1992) and the *Diagnostic and Statistical Manual of Mental Disorders* of the American Psychiatric Association (DSM-III-R and DSM-IV) (APA, 1987, 1994). Both DSM and ICD differentiate between childhood autism (ICD-10) resp. autistic disorder (DSM-IV), childhood schizophrenia, and early childhood dementia subsumed under the headline "Other childhood disintegrative disorder" resp. "Childhood disintegrative disorder" (DSM-IV).

Early descriptions

Hermann Emminghaus (1887) wrote the first textbook on child psychiatry, *Psychic Disturbances of Childhood*. This text described childhood psychosis as "cerebral neurasthenia" and defined this disorder as "neurosis of the brain characterized by a reduction of cognitive (intellectual) abilities, mood changes, sleep disturbances and manifold anomalies of innervation with a subacute or chronic course and different states of outcome" (p. 134). He also believed that neuropathic children are predisposed to psychotic states and that the etiology of the disorders lies in disturbances of the blood vessels of the cortex.

Emminghaus was also the first (to our knowledge) to introduce a developmental perspective into child psychiatry, with special focus on psychoses. He writes, after complaining that there is no systematic and general symptomatology of childhood psychoses, that it is the task of psychopathology to study the anomalies of the mind through all developmental stages and to differentiate normal from pathologic psychic processes. At the beginning of this century, Kraepelin (1913) distinguished two kinds of endogenous psychoses: dementia praecox and manic-depressive psychoses. Kraepelin went on to develop further differentiations, but his successors continued to use this simplistic dichotomy.

The term "schizophrenia" was introduced by Eugen Bleuler (1911) who spoke of the "group of schizophrenias", different forms of schizophrenia that had to be distinguished from each other. Kraepelin believed that some children classified as mentally handicapped actually had schizophrenia. Karl Leonhard (1986) recently identified a very early manifestation of schizophrenia, the so-called early infantile catatonia. Leonhard believes that this form of childhood schizophrenia is regularly misdiagnosed as severe mental handicap.

August Homburger (1926) stated that childhood schizophrenia is characterized by withdrawal, negativism, and strange and unexpected behavior. Today, we call these "negative" symptoms. He also stated that delusions are rare, especially in young children. Homburger believed that schizophrenia had at least two manifestations: a slow retarded hebephrenic form with cognitive deterioration and an acute catatonic form.

According to Homburger, children also manifest premorbid characteristics and can be divided into three groups on the basis of these characteristics: (i) children with a *premorbid normal development*, good intellectual functions, and no character anomalies; (ii) children with *premorbid mental retardation*; and (iii) children who have *normal intellectual functions* but have character anomalies and display some types of strange behavior.

Jakob Lutz (1937–38) described childhood schizophrenia as a distinct entity, separate from adult schizophrenia. Leo Kanner (1943) and Hans Asperger (1944) delineated two well-known autistic syndromes – early infantile autism and autistic personality disorder – out of the pool of schizophrenic psychoses. Kanner (1943, 1957) and James Anthony (1962) proposed three groups of psychoses, with and without relationship to schizophrenia, which will be discussed later.

Finally, Leonhard (1986) proposed some ideas that are pertinent to our discussion. First, he believes that we should not speak of schizophrenia, but of the group of schizophrenic psychoses, a group that includes several disorders. A unique etiology of schizophrenia is therefore an illusion. By the group of schizophrenic psychoses, Leonhard does not refer to the traditional subdivisions of hebephrenic, paranoid, catatonic, and so on, but to a special subdivision of schizophrenic disorders consisting of unsystematic and systematic schizophrenias. Unsystematic schizophrenias and systematic schizophrenias differ in symptoms, course, and prognosis. Unsystematic schizophrenias are characterized by predominantly affective symptoms (e.g., extreme anxiety states, delusions, hallucinations, ideas of reference). The course is acute, sometimes periodic, and has good remissions. Unsystematic schizophrenias have more in common with affective psychoses than with systematic schizophrenias. Systematic schizophrenias are characterized predominantly by cognitive dysfunctions and disturbances of voluntary functions. The primary dysfunction is in the basic cognitive processes. Leonhard's systematic schizophrenias have nothing to do with systematic or systematized symptomatology, but with disturbances in the brain that result in a defect. The course is chronic, without recovery to the former cognitive level, and the prognosis is poor. Leonhard argues that the cause may lie in disorders of cerebral systems. Leonhard distinguishes *early infantile catatonia* as a special form of childhood schizophrenia. The clinical picture is characterized by motor symptoms, absence of language development or very poor language ability, circumscribed intellectual impairments, negativism (sometimes) periodic course, and predominance of the male sex.

General criteria for the classification of psychotic disorders in children and adolescents

Fig. 2.1 shows some general criteria for the classification of psychotic disorders in childhood and adolescence. Though classification according to etiologic principles would be preferable, our current knowledge does not allow such an approach. Therefore, modern classification systems base their definitions on the symptomatology of the disorders. In childhood and adolescence, however, age and developmental stage play a very important role in the classification of schizophrenia.

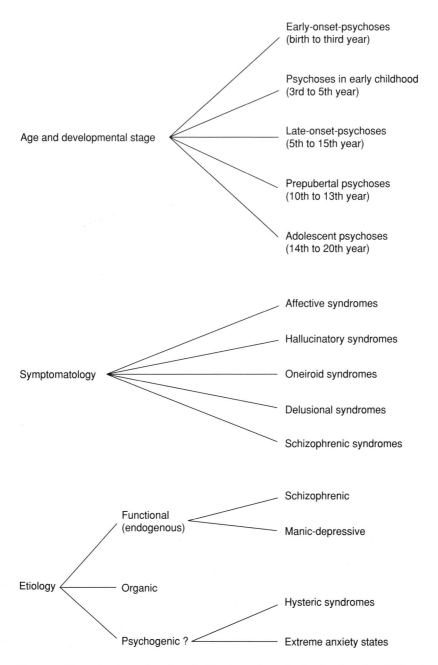

Fig. 2.1. General criteria for the classification of psychotic disorders in childhood and adolescence.

Psychotic disorders in childhood and adolescence and their relation to schizophrenia

Several studies have shown that age and developmental stage are the most influential factors in the clinical picture of childhood psychoses (Anthony, 1958, 1962; Stutte, 1960, 1969; Kolvin, 1971; Kolvin et al., 1971a,b,c,d,e; Werry, 1979; Bettes & Walker, 1987). Most researchers agree that at least four groups of psychoses in childhood and adolescence can be differentiated by age and developmental stage. This subdivision was first proposed by Anthony (1958, 1962) and is demonstrated in Table 2.1.

The first group of psychoses comprises different psychotic syndromes, all of which have a slow beginning and chronic course, and manifest themselves before the third year of life. Except for early infantile catatonia, they have no connection to schizophrenia.

The second group includes different psychotic states, most of which have an acute beginning and different regressive behaviors that manifest themselves between the third and fifth years of life. The connection with schizophrenia is questionable, again with the exception of the early infantile catatonia described by Leonhard (1986), who believes that a connection to schizophrenia is likely.

The third group of psychoses are the late-onset psychoses of late childhood to prepuberty, which have a fluctuating or subacute course and a clear relationship to schizophrenia of adolescence and adulthood. A good example here is the prepubertal schizophrenia described by Stutte (1969) and Eggers (1973).

In his review, Werry (1992) distinguishes between early-onset schizophrenia beginning in childhood or adolescence (before age 16 or 17) and very early-onset schizophrenia (onset before age 13). Werry separates the latter group because that definition is more precise than the term "prepubertal." The age of puberty varies, and most studies that have used the term "prepubertal schizophrenia" have not considered the pubertal stages. Werry states further that a review of the studies of childhood schizophrenia is complicated by the fact that, before ICD-9 and DSM-III, all psychotic disorders of childhood were aggregated into the single category of childhood schizophrenia. So, in many articles, it is impossible to differentiate between early infantile autism, childhood schizophrenia, and other psychoses.

The fourth group of psychoses is adolescent schizophrenia, which manifests at puberty and adolescence and is clearly related to schizophrenia. Psychoses manifested during adolescence may or may not have precursor symptoms in childhood (Rutter, 1967; Remschmidt, 1975a,b). This subdivision according to

Table 2.1. Psychotic syndromes in childhood and adolescence and their relation to schizophrenia[a]

Clinical syndrome	Age at manifestation and course	Relation to schizophrenia
Group 1 (Anthony, 1958, 1962) Autism (Kanner, 1943) Pseudodefective psychosis (Bender, 1947, 1959) "No-onset" type (Despert, 1938)	Early manifestation until third year of life and chronic course	No relation to schizophrenia
Early infantile catatonia (Leonhard, 1986)	Manifestation before third year of life possible	Relation to schizophrenia likely
Group 2 (Anthony, 1958, 1962) Dementia infantilis (Heller, 1908) Dementia praecocissima (DeSanctis, 1908) Pseudoneurotic schizophrenia (Bender, 1947, 1959) "Acute-onset" type (Despert, 1938) Symbiotic psychosis (Mahler et al., 1949; Mahler, 1952) Asperger syndrome (Asperger, 1944, 1968)	Manifestation between third and fifth year of life with acute course and regressive behavior	Relation to schizophrenia questionable
Early infantile (Leonhard, 1986)	Most frequent manifestation within the first 6 years of life	Relation to schizophrenia likely
Group 3 (Anthony, 1958, 1962) Psychoses (late-onset psychoses) (Kolvin, 1971) Pseudopsychopathic schizophrenia (Bender, 1959)	Late-onset psychoses (late childhood and prepuberty) with fluctuating, subacute course	Relation to schizophrenia of adolescence and also adulthood (Anthony, 1958, 1962; Eisenberg, 1957; Rimland, 1964; Rutter, 1967)
Prepuberal schizophrenia (Stutte, 1969; Eggers, 1973)	Manifestation in prepuberty	Clear relation to schizophrenia
Group 4 Adolescent schizophrenia	Manifestation during puberty and adolescence	Clear relation to schizophrenia

[a]Adapted from Remschmidt (1988).

premorbid personality and psychosocial adaptation also seems to be important in positive and negative schizophrenia in adolescence, because there is a relationship between poor premorbid adjustment and negative schizophrenia in adulthood (Andreasen & Olsen, 1982).

The concept of positive and negative schizophrenia in children and adolescents

The concept of positive and negative symptoms in schizophrenia has been widely used in general psychiatry, but has rarely been applied to schizophrenia in childhood and adolescence (Remschmidt et al., 1991). One of the few studies that applied this concept to childhood schizophrenia was carried out by Bettes and Walker (1987). They analyzed a sample of 1084 children with psychotic symptoms, who were selected from a total sample of 11 478 children and adolescents, ages 5–18, from all State-supported inpatient and outpatient facilities in Erie County, NY, and the New York city area. The presence or absence of 31 symptoms, including psychotic symptoms, were recorded at intake by a psychiatrist, a psychologist, or a social worker. The authors found a strong effect of age on the manifestation of positive and negative symptoms. Positive symptoms increased linearly with age, while negative symptoms occurred most frequently in early childhood and late adolescence. This was true for both the total sample of children and the subsample of children with psychotic diagnoses. Bettes and Walker found few sex differences and a correlation between symptoms and IQ: children with high IQs showed more positive and fewer negative symptoms than low-IQ children.

Bettes and Walker (1987) offered three interpretations of their results:

(i) Positive and negative symptoms may represent different psychiatric conditions with different underlying causes. This association has been proposed by Crow (1980) for adult schizophrenia.

(ii) The two symptom types may be associated with different stages of the course of schizophrenia. For instance, negative symptoms could be associated with advanced stages of the disorder. But, as the authors state, this interpretation does not explain the simultaneous increase of both positive and negative symptoms during adolescence.

(iii) Finally, "the clinical manifestation of psychosis in the vulnerable child varies as a function of environmental demands as well as characteristics of the individual. Positive symptoms, particularly those that are based on ideational excess (e.g., paranoia, delusion, grandiosity), may increase in likelihood as cognitive capacity increases. This would explain the linear increase in positive symptoms with age, as well as the lower rate of positive symptomatology in low-IQ children. Alternatively, positive symptoms may be subserved by certain biochemical processes that are triggered during puberty" (p. 565).

In a study of a sample of 113 consecutively admitted adolescents with schizophrenia (58 male, 55 female; mean age 18.3 ± 2 years), Remschmidt et al. (1991) investigated the course of positive and negative symptoms during inpatient treatment using the Andreasen scales (Andreasen, 1982; Andreasen & Olsen, 1982) and an own-rating scale for positive and negative symptoms. In terms of these ratings, the symptomatology of each patient at the beginning and at the end of the inpatient treatment episode was classified into three types: type I (positive schizophrenia), type II (negative schizophrenia), or type III (mixed type). With respect to positive and negative symptomatology, an index was calculated for each patient, so that all patients could be placed on a continuous scale with the extremes +1 and −1, representing the positive and negative end of the schizophrenic symptomatology spectrum, respectively. By comparing the symptomatology at the beginning and at the end of the treatment episode, the following results were obtained: a comparison of positive and negative symptoms revealed a reduction of the number of symptoms with time, but also a clear symptom shift in the direction of negativity. This may be due to the fact that negative symptoms at the beginning of the episode could be hidden by positive symptoms and probably become evident after the disappearance of positive symptoms due to neuroleptic therapy. This notion was put forward by Angst et al. (1989) with regard to schizophrenia in adults, but may also be true for adolescents. Another interpretation is, however, that a high proportion of the patients became chronic. An argument for this interpretation is the fact that, only among type I-schizophrenia patients, a higher proportion (40%) did reach the state of remission. One must, however, bear in mind that the sample was not representative for schizophrenic adolescents with the first manifestation of the disorder. In spite of the fact that all patients were consecutively admitted, the sample comprised a remarkable subgroup of patients who had already been hospitalized. But the study demonstrates nevertheless that the concept of positive and negative symptoms can also be used in adolescent schizophrenia and that we cannot look upon positive and negative symptoms as stable traits of schizophrenic psychoses. They are rather dynamic symptoms that change remarkably during treatment and during the course of the disorder. As far as the direction of change is concerned, the change seems to occur more or less in one direction, namely the negative one.

Premorbid characteristics

About 50% of children and adolescents with schizophrenia show an uncharacteristic symptomatology in their premorbid personality (Stutte, 1969). They have been described as withdrawn, shy, introverted, sensitive, and anxious. It is not clear whether these personality characteristics directly predispose them to schizophrenia, or whether they enhance the vulnerability of those children to adverse experiences in general. Beyond that, there is a large body of evidence for neurobiological and neurodevelopmental deficits in schizophrenic children and adolescents prior to the manifestation of their disorder. These are described in other chapters of this book. Here, we refer only to some behavioral symptoms that may precede the manifestation of the schizophrenic disorder.

Remschmidt et al. (1994) have studied a group of 61 children and adolescents with schizophrenia and have tried to investigate, retrospectively, premorbid symptoms of these children and adolescents. They developed a checklist of premorbid symptoms that could be classified as either "introversive" or "extraversive." Examples of introversive symptoms are mutism, mental slowness, social isolation, general anxieties, specific anxieties, and obsessive–compulsive symptoms. The extraversion dimension comprised items such as hyperactive and dissocial behavior, aggression, and school refusal. According to this categorization, there was no difference between the two groups with first manifestation prior to 14 years ($n = 11$) and the group with first manifestation beyond 14 years of age ($n = 50$). However, they found more introversive than extraversive symptoms in both age groups. The checklist also allowed children to be classified according to four subgroups of premorbid disturbances: developmental disorders, conduct disorders, learning disabilities, and emotional disorders. In all cases, it was attempted to obtain information on premorbid behavior through a careful analysis of the case histories and through information from parents. There were no remarkable differences between the two groups mentioned above, but there was a general trend for developmental disorder to appear first, followed by conduct disorder, emotional disorder, and learning disabilities.

In the same study, the occurrence of positive and negative symptoms as "precursor symptoms of schizophrenia" was studied by the application of a semistructured instrument for the retrospective assessment of the onset of schizophrenia (IRAOS; Häfner et al., 1990). This instrument was modified for the investigation of children and adolescents and their parents. Fig. 2.2 shows the cumulative frequency of positive and negative symptoms before the index admission. While many patients show both negative and positive symptoms

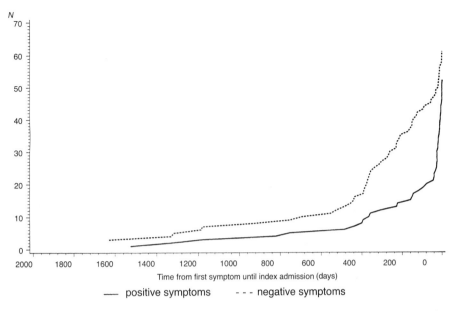

Fig. 2.2. Retrospective assessment of positive and negative symptoms in 61 children and adolescents with schizophrenia.

before the index admission for inpatient treatment, both categories of symptoms become more frequent and converge at the time of the index admission. These results underline the findings in earlier studies that age and developmental stage are decisive variables for the symptomatology of schizophrenic states in childhood and adolescence.

Classification according to ICD-10

In ICD-10, schizophrenia is defined as a disorder

"characterized in general by fundamental and characteristic distortions of thinking and perception, and by inappropriate or blunted affect. Clear consciousness and intellectual capacity are usually maintained, although certain cognitive deficits may evolve in the course of time. The disturbance involves the most basic functions that give the normal person a feeling of individuality, uniqueness, and self-direction" (WHO, 1992, p. 86).

This is only the first part of the definition that includes further hallucinations, disturbances of thinking, mood disturbances, and several other symptoms.

For practical purposes, the symptom characteristic of schizophrenia are divided into several groups, demonstrated in Table 2.2.

Table 2.2. Groups of symptoms with special importance for the diagnosis of schizphrenia (according to ICD-10)

(i)	Thought echo, thought insertion or withdrawal, and thought broadcasting;
(ii)	delusions of control, influence, or passivity, clearly referred to body or limb movements or specific thoughts, actions, or sensations; delusional perception;
(iii)	hallucinatory voices giving a running commentary on the patient's behavior, or discussing the patient among themselves, or other types of hallucinatory voices coming from some part of the body;
(iv)	persistent delusions of other kinds that are culturally inappropriate and completely impossible, such as religious or political identity, or superhuman powers and abilities (e.g., being able to control the weather, or being in communication with aliens from another world);
(v)	persistent hallucinations in any modality, when accompanied either by fleeting or half-formed delusions without clear affective content, or by persistent overvalued ideas, or when occurring every day for weeks or months on end;
(vi)	breaks or interpolations in the train of thought, resulting in incoherence or irrelevant speech, or neologisms;
(vii)	catatonic behavior, such as excitement, posturing, or waxy flexibility, negativism, mutism, and stupor;
(viii)	"negative" symptoms such as marked apathy, paucity of speech, and blunting or incongruity of emotional responses, usually resulting in social withdrawal and lowering of social performance; it must be clear that these are not due to depression or to neuroleptic medication;
(ix)	a significant and consistent change in the overall quality of some aspects of personal behavior, manifest as loss of interest, aimlessness, idleness, a self-absorbed attitude, and social withdrawal.

The diagnostic guidelines require two conditions for the diagnosis of schizophrenia:

– At least one very clear symptom (and usually two or more, if less clearcut) that belong to anyone of the groups listed as (i) to (iv), or symptoms from at least two of the groups referred to as (v) to (viii).

– These symptoms must have been clearly present for most of the time during a period of 1 month or more.

Conditions of a duration of less than 1 month should be diagnosed as acute schizophrenia-like disorder (F23.2). It can be questioned whether the symptom catalogue mentioned in Table 2.2 with the diagnostic guidelines is appropriate for children with very early-onset schizophrenia (prior to the age of 13 years). This has to be tested by further research.

Table 2.3. Schizophrenia, schizotypical and delusional disorders (ICD-10)

Schizophrenia
    Paranoid schizophrenia
    Hebephrenic schizophrenia
    Catatonic schizophrenia
    Undifferentiated schizophrenia
    Postschizophrenic depression
    Residual schizophrenia
    Simple schizophrenia

The course can also be classified using additional categories.
Schizo-typical disorder
Persistent delusional disorders
Acute and transient psychotic disorders
Induced delusional disorder
Schizo-affective disorder
    with subtypes: manic, depressive, and mixed

Table 2.3 gives an overview over the ICD-10 classification of schizophrenia, schizotypical, and delusional disorders.

As the table demonstrates, there are six groups of disorders, five of them outside the core syndrome, and some of them with a questionable relationship to schizophrenia. Schizophrenia itself (F20) is divided into several subtypes, derived from clinical experiences of adult schizophrenia being less clearly diagnosable in childhood and early adolescence.

As far as the subtypes of schizophrenia are concerned, the course can be classified by a special coding, as continuous, episodic with progressive deficit, episodic with stable deficit, episodic remittent, incomplete remission, and complete remission.

Schizotypical disorder (F21)

This category is not clearly demarcated neither from simple schizophrenia nor from schizoid personality disorder and is therefore not recommended for general use. If used at all, one must be sure that the individual never met the criteria for schizophrenia itself. However, there seems to be a connection to schizophrenia insofar as schizophrenia is frequently found in first-degree relatives of the subjects. With regard to terminology, schizotypical disorder includes: borderline schizophrenia, latent schizophrenia, and pseudoneurotic schizophrenia. These descriptions can be found in the literature, but they should not be used owing to unprecise definition.

Persistent delusional disorders (F22)

Under this heading, a group of disorders is subsumed characterized by long-standing delusions without other symptoms characteristic of schizophrenia and without the presence of organic factors. The relationship to schizophrenia is uncertain. The diagnostic guidelines require the presence of delusions for at least 3 months without any evidence of brain disease or schizophrenic symptoms.

The condition includes paranoia, but excludes paranoid schizophrenia (F20.0) and paranoid personality disorder (F60.0).

Acute and transient psychotic disorders (F23)

These are very ill-defined clinical conditions that can be characterized by three features:
an acute onset within 2 weeks,
  - the presence of typical syndromes characterized by rapidly changing and variable states, and by the presence of typical schizophrenic symptoms, and
  - the presence of associated acute stress, e.g., within two weeks after a stressful experience (bereavement, unexpected loss of a parent, abuse).
It is further characteristic of these conditions that complete recovery usually occurs within 2 to 3 months, often also within a few weeks or even days without the development of persistent or disabling states.

Induced delusional disorder (F24)

The main characteristic of this disorder is the induction of delusional symptoms from a person who suffers from a genuine psychotic disorder to another one. The ill person usually suffers from a schizophrenic disorder, and the individual delusions are induced and usually dependent of the person with the genuine psychosis. The two persons usually share a common delusion or delusional system.

This condition is well known in the literature and is described as "folie à deux" or as "symbiotic psychosis."

Schizo-affective disorders (F25)

They are characterized by the presence of both affective and schizophrenic symptoms within the same episode of illness, mostly simultaneously, but at least following each other within a few days. There are three major types that can be differentiated from each other: schizo-affective disorder, manic type (F25.0), schizo-affective disorder, depressive type (F25.1), and schizo-affective

Table 2.4. Diagnostic criteria for schizophrenia (DSM-IV, abbreviated)

A. *Characteristic symptoms:* Two (or more) of the following, each present for a significant portion of time during a 1-month period

   (1) Delusions

   (2) Hallucinations

   (3) Disorganized speech

   (4) Grossly disorganized or catatonic behavior

   (5) Negative symptoms, i.e., affective flattening, alogia or avolition

B. Social/occupational dysfunction

C. *Duration:* Continuous signs persist for at least 6 months. 6-month period must include at least 1 month of symptoms that meet criterion A

D. *Schizoaffective and mood disorder exclusion*

E. *Substance/general medical condition exclusion*

F. *Relationship to a pervasive developmental disorder:* If there is a history of autism or another PDD additional diagnosis of schizophrenia only if prominent delusions or hallucinations are also present for at least a month

---

disorder, mixed type (F25.2). These types of disorders can be found in children and adolescents and have been described clearly.

The ICD-10 system has improved the diagnostic assessment of schizophrenia in all age groups; however, not all categories can be applied to children and adolescents, and empirical studies in younger age groups are rare. Compared with DSM-IV, one major difference concerns the requirement of a period of at minimum 1 month of presence of schizophrenic symptoms, whereas DSM-IV requires the presence of symptoms for at least for 6 months. With regard to these differences, some disorders may be diagnosed as schizophrenia, according to the ICD-10 criteria, but not to those of DSM-IV.

Classification according to DSM-IV

In DSM-IV, schizophrenia is characterized as a disturbance that lasts for at least 6 months and includes at least 1 month of active-phase symptoms (i.e., two [or more] of the following: delusions, hallucinations, disorganized speech, grossly disorganized or catatonic behavior, negative symptoms). Table 2.4 describes the DSM-IV diagnostic criteria for schizophrenia.

Table 2.5 gives an overview of the classification of schizophrenia and other psychotic disorders according to DSM-IV and ICD-10. As the table demonstrates, many categories correspond with those of ICD-10. There are, however, some differences. These concern the subtypes of schizophrenia and the

Table 2.5. Comparison of the ICD-10 and DSM-IV-classification of schizophrenia and related disorders

Schizophrenia, schizotypical, and delusional disorders (ICD-10)	Schizophrenia and other psychotic disorders (DSM-IV)
Schizophrenia	*Schizophrenia*
Paranoid schizophrenia	Paranoid type
Hebephrenic schizophrenia	Disorganized type
Catatonic schizophrenia	Catatonic type
Undifferentiated schizophrenia	Undifferentiated type
Post-schizophrenic depression	
Residual schizophrenia	Residual type
Simple schizophrenia	
Classification of course possible	Classification of course possible
Schizotypical disorder	Schizophreniform disorder
Persistent delusional disorder	Delusional disorder
Acute and transient psychotic disorder	Brief psychotic disorder
Induced delusional disorder	Shared psychotic disorder (folie à deux)
Schizoaffective disorder with subtype: manic, depressive, and mixed	Schizoaffective disorder
	Bipolar subtype, depressive subtype
	Psychotic disorder due to a general medical condition
	Substance-induced psychotic disorder

inclusion of psychotic disorders due to general medical conditions and in substance-induced psychotic disorder. These disorders are classified in ICD-10 under other categories.

The *schizophreniform* disorder is somewhat different compared with schizotypical disorder in ICD-10. The diagnosis of schizophreniform disorder requires the identical criteria of schizophrenia (criterion A), except for two differences: The total duration of the illness is at least 1 month, but less than 6 months (criterion B), and impaired social or occupational functioning during some part of the illness is not required. The delusional disorder corresponds more or less with the category "persistent delusional disorder" of ICD-10, and "brief psychotic disorder" is somewhat identical with the ICD-10 category "acute and transient psychotic disorder," whereas the "shared psychotic disorder" of the DSM-IV corresponds with "induced delusional disorder" of ICD-10.

Conclusions

Since the descriptions of Homburger (1926) and Lutz (1937/38), there is no doubt about the existence of schizophrenic psychoses in childhood. According to Bleuler (1911) and Lutz (1937/38) about 4% of schizophrenic psychoses begin before the 15th year of life and 0.5 to 1% before the 10th year of life. There is a remarkable increase in frequency during adolescence and with increasing age the symptomatology becomes quite similar to that of adult patients. These results are important for the classification which is much easier during adolescence as compared to childhood. It is not clear if the criteria of the current classification systems (ICD-10 and DSM-IV) are appropriate for schizophrenic disorders in younger children, e.g., below the age of 10 or 12 years. Many of these children suffer from early developmental disorders, cognitive and emotional disturbances that complicate an adequate classification within the system that primarily was constructed for the adult type of schizophrenia. On the other hand, our knowledge about the relationship between the different developmental, cognitive and emotional disorders and the later manifestation of schizophrenia is poor and not at all unequivocal. Fortunately, most of the children with these developmental cognitive and behavioral disorders do not develop schizophrenia, and some grow out of these disorders without having long-lasting psychopathological symptoms. The concept of positive and negative symptoms can be applied to childhood and adolescent schizophrenia, but is, as such, also no key issue for a more reliable and valid classification of the disorder in this age group. Perhaps, there are two types of childhood and adolescent schizophrenia: one type that can clearly be diagnosed using the prototype of adult symptomatology without remarkable developmental precursors and another one, complicated by an additional and complex developmental disorder that may modify the expression of symptoms in an age- and developmental stage-appropriate way. This hypothesis has to be tested by careful prospective longitudinal studies. For practical purposes, the current classification systems can be used, but we should always be aware that they reflect our current knowledge and do not describe clearcut nosological entities. That is the reason why they have to be continuously improved by well-conceptualized empirical studies.

REFERENCES

American Psychiatric Association (1987). *Diagnostic and Statistical Manual of Mental Disorders*. 3rd edn, revised (DSM-III-R). Washington, DC: APA.

American Psychiatric Association (1994). *Diagnostic and Statistical Manual of Mental Disorders*. 4th edn (DSM-IV). Washington, DC: APA.

Andreasen, N.C. (1982). Negative symptoms in schizophrenia: Definition and rehabilitation. *Archives of General Psychiatry*, **39**, 784–8.

Andreasen, N.C. & Olsen, S. (1982). Negative and positive schizophrenia: Definition and validation. *Archives of General Psychiatry*, **39**, 789–94.

Angst, J., Stassen, H.H., & Woggon, B. (1989). Effects of neuroleptics on positive and negative symptoms and deficit state. *Psychopharmacology (Berlin)*, **99**, 41–6.

Anthony, E.J. (1958). An experimental approach to the psychopathology of childhood autism. *British Journal of Medical Psychology*, **31**, 211–25.

Anthony, E.J. (1962). Low-grade psychosis in childhood. In *Proceedings of London Conference on Scientific Study of Mental Deficiency*, Vol. 2, ed. B.W. Richards, pp. 398–410. Dagenham: May and Baker.

Asperger, H. (1944). Die "autistischen Psychopathen" im Kindesalter. *Archiv für Psychiatrie und Nervenkrankheiten*, **117**, 76–136.

Asperger, H. (1968). Zur Differentialdiagnose des kindlichen Autismus. *Acta Paedopsychiatrica*, **35**, 136–46.

Bender, L. (1947). Childhood schizophrenia: clinical study of one hundred schizophrenic children. *American Journal of Orthopsychiatry*, **17**, 40–56.

Bender, L. (1959). The concept of pseudopsychopathic schizophrenia in adolescence. *American Journal of Orthopsychiatry*, **29**, 491–509.

Bettes, B.A. & Walker, E. (1987). Positive and negative symptoms in psychotic and other psychiatrically disturbed children. *Journal of Child Psychology and Psychiatry and Allied Disciplines*, **28**, 555–68.

Bleuler, E. (1911). Dementia praecox oder Die Gruppe der Schizophrenien. In *Handbuch der Psychiatrie*, special part, section 4, ed. G. Aschaffenburg, pp. 1–420. Leipzig: Deuticke.

Crow, T.J. (1980). Molecular pathology of schizophrenia: more than one disease process? *British Medical Journal*, **280**, 66–8.

DeSanctis, S. (1908). Dementia praecocissima catatonica. *Folia Neurobiologica*, **1**, 9–12.

Despert, J.L. (1938). Schizophrenia in children. *Psychiatric Quarterly*, **12**, 366–71.

Eggers, C. (1973). *Verlaufsweisen kindlicher und präpuberaler Schizophrenien*. Berlin: Springer.

Emminghaus, H. (1887). *Die psychischen Störungen des Kindesalters*. Tübingen: Laupp.

Eisenberg, L. (1957). The course of childhood schizophrenia. *Archives of Neurology and Psychiatry*, **78**, 69–83.

Group for the Advancement of Psychiatry (1966). *Psychopathological Disorders in Childhood: Theoretical Considerations and a Proposed Classification*. New York, NY: The Group.

Häfner, H., Riecher, A., Maurer, K., Meissner, S., Schmidtke, A., Fätkenheuer, B., Löffler, W., & der Heiden, W. (1990). Instrument for the retrospective assessment of the onset of schizophrenia (IRAOS). *Zeitschrift für Klinische Psychologie*, **19**, 230–55.

Heller, T. (1908). Über Dementia infantilis (Verblödungsprozeß im Kindesalter). *Zeitschrift für die Erforschung und Behandlung des jugendlichen Schwachsinns auf wissenschaftlicher Grundlage*, **2**, 17–28.

Homburger, A. (1926). *Vorlesungen über Psychopathologie des Kindesalters*. Berlin: Springer (Wiss Buchgesellschaft, Dormstadt, 1967).

Kallman, F.J. & Roth, B. (1956). Genetic aspects of pre-adolescent schizophrenia. *American Journal of Psychiatry*, **112**, 599–606.

Kanner, L. (1943). Autistic disturbances of affective contact. *Nervous Child*, **2**, 217–50.

Kanner, L. (1957). *Child psychiatry*. 3rd edn. Oxford: Blackwell.

Kolvin, I. (1971). Studies in the childhood psychoses: I. Diagnostic criteria and classification. *British Journal of Psychiatry*, **118**, 381–4.

Kolvin, I., Garside, R.F., & Kidd, J.S.H. (1971a). Studies in the childhood psychoses: IV. Parental personality and attitude and childhood psychoses. *British Journal of Psychiatry*, **118**, 403–6.

Kolvin, I., Humphrey, M., & McNay, A. (1971b). Studies in the childhood psychoses: VI. Cognitive factors in childhood psychoses. *British Journal of Psychiatry*, **118**, 415–19.

Kolvin, I., Ounsted, C., Humphrey, M., & McNay, A. (1971c). Studies in the childhood psychoses: II. The phenomenology of childhood psychoses. *British Journal of Psychiatry*, **118**, 385–95.

Kolvin, I., Ounsted, C., Richardson, L.M., & Garside, R.F. (1971d). Studies in the childhood psychoses: III. The family and social background in childhood psychoses. *British Journal of Psychiatry*, **118**, 396–402.

Kolvin, I., Ounsted, C., & Roth, M. (1971e). Studies in the childhood psychoses: V. Cerebral dysfunction and childhood psychoses. *British Journal of Psychiatry*, **118**, 407–14.

Kraepelin, E. (1913). *Psychiatrie*. 8th edn, Vol. 3, Part 2. Leipzig: Barth.

Leonhard, K. (1986). *Aufteilung der endogenen Psychosen und ihre differenzierte Ätiologie*. 2nd edn. Berlin: Akademie-Verlag.

Lourie, R.S., Pacella, B.L., & Piotrowski, Z.A. (1943). Studies on the prognosis in schizophrenic-like psychoses in children. *American Journal of Psychiatry*, **99**, 542–52.

Lutz, J. (1937/38). Über die Schizophrenie im Kindesalter. *Schweizer Archiv für Neurologie, Neurochirurgie und Psychiatrie*, **39**, 335–72 and **40**, 141–63.

Mahler, M.S. (1952). On child psychosis and schizophrenia: Autistic and symbiotic infantile psychosis. *Psychoanalytic Study of the Child*, **7**, 286–305.

Mahler, M.S., Ross, J.R., & de Fries, Z. (1949). Clinical studies in benign and malignant cases of childhood psychosis (schizophrenia-like). *American Journal of Orthopsychiatry*, **19**, 2952–304.

Remschmidt, H. (1975a). Neuere Ergebnisse zur Psychologie und Psychiatrie der Adoleszenz. *Zeitschrift für Kinder- und Jugendpsychiatrie*, **3**, 67–101.

Remschmidt, H. (1975b). Psychologie und Psychopathologie der Adoleszenz. *Monatsschrift für Kinderheilkunde*, **123**, 316–23.

Remschmidt, H. (1998). Schizophrene Psychosen im Kindes- und Jugendalter. In *Psychiatrie der Gegenwart*, 3rd edn., vol. 7, ed. K.P. Kisker, H. Lauter, J.E. Meyer, C. Müller, & E. Strömgren, pp. 89–117. Berlin; Springer.

Remschmidt, H., Martin, M. Schulz, E., Gutenbrunner, C., & Fleischhaker, C. (1991). The concept of positive and negative schizophrenia in child and adolescent psychiatry. In *Negative Versus Positive Schizophrenia*, ed. A. Marneros & N.C. Andreasen, pp. 219–42. Berlin–Heidelberg: Springer.

Remschmidt, H., Schulz, E., Martin, M., Warnke, A., & Trott, G-E. (1994). Childhood-onset schizophrenia: history of the concept and recent studies. *Schizophrenia Bulletin*, **20**, 727–45.

Rimland, B. (1964). *Infantile Autism: The Syndrome and its Implications for a Neural Theory of Behavior*. New York, NY: Appleton-Century-Crofts.

Rutter, M. (1967). Psychotic disorders in early childhood. In *Recent Developments in Schizophrenia*, ed. A.J. Coppen & A. Walk, pp. 133–58. Ashford: Headly Brothers Ltd.

Rutter, M. & Lockyer, L. (1967). A five to fifteen-year follow-up study of infantile psychosis: I. Description of sample. *British Journal of Psychiatry*, **113**, 1169–82.

Rutter, M., Lockyer, L. & Greenfield, D. (1967). A five to fifteen-year follow-up study of infantile psychosis: II. Social and behavioural outcome. *British Journal of Psychiatry*, **113**, 1183–99.

Stutte, H. (1960). Kinderpsychiatrie und Jugendpsychiatrie. In *Psychiatrie der Gegenwart*, Vol. II, ed. H.W. Gruhle, R. Jung, W. Mayer-Gross & M. Müller, pp. 952–1087. Berlin: Springer.

Stutte, H. (1969). Psychosen des Kindesalters. In *Neurologie–Psychologie–Psychiatrie (Handbuch der Kinderheilkunde)*, Vol. VIII/1, ed. F. Schmidt & H. Asperger, pp. 908–38. Berlin: Springer.

Werry, J.S. (1979). The childhood psychoses. In *Psychopathological Disorders of Childhood*, 2nd edn, ed. H.C. Quay & J.S. Werry, pp. 43–89. New York: John Wiley.

Werry, J.S. (1992). Child and adolescent (early onset) schizophrenia: a review in light of DSM-III-R. *Journal of Autism and Developmental Disorders*, **22**, 601–24.

World Health Organization (WHO) (1992). *International Statistical Classification of Disease and Related Health Problems*. Vol I, 10th revision. Geneva: The Organization.

3

Epidemiology of early onset schizophrenia

Christopher Gillberg

Introduction

The diagnosis of schizophrenia is rarely made in childhood, and it seems almost certain that prepubertal onset of schizophrenia is rare. However, for decades, the disorders now subsumed under the label of autism spectrum disorders (Wing, 1996b) or pervasive developmental disorders (APA, 1994) – themselves relatively rare conditions – were referred to as "childhood schizophrenia" (Bender, 1969), leading to difficulty in separating out "true" cases of schizophrenia in older studies. Only after the publication by Kolvin of a study showing two fairly distinct peaks for age of onset of prepubertal "psychosis" (Kolvin, 1971) did the current emphasis of a split between early childhood autism and later onset cases of schizophrenia begin to develop (Rutter, 1978). It has been – almost universally – agreed for two decades that childhood autism and schizophrenia are qualitatively different conditions and that early onset pervasive developmental disorders (such as Kanner's variant of autism) do not represent precursors of schizophrenia (Gillberg, 1990). However, in the most recent past, the emergence of the concept of Asperger syndrome (Wing, 1981) and the upsurge in publications on early onset schizophrenia – and particularly on the antecedents of disorders diagnosed as childhood schizophrenia (Watkins et al., 1988) – have led to a reopening of the debate as to whether or not autism spectrum disorders (of which Asperger syndrome is believed to constitute one part) should be seen as totally distinct from schizophrenia with prepubertal (or later) onset. All these issues need to be taken into account when considering matters to do with the epidemiology of early onset schizophrenia.

This chapter reviews what limited evidence there is in respect of early onset schizophrenia. Early onset schizophrenia will be subdivided into "very early onset schizophrenia" (with documented major signs of schizophrenia at or under the age of 12 years) and "adolescent onset schizophrenia" (with documented major signs becoming apparent only in the teenage period, i.e., the 13–19-year age range). Findings from neighboring areas, particularly

Kanner syndrome (childhood autism) and Asperger syndrome, will also be briefly surveyed so as to provide a fuller background against which the scope of the problem of childhood schizophrenia might be interpreted.

Childhood autism

It now seems clear that the behavioral syndrome of autism as originally described by Kanner – and comprising the triad of impairments of reciprocal social interaction, communication and imagination/behavior – is more common than was once widely held. Recent estimates range from 5 to 12 in 10 000 children surviving the first years of life (Wing, 1993; Gillberg, 1995) and some studies indicate that the prevalence may be even higher (Ishii & Takahashi, 1982; Tanoue et al., 1988; Wing, 1996a; Arvidsson et al., 1997). The vast majority of individuals with childhood autism are also mentally retarded and test reliably in the IQ ranges under 70. Boys are diagnosed as having childhood autism two to four times as often as girls, and the male : female ratio is higher still among those with the highest IQ levels (Wing, 1996b). There is a strong association of autism with epilepsy (Rutter, 1970) and with known medical syndromes (Gillberg & Coleman, 1996). High social class is probably not specifically linked with autism (Schopler et al., 1979).

There appears to be no over-representation of classic schizophrenic symptoms (auditory hallucinations, delusions and schizophrenic-type thought disorder) among individuals diagnosed in the first 5 to 10 years of life as having childhood autism (Howlin, 1997). Nevertheless, rare instances of autism and schizophrenia do occur, and it appears that individuals diagnosed with early onset schizophrenia quite often have some marked autistic symptoms in their premorbid history (Watkins et al., 1988).

Asperger syndrome

Once hypothesized to be a very rare disorder (LeCouteur & Rutter, 1988), it is now believed that Asperger syndrome is more common than classical childhood autism – as would be expected if it is seen to represent a milder variant of autism or simply equivalent to "very high-functioning autism." Three epidemiological studies suggest that the prevalence in school-age children is in the range of 26–36 in 10 000 (Gillberg & Gillberg, 1989; Ehlers & Gillberg, 1993; Gunnarsdóttir & Magnússon, 1994). The male : female ratio appears to be even higher in Asperger syndrome than in autism (Wing, 1981), even though it has not exceeded 4 : 1 in the population studies. Medical syndromes and epilepsy are sometimes associated with Asperger syndrome, but at a considerably lower rate than in classic childhood autism (Gillberg, 1991). Pre- and perinatal premorbid problems, on the other hand, may be at least as frequent in Asperger syndrome as in classic autism (Gillberg, 1989). It is possible, although population-based evidence is lacking, that Asperger syndrome may be more frequently diagnosed among children belonging in higher social classes (Gillberg, 1989).

The syndrome – comprising the core triad of symptoms seen in classical childhood autism – is diagnosed in individuals with no or only mild general cognitive problems (Wing, 1981; Gillberg, 1985; Gillberg & Gillberg, 1989). There is some disagreement as to whether delayed development of language and of decreased curiosity about the environment can occur in cases receiving this diagnosis (Wing, 1991; WHO, 1993; APA, 1994; Ehlers & Gillberg, 1993). The higher IQ in this group of individuals as compared with those who receive a diagnosis of childhood autism, particularly the higher verbal IQ (Ehlers et al., 1997), leads to a situation in which the severe restriction of empathy and of reciprocal social interaction – typical of both diagnostic groups – is often perceived by clinicians as more subtle. The diagnosis is often made much later than childhood autism, and usually not until well into the school years.

There is no consensus with regard to the scope of a possible overlap of Asperger syndrome and schizophrenia. Lorna Wing (1981) believes that it is only rarely associated with schizophrenia, in a fashion which might suggest chance co-occurrence. Sula Wolff (1995) – in comparing schizoid personality in childhood with Asperger syndrome – on the other hand, suggests that there might indeed be meaningful overlap of the two syndromes, a view also held by Chris Frith (1991). The *symptoms* of Asperger syndrome certainly suggest a location of the condition "in the 'no man's land' of classification between autism, on the one hand, and schizophrenia on the other" (Kay & Kolvin, 1987; Kolvin & Bernie, 1990). Much of the debate on whether or not Asperger syndrome is in some way related to schizophrenia would probably be resolved if schizophrenia was not conceptualized as a single diagnostic entity. For instance, Wing and Shah (1994) have reported several cases of autism and Asperger syndrome developing into catatonia, a symptom/syndrome regarded by many to be one variant of schizophrenia. The development of catatonia in high-functioning autism has also been observed by our group (E. Billstedt, unpublished data). Further, it appears that a considerable proportion of all inidividuals with the diagnosis of Asperger syndrome may have "micro-psycho-tic" episodes in adult life, particularly in situations perceived by themselves as very stressful. Such cases may be misdiagnosed as having schizophrenia or, at least, "schizophreniform psychosis." This would seem to be particularly likely in cases showing Lorna Wing's "active but odd" style of social interaction (Wing, 1989). In my own clinic I have followed several young people with Asperger syndrome into early adult life, and a few of them have developed striking paranoid features. In one instance these were diagnosed by an adult psychiatrist as "paranoid schizophrenia." In other words, it seems clear that individuals with Asperger syndrome often develop adult psychiatric symptoms, some of which are seen in the syndromes subsumed under the general label of "schizophrenia." However, typical auditory hallucinations and schizophrenia-type thought disorder, appear to be rare.

Disintegrative disorder and Rett syndrome variants

Heller syndrome or childhood onset disintegrative disorder is a very rare condition, affecting no more than 11 in 1 000 000 children (Burd et al., 1987). The male : female ratio is similar to that encountered in childhood autism and Asperger syndrome (Volkmar, 1992).

In most instances this disorder would not be confused with childhood schizophrenia, and the symptoms, after a period of hyperactivity, regression and confusion in connection with onset/setback around 3–4 years of age, are strikingly reminiscent of those seen in classic chilhood autism, not of schizophrenia. However, in those few instances of Heller syndrome with slightly later onset, it is possible that differential diagnosis *vis-à-vis* schizophrenia may sometimes be difficult.

There is also a small number of girls with variants of Rett syndrome (Hagberg & Gillberg, 1993), particularly the preserved speech variant (Zappella et al., 1997), that may present with symptoms that might well be confused with schizophrenia early in the course of the disorder. Rett syndrome variants are more common than previously believed, but probably occurring at a rate under 1 in 10 000 girls.

Landau–Kleffner syndrome and the syndrome of electrical status epilepticus during sleep

Disruption of normal language development sometimes co-occurs with the appearance of epileptogenic discharge on the EEG (particularly during sleep) or overt epileptic seizures in children aged 3–10 years. This group of disorders is often referred to as Landau–Kleffner syndrome (Mouridsen, 1995). A related concept is the so-called electrical status epilepticus during sleep (ESES), also known as continuous spike wave activity during slow sleep (CSWSS). These disorders are all rare, although their actual prevalence has never been established. Occasionally, they may cause considerable differential diagnostic problems in relation to early onset schizophrenia, especially in the case of ESES (Kyllerman et al., 1996).

Very early onset schizophrenia (12 years or under)

There is a paucity of studies of very early onset schizophrenia. No study particularly geared to the estimation of prevalence of very early onset schizophrenia has been published. If the syndrome is as rare as currently hypothesized, this should come as no surprise, given the difficulty of recruiting cases for studies of rare disorders.

Population studies

Using data from a general population survey of autism and other severe neuropsychiatric disorders with early childhood onset published in Gillberg (1984) and Gillberg and Steffenburg (1987), the prevalence of very early onset schizophrenia was estimated at 1.6 per 100 000 in the general population of children in western Sweden in 1980. This rate was calculated on the basis of two cases of "childhood schizophrenia" (meeting DSM-III-criteria (APA, 1980) for schizophrenia and with onset of symptoms before age 10 years) ascertained in a study geared to finding all individuals with classic autism. These two individuals (males) recruited at population screening plus one more individual (female) referred to a specialized child neuropsychiatric service (with nationwide coverage in respect of diagnostic work-up in "child psychosis") constitute all those with schizophrenia with prepubertal onset ever diagnosed (over a 25-year period) by the present author in Sweden (out of a total of more than 2000 prepubertal children evaluated for neurodevelopmental or neuropsychiatric disorders). Also, no cases of early onset schizophrenia were found in two more recent population studies of autism spectrum disorders in the western Swedish region (Steffenburg & Gillberg, 1986; Gillberg et al., 1991). This suggests that the true rate of very early onset schizophrenia may actually be even lower than 1.6 in 100 000 children. It is also of some interest that one of the boys had many autistic-like symptoms in early childhood, although never qualifying for a diagnosis of childhood autism, and that a girl, in addition to meeting full symptom criteria for schizophrenia, also met symptom criteria for childhood autism.

On the basis of data obtained in a study of autism prevalence in North Dakota (Burd et al., 1987), it can be estimated that 1.9 in 100 000 children in the general population had very early onset schizophrenia.

Thus, the only two population studies that have mentioned cases of very early onset schizophrenia have both come up with data showing the disorder to be extremely rare.

Clinical studies

Kolvin (1971) estimated that the rate of late onset child psychosis was about 70% of that for classic autism, and corresponded to about 30 per 100 000 school children. However, it is unclear what proportion of this rate was contributed by very early onset schizophrenia, and how many could have been cases of Heller syndrome/disintegrative disorder of childhood (Volkmar, 1992). It seems that very early onset ("childhood") schizophrenia is almost never diagnosed in Europe. Eggers (1978), performing an outcome study in Germany, had to cover a period of 30 years in order to come up with 40 cases, many of which had onset of major symptoms after the age of 10 years (but before age 13 years).

Equally, it appears that very early onset schizophrenia is diagnosed very rarely in New Zealand. Werry found only nine cases of schizophrenia under the age of 16 years over a 10-year period in a unit serving an at-risk population of 130 000, and only two of these had onset at 12 years or under. There were also a few cases with schizo-phreniform disorder, including a boy with suspected Sydenham chorea who developed florid psychotic symptoms around age 6 years (and who had a good outcome). It is notable that a significant number of the cases, originally diagnosed as having schizophrenia, on follow-up several years later were instead diagnosed as suffering from bipolar disorder (Werry et al., 1991).

In marked contrast, over a 10-year period, several authors from one of the many child psychiatric services in New York City – the Child Psychiatry Department at Bellevue Hospital, New York University – have reported on at least 56 individuals with very early onset schizophrenia (Green et al., 1984; Spencer et al., 1992). Although catchment areas and population rates cannot be readily compared to those reported by other authors, it does seem that the diagnosis of schizophrenia with very early onset may have been made more commonly in this setting than in those previously described.

Male:female ratios

Male:female ratios tend to be 2:1 or higher in the very early onset group (Werry, 1992), even though one study found no indication of a high male:female ratio (Eggers, 1978).

Onset

Onset is usually insidious (or even "chronic") as reported by at least three different groups (Kolvin, 1971; Green et al., 1992; Asarnow & Ben-Meir, 1988). The youngest age of onset reported in the literature is 3 years in one case (Russell et al., 1989) and 5 years in a few other cases (Green et al., 1992; Caplan et al., 1989).

Age and developmental trends

Given the considerable difficulty of evaluating symptoms such as delusions and thought disorder in children with mental ages under about 6 years, and in mute or language-disordered children regardless of mental age, it would seem that a diagnosis of schizophrenia in a child under about 6 years would have to be preliminary for a few years, if at all accepted in this age group (Werry, 1992). There is some evidence for age-dependent variation in symptoms as children grow older (Asarnow, 1994). Well-formulated delusions are very rare – if at all possible to ascertain – in the youngest age group, while hallucinations and disorganized thinking may be characteristic of children 6 years of age or older (Caplan et al., 1990), and particularly in those over 8 or 9 years of age (Garralda, 1984a,b; Watkins et al., 1988).

Intelligence

Mean IQ is probably lower than in the general population, and about 10–20% score about 70 or under (Eggers, 1978; Green et al., 1992; Werry et al., 1991; Werry, 1992). Mental retardation is considered a premorbid feature and not a consequence of schizophrenia (Aylward et al., 1984). However, because of the small number of cases of very early onset schizophrenia reported so far, and the trend for some authors to exclude cases scoring in the mentally retarded range (Bettes & Walker, 1987; Russell et al., 1989), it is not possible to draw any definite conclusions in respect of IQ (or test profiles) in the youngest age group with schizophrenia.

Pre- and comorbid problems

In respect of premorbid and comorbid conditions (other than low IQ), there is growing evidence that childhood schizophrenia is associated with other diagnoses in a developmentally complex fashion (Asarnow, 1994). A premorbid history suggestive of pervasive developmental disorder (or "autism spectrum disorder") is quite common (Watkins et al., 1988; Asarnow et al., 1988) and comorbid problems of conduct, oppositional defiant disorder, schizoid and schizotypal personality features and depression are all fairly common. Children who are diagnosed as having schizophrenia in the 6–12-year-old age period frequently have shown early language abnormality and delay, motor delay and hypotonia, unusual responses to the environment and sometimes a lack of responsiveness in infancy. Hyperactivity and attention deficits are very common also (Asarnow et al., 1991; Asarnow, 1994). This clinical picture is consistent with the descriptions of so-called DAMP (deficits in attention, motor control and perception) given by Scandinavian researchers (Gillberg et al., 1982; Hellgren et al., 1994; Gillberg, 1995; Landgren et al., 1996), a phenomenological syndrome showing considerable overlap both with the DSM categories of ADHD (attention deficit hyperactivity disorder) and developmental coordination disorder (Kadesjö & Gillberg, 1997). In a study of adolescent onset schizophrenia (Hellgren et al., 1987), premorbid DAMP was more common than in a non-schizophrenia comparison group matched for sex, age and maternity clinic (see below). Affective change with mood swings is also common both as a prodrome and as a comorbid problem. It has been estimated that about 10% of all severe cases of depression occuring in early childhood constitute precursors of schizophrenia (Nissen, 1981).

Outcome

There is very little evidence with respect to outcome of very early onset schizophrenia with little in the way of clearly longitudinal data available. A tendency for cases diagnosed with schizophrenia in the prepubertal period to be rediagnosed with bipolar disorder a few years later has been noted by one group in New Zealand (Werry, 1992). However, another group – in Canada – found a high degree of diagnostic stability from childhood to early adult life in respect of very early onset schizophrenia (although this conclusion was based on only five cases) (Maziade et al., 1996).

Children with severe DAMP (see above) often have some autistic features or "psychotic behavior" (Gillberg, 1983), and some meet symptom criteria for Asperger syndrome (Hellgren et al., 1994). It is possible that some of these children would have been diagnosed as having very early onset schizophrenia by US groups studying this particular disorder. This was supported by an unpublished clinical study of very early onset psychosis and schizophrenia cases performed at the NYU Medical Center. The majority of a group of ten children diagnosed by US research clinicians as having psychosis and schizophrenia in the Department of Child Psychiatry at Bellevue Hospital in the spring of 1993 were given clinical diagnoses of DAMP and ADHD with or without autistic features by the present author. Long-term follow-up of children with DAMP indicate that a substantial minority develop severe affective disorder (including bipolar disorder) in adolescence and that some become antisocial. However, the rate of schizophrenia in adolescence or early adulthood does not appear to be raised much above the level expected in the general population (Hellgren et al., 1994). This would be in line with Werry's finding that young children suspected of having very early onset schizophrenia turn out to have bipolar disorder in the longer term (Werry, 1992).

Adolescent onset schizophrenia (13–19 years of age)

There have been few epidemiological studies specifically of adolescent onset schizophrenia. Most of the data on the epidemiology of schizophrenia in the adolescent age group derive from studies that include only a small subgroup of adolescents and young adults.

Some estimates of the incidence of schizophrenia suggest that it occurs about 50 times less often before age 15 years than after it (Beitchman, 1985).

Population-based studies

One Swedish study was aimed explicitly at estimating the rate of teenage onset psychotic disorders (including schizophrenia). All psychiatric inpatients in one birth cohort were screened for schizophrenia and schizophreniform disorder, and for other psychotic disorders with onset of symptoms in the 13–19-year age period. The accumulated prevalence for DSM-III (APA, 1980) schizophrenia was 0.23%. This figure means that, out of all 20-year-old individuals living in Göteborg, Sweden in the early 1980s, 0.23% had been admitted to a psychiatric clinic for schizophrenia commencing in the teenage period (13 to 19 years of age). About half of this prevalence was contributed by cases with onset at or under 16 years of age.

In a Scottish national sample, the *incidence* of schizophrenia in the 15–19-year-old age range dropped from 2.0 in 10 000 to 1.0 in 10 000 in males and from 1.4 to 0.5 in females from the late 1960s to the late 1980s (Takei et al., 1996). The authors interpreted the decline as showing the diminishing influence of environmental factors operating early in life.

Clinical studies

Among adolescent (12–19-year-old) psychiatric outpatients in a Scottish study, only about 1% were diagnosed as having psychosis (Evans & Acton, 1972).

In an inpatient psychiatric unit, 5% of 11–18-year-olds had psychosis, and about 60% of these had schizophrenia or schizo-affective disorder (Steinberg et al., 1981).

Male: female ratio

The male: female ratio in the Swedish study (of 13–19-year-olds) was 1.9:1. In the Scottish study (of 15–19-year-olds), it varied from 1.4:1 to 2.2:1 depending on birth cohort. In older individuals, and in clinical samples of adolescent onset schizophrenia, male: female ratios tend to approach 1:1 (Werry, 1992).

Onset

There is a steep increase in the frequency of the diagnosis of schizophrenia from about 13 years of age, and then a gradual increase each year up until about age 18 years (Gillberg et al., 1986). Onset in this group as compared to the very early onset group is more likely to be acute (Werry, 1992), although this was not found by Kolvin (1971).

Age and developmental trends

Four of the 25 affected individuals diagnosed as having teenage onset schizophrenia had been examined by child psychiatrists in early childhood, long before the onset of schizophrenic symptoms. They had received diagnoses of "psychosis", "possible schizophrenia", "attention deficit disorder with emotional disorder" and "emotional disorder". All four had been considered much improved before the teenage period, had not been in treatment or counselling for several years, and had functioned relatively well in normal schools.

Intelligence

There is little evidence that IQ differs from the general population norm in cases of adolescent onset schizophrenia. In the Swedish population study, there was a tendency towards an increased rate of subnormal IQ in the schizophrenia group. Special education had been given premorbidly significantly more often in the schizophrenia group than in an age-, sex- and school-matched group. However, there were no cases of clearcut mental retardation among the 25 cases identified. In a population study of all 149 13–17-year-olds with IQ levels of 70 or under in Göteborg, Sweden, performed in 1984, two individuals (one with severe and one with mild mental retardation) met full criteria for schizophrenia according to the DSM-III. This corresponds to a population rate of adolescent onset schizophrenia with mental retardation of about 1.34%, which is higher than in the general population sample (where it was 0.23%), again suggesting that there is a weak–moderate association of schizophrenia with low IQ in adolescence.

Pre- and comorbid problems

About one in eight of the whole group with schizophrenia had a premorbid history suggestive of DAMP (see above). However, DAMP is a common problem, affecting several percent of all school age children. Thus, the proportion of this group who develops schizophrenia in adolescence is low (Hellgren et al., 1994) – given the low base rate of adolescent onset schizophrenia in the general population.

Outcome

On follow-up at age 30 years of the Swedish sample, 35% of those with a diagnosis of schizophrenia in teenage had received this diagnosis again on repeated inpatient treatment in the 20–30-year age period (Gillberg, IC et al., 1993). An additional 13% were diagnosed as having chronic alcoholism, and a further 13% were given diagnoses of paranoid reaction with Asperger syndrome, borderline personality disorder and atypical psychosis. In addition to these 61% of the original group, 17% had received a full pension without having been diagnosed as having a specific psychiatric disorder (although the diagnosis of schizophreniform disorder or schizophrenia had been considered in all the cases). Thus, 50 to 60% of the original group were still considered to be in the schizophrenia spectrum disorder diagnostic category more than 10 years after onset of psychotic symptoms in teenage. None was diagnosed as having a major affective disorder. However, among the group with diagnoses of teenage onset unipolar or bipolar psychotic disorders, 1 out of 15 had "changed" from affective disorder to "schizophrenia" at age 30 years. All the individuals with schizophrenia diagnosed in the teenage period were still alive at follow-up at age 30 years. This findings contrasts with the risk of 5–15% suicide or accidental death directly due to psychosis reported in clinical studies (Eggers, 1978; Werry et al., 1991). Only about 20% of the group were relatively well functioning at age 30 years and had not received a full pension, were not undergoing psychiatric treatment and were not known to have offended.

In the Canadian study (Maziade et al., 1996), which included 36 cases with adolescent onset schizophrenia, there was even greater stability over time in respect of the diagnosis of schizophrenia made in the teenage period, with about 90% receiving this diagnosis again in connection with follow-up at a mean age of 28 years. Outcome, if anything, was even worse than in the Swedish sample.

Conclusions

It seems reasonable to subdivide early onset schizophrenia into those with onset at or under age 12 years ("very early onset") and those with onset in the teenage period (13–19 years) ("adolescent onset"). A case could also be made for subdividing according to onset of puberty, but this has not been possible on the basis of data published to date, given that details in respect of pubertal development have not been mentioned. Onset tends to be insidious in the youngest group and more often acute in the adolescent group. Males predominate strongly in the youngest age group, but less markedly so in those with adolescent onset. Very early onset schizophrenia appears to be extremely rare with only one or two cases in 100 000 children, but the evidence on which this conclusion is based is minimal. Standards for diagnosing schizophrenia in the US as compared with the rest of the world could be slightly different, and might account for the impression of a higher rate of diagnosed disorder, at least in some centres. Adolescent onset schizophrenia is not an extremely rare diagnosis and, according to one population study, affects 0.23% of the general population, and, according to another population study, 1.34% of the general population of teenagers with mental retardation. There is a high degree of pre- and comorbid problems suggestive of autism spectrum disorders (particularly in the very early onset group) and of attention dysfunction and developmental coordination disorders – including the syndrome of DAMP. Outcome is psychosocially poor, although a subgroup of about 20% may have relatively good outcomes with acceptable social functioning around 30 years of age. The stability of a diagnosis of early onset schizophrenia is relatively good, but not perfect. There appears to be a particular risk of misdiagnosing schizophrenia in bipolar disorders with very early onset.

There is now a great need for collaborative cross-cultural research aiming to establish with better precision the epidemiology of early onset schizophrenia – both the prepubertal and adolescent variants.

REFERENCES

American Psychiatric Association (1994). *Diagnostic and Statistical Manual of Mental Disorders*, 4th edn (DSM-IV). Washington, DC: APA.

American Psychiatric Association (1980). *Diagnostic and Statistical Manual of Mental Disorders*, 3rd edn (DSM-III). Washington, DC: APA.

Arvidsson, T., Danielsson, B., Forsberg, P., Gillberg, C., Johansson, M., & Källgren, G. (1997).

Autism in 3–6-year-old children in a suburb of Göteborg, Sweden. *Autism*, **1**, 163–73.

Asarnow, J.R. (1994). Annotation: childhood-onset schizophrenia. *Journal of Child Psychology and Psychiatry*, **35**, 1345–71.

Asarnow, J.R. & Ben-Meir, S. (1988). Children with schizophrenia spectrum and depressive disorders: a comparative study of premorbid adjustment, onset pattern and severity of impairment. *Journal of Child Psychology and Psychiatry and Allied Disciplines*, **29**, 477–88.

Asarnow, J.W., Goldstein, M.J., & Ben-Meir, S. (1988). Parental communication deviance in childhood onset schizophrenia spectrum and depressive disorders. *Journal of Child Psychology and Psychiatry*, **29**, 825–38.

Asarnow, J.R., Asarnow, R.F., Hornstein, N., & Russell, A.T. (1991). Childhood-onset schizophrenia: developmental perspectives on schizophrenic disorders. In *Schizophrenia: A Life Course Developmental Perspective*, ed. E.F. Walker, pp. 92–122. New York: Academic Press.

Aylward, E., Walker, E., & Bettes, B. (1984). Intelligence in schizophrenia: meta-analysis of the research. [Review] [96 refs]. *Schizophrenia Bulletin*, **10**, 430–59.

Beitchman, J.H. (1985). Childhood schizophrenia. A review and comparison with adult-onset schizophrenia. *Psychiatric Clinics of North America*, **8**, 793–814.

Bender, L. (1969). A longitudinal study of schizophrenic children with autism. *Hospital and Community Psychiatry*, **20**, 230–7.

Bettes, B.A. & Walker, E. (1987). Positive and negative symptoms in psychotic and other psychiatrically disturbed children. *Journal of Child Psychology and Psychiatry and Allied Disciplines*, **28**, 555–68.

Burd, L., Fisher, W., & Kerbeshian, J. (1987). A prevalence study of pervasive developmental disorders in North Dakota. *Journal of the American Academy of Child and Adolescent Psychiatry*, **26**, 704–10.

Caplan, R., Guthrie, D., Fish, B., Tanguay, P.E., & David-Lando, G. (1989). The Kiddie Formal Thought Disorder Rating Scale: clinical assessment, reliability, and validity. *Journal of the American Academy of Child and Adolescent Psychiatry*, **28**, 408–16.

Caplan, R., Perdue, S., Tanguay, P., & Fish, B. (1990). Formal thought disorder in childhood onset schizophrenia and schizotypal personality disorder. *Journal of Child Psychology and Psychiatry and Allied Disciplines*, **31**, 1103–14.

Eggers, C. (1978). Course and prognosis of childhood schizophrenia. *Journal of Autism and Childhood Schizophrenia*, **8**, 21–36.

Ehlers, S. & Gillberg, C. (1993). The epidemiology of Asperger syndrome. A total population study. *Journal of Child Psychology and Psychiatry*, **34**, 1327–50.

Ehlers, S., Nydén, A., Gillberg, C., Dahlgren-Sandberg, A., Dahlgren, S-O., Hjelmquist, E., & Odén, A. (1997). Asperger syndrome, autism and attention disorders: a comparative study of the cognitive profile of 120 children. *Journal of Child Psychology and Psychiatry*, **38**, 207–17.

Evans, J. & Acton, W.P. (1972). A psychiatric service for the disturbed adolescent. *British Journal of Psychiatry*, **120**, 429–32.

Frith, C. (1991). *Schizophrenia and Youth*, ed. C. Eggers, pp. 80–7. Berlin: Springer.

Garralda, M.E. (1984a). Hallucinations in children with conduct and emotional disorders: I. The clinical phenomena. *Psychological Medicine*, **14**, 589–96.

Garralda, M.E. (1984b). Hallucinations in children with conduct and emotional disorders: II. The follow-up study. *Psychological Medicine*, **14**, 597–604.

Gillberg, C. (1983). Psychotic behaviour in children and young adults in a mental handicap hostel. *Acta Psychiatrica Scandinavica*, **68**, 351–8.

Gillberg, C. (1984). Infantile autism and other childhood psychoses in a Swedish urban region. Epidemiological aspects. *Journal of Child Psychology and Psychiatry*, **25**, 35–43.

Gillberg, C. (1985). Asperger's syndrome and recurrent psychosis – a case study. *Journal of Autism and Developmental Disorders*, **15**, 389–97.

Gillberg, C. (1989). Asperger syndrome in 23 Swedish children. *Developmental Medicine and Child Neurology*, **31**, 520–31.

Gillberg, C. (1990). Autism and pervasive developmental disorders: published erratum appears in *Journal of Child Psychology and Psychiatry* (1991) *32*(1), 213. *Journal of Child Psychology and Psychiatry*, **31**, 99–119.

Gillberg, C. (1991). Clinical and neurobiological aspects of Asperger syndrome in six family studies. In *Autism and Asperger Syndrome*, ed U. Frith, pp. 122–46. Cambridge: Cambridge University Press.

Gillberg, C. (1995). *Clinical Child Neuropsychiatry*. 366 pp. Cambridge and New York: Cambridge University Press.

Gillberg, C. & Coleman, M. (1996). Autism and medical disorders. A review of the literature. *Developmental Medicine and Child Neurology*, **38**, 191–202.

Gillberg, C. & Steffenburg, S. (1987). Outcome and prognostic factors in infantile autism and similar conditions: a population-based study of 46 cases followed through puberty. *Journal of Autism and Developmental Disorders*, **17**, 273–87.

Gillberg, C., Rasmussen, P., Carlström, G., Svenson, B., & Waldenström, E. (1982). Perceptual, motor and attentional deficits in six-year-old children. Epidemiological aspects. *Journal of Child Psychology and Psychiatry*, **23**, 131–44.

Gillberg, C., Wahlström, J., Forsman, A., Hellgren, L., & Gillberg, I.C. 1986. Teenage psychoses – epidemiology, classification and reduced optimality in the pre-, peri- and neonatal periods. *Journal of Child Psychology and Psychiatry*, **27**, 87–98.

Gillberg, C., Steffenburg, S., & Schaumann, H. (1991). Is autism more common now than 10 years ago? *British Journal of Psychiatry*, **158**, 403–9.

Gillberg, I.C. & Gillberg, C. (1989). Asperger syndrome – some epidemiological considerations: a research note. *Journal of Child Psychology and Psychiatry*, **30**, 631–8.

Gillberg, I.C., Hellgren, L., & Gillberg, C. (1993). Psychotic disorders diagnosed in adolescence. Outcome at age 30 years. *Journal of Child Psychology and Psychiatry*, **34**, 1173–85.

Green, W.H., Campbell, M., Hardesty, A.S., Grega, D.M., Padron-Gayol, M., Shell, J., & Erlenmeyer-Kimling, L. (1984) A comparison of schizophrenic and autistic children. *Journal of the American Academy of Child Psychiatry*, **23**, 399–409.

Green, W., Padron-Gayol, M., Hardesty, A.S., & Bassiri, M. (1992). Schizophrenia with childhood onset: a phenomenological study of 38 cases. *Journal of the American Academy of Child and Adolescent Psychiatry*, **35**, 968–76.

Gunnarsdóttir, K. & Magnussón, P. (1994) The epidemiology of autism and Asperger syndrome in Iceland. A pilot study. *Nordic Conference on Autistic Disorders, Epidemiology, Biology, Diagnostic Aspects.* Oslo, Norway.

Hagberg, B. & Gillberg, C. (1993). Rett variants – rettoid phenotypes. In *Rett Syndrome – Clinical and Biological Aspects*, ed. B. Hagberg, pp. 40–60. London: MacKeith Press.

Hellgren, L., Gillberg, C., & Enerskog, I. (1987). Antecedents of adolescent psychoses: a population-based study of school health problems in children who develop psychosis in adolescence. *Journal of the American Academy of Child and Adolescent Psychiatry*, **26**, 351–5.

Hellgren, L., Gillberg, I.C., Bågenholm, A., & Gillberg, C. (1994). Children with Deficits in Attention, Motor control and Perception (DAMP) almost grown up: psychiatric and personality disorders at age 16 years. *Journal of Child Psychology and Psychiatry*, **35**, 1255–71.

Howlin, P. (1997). Prognosis in autism: do specialist treatment affect long-term outcome? *European Child and Adolescent Psychiatry*, **6**, 55–72.

Ishii, T. & Takahashi, O. (1982). Epidemiology of autistic children in Toyota City, Japan. Prevalence. *World Child Psychiatry Conference.* Dublin.

Kadesjö, B. & Gillberg, C. (1997). Attention deficit and clumsiness in Swedish 7-year-old children. *Developmental Medicine and Child Neurology*, **40**, 796–811.

Kay, P. & Kolvin, I. (1987). Childhood psychoses and their borderlands. *British Medical Bulletin*, **43**, 570–86.

Kolvin, I. (1971). Studies in the childhood psychoses. *British Journal of Psychiatry*, **118**, 381–419.

Kolvin, I. & Bernie, T.P. (1990). Childhood schizophrenia. In *Handbook of Studies of Child Psychiatry*, ed. B. Tonge, G.D. Burrows, & J.S. Werry, pp. 123–35. Amsterdam: Elsevier.

Kyllerman, M., Nydén, A., Praquin, N., Rasmussen, P., Wetterquist, A-K., & Hedström, A. (1996). Transient psychosis in a girl with epilepsy and continuous spikes and waves during slow sleep (CSWS). *European Child and Adolescent Psychiatry*, **5**, 216–21.

Landgren, M., Kjellman, B., & Gillberg, C. (1996). ADHD, DAMP and other neurodevelopmental/neuropsychiatric disorders in six-year-old children. Epidemiology and comorbidity. *Developmental Medicine and Child Neurology*, **38**, 891–906.

Le Couteur, A. & Rutter, M. (1988). Fragile X in female autistic twins [letter]. *Journal of Autism and Developmental Disorders*, **18**, 458–60.

Maziade, M., Bouchard, S., Gingras, N., Charron, L., Cardinal, A., Roy, M., Gauthier, B., Tremblay, G., Cote, S., Fournier, C., Boutin, P., Hamel, M., Merette, C., and Martinez, M. (1996). Long-term stability of diagnosis and symptom dimensions in a systematic sample of patients with onset of schizophrenia in childhood and early adolescence. II Postnegative distinction and childhood predictors of adult outcome. *British Journal of Psychiatry*, **169**, 371–8.

Mouridsen, S.E. (1995). The Landau–Kleffner syndrome: a review. *European Child and Adolescent Psychiatry*, **4**, 223–8.

Nissen, G. (1981). [Classification of childhood depression]. [German] Zur Klassifikation der Depressionen im Kindesalter. *Acta Paedopsychiatrica*, **46**, 275–84.

Russell, A.T., Bott, L., & Sammons, C. (1989). The phenomenology of schizophrenia occurring in childhood. *Journal of the American Academy of Child and Adolescent Psychiatry*, **28**, 399–407.

Rutter, M. (1970). Autistic children: infancy to adulthood. *Seminars in Psychiatry*, **2**, 435–50.

Rutter, M. (1978). Diagnosis and definition of childhood autism. *Journal of Autism and Childhood Schizophrenia*, **8**, 139–61.

Schopler, E., Andrews, C.E., & Strupp, K. (1979). Do autistic children come from upper-middle-class parents? *Journal of Autism and Developmental Disorders*, **9**, 139–52.

Spencer, E.K., Kafantaris, V., Padron-Gayol, M.V., Rosenberg, C.R., & Campbell, M. (1992). Haloperidol in schizophrenic children: early findings from a study in progress. *Psychopharmacology Bulletin*, **28**, 183–6.

Steffenburg, S. and Gillberg, C. (1986). Autism and autistic-like conditions in Swedish rural and urban areas: a population study. *British Journal of Psychiatry*, **149**, 81–7.

Steinberg, D., Galhenage, D.P., & Robinson, S.C. (1981). Two years' referrals to a regional adolescent unit: some implications for psychiatric services. *Social Science and Medicine – Part E, Medical Psychology*, **15**, 113–22.

Takei, N., Lewis, G., Sham, P.C., & Murray, R.M. (1996). Age-period-cohort analysis of the incidence of schizophrenia in Scotland. *Psychological Medicine*, **26**, 963–73.

Tanoue, Y., Oda, S., Asano, F., & Kawashima, K. (1988). Epidemiology of infantile autism on Southern Ibaraki, Japan: differences in prevalence rates in birth cohorts. *Journal of Autism and Developmental Disorders*, **18**, 155–66.

Volkmar, F.R. (1992). Childhood disintegrative disorder: issues for DSM-IV. *Journal of Autism and Developmental Disorders*, **22**, 625–42.

Watkins, J.M., Asarnow, R.F., & Tanguay, P.E. (1988). Symptom development in childhood onset schizophrenia. *Journal of Child Psychology and Psychiatry*, **29**, 865–78.

Werry, J.S. (1992). Child and adolescent (early onset) schizophrenia: a review in light of DSM-III-R. *Journal of Autism and Developmental Disorders*, **22**, 601–24.

Werry, J.S., McClellan, J.M., & Chard, L. (1991). Childhood and adolescent schizophrenic, bipolar, and schizoaffective disorders: a clinical and outcome study. *Journal of the American Academy of Child and Adolescent Psychiatry*, **30**, 457–65.

WHO (1993). *The ICD-10 Classification of Mental and Behavioural Disorders. Clinical Descriptions and Guidelines*. Geneva: WHO.

Wing, L. (1981). Asperger's syndrome: a clinical account. *Psychological Medicine*, **11**, 115–29.

Wing, L. (1989). Autistic adults. *Diagnosis and Treatment of Autism*, ed. C. Gillberg, pp. 419–32. New York: Plenum Press.

Wing, L. (1991). The relationship between Asperger's syndrome and Kanner's autism. In *Autism and Asperger syndrome*, ed. U. Frith, pp. 93–121. Cambridge: Cambridge University Press.

Wing, L. (1993). The definition and prevalence of autism: a review. *European Child and Adolescent Psychiatry*, **2**, 61–74.

Wing, L. (1996a). Autism spectrum disorder. *British Medical Journal*, **312**, 327–8.

Wing, L. (1996b). *The Autism Spectrum*. London: Constable.

Wing, L. & Shah, A. (1994). Catatonic features in autism. Paper given at the "Autism on the Agenda" Conference. Leeds, UK.

Wolff, S. (1995). Schizoid personality, Asperger's syndrome and autism. *Nordic Conference on*

Autistic Disorders – What goes on in the mind? Understanding underlying mechanisms – language and cognition. Oslo, Norway.

Zappella, M., Gillberg, C., & Ehlers, S. (1997). Rett Syndrome Variants? Preserved speech in 30 girls with autistic behavior and many features of Rett Syndrome. *Journal of Autism and Developmental Disorders*, **28**, 519–26.

4

Childhood schizophrenia: developmental aspects

Fred R. Volkmar

Introduction

Changes in our understanding of childhood onset schizophrenia over the past century have increasingly reflected an awareness of the importance of developmental factors in the diagnosis of this, and indeed all, psychotic conditions of childhood. There have been marked changes in the way schizophrenia of childhood onset is conceptualized and diagnosed (Werry, 1996). Early notions of a fundamental continuity of schizophrenia over the life span have been modified as data have suggested important differences, as well as similarities, in the manifestation of this condition at different ages (Volkmar, 1996a).

In his ground-breaking work on schizophrenia, Kraepelin noted (e.g., 1907) that the condition had its onset in childhood in some cases. Attempts were made, e.g., De Sanctis (1906), to denote childhood onset psychosis specifically but, with a few exceptions, e.g., Potter (1933), the terms childhood psychosis and childhood schizophrenia became interchangeable. This occurred even though psychotic conditions were much less common than in adults and were even more difficult to characterize. Differences in diagnostic approaches and theory also led to the over- (or under-) emphasis of certain aspects of the condition, e.g., the centrality of a deteriorating course, of disturbances in thinking or other specific pathognomonic symptoms were variously emphasized.

Initial attempts to understand psychotic processes were often developmental in nature, e.g., Freud and his early followers assumed a basic continuity between psychotic processes and early development in which the psychotic process was assumed to represent regression to earlier and "primitive" levels of functioning. This led early clinicians and investigators to equate early developmental and psychotic phenomena, e.g., infants were thought to "hallucinate" as a way of fulfilling wishes and to exhibit an early "autistic" phase. A large body of data now questions such assumptions (see Volkmar, 1996b).

The introduction, by Leo Kanner, of the concept of early infantile autism (1943) contributed to diagnostic confusion. Initially, although Kanner emphasized ways in which this condition differed from schizophrenia, his use of the word "autism" suggested a point of similarity. Bender (1947) and her students advocated for a rather broad and inclusive view of childhood schizophrenia; other early attempts to draw meaningful distinctions within the "psychotic" conditions of childhood (e.g., Creak, 1963) were also very broad and inclusive reflecting a fundamental assumption of continuity based on severity. In the first two editions of the American Psychiatric Association's *Diagnostic and Statistical Manual*, only the concept of childhood schizophrenia was officially recognized.

By the 1970s, various lines of evidence began to question the broad view of childhood schizophrenia, and suggested the importance of developmental factors in characterizing the disorder and of making distinctions within the "childhood psychoses." For example, the work of Kolvin (1971) and Rutter (1972) revealed important distinctions which could be made within the broad group of "psychotic" children. Thus, clinical features such as later age of onset, the presence of specific clinical signs, and positive family history served to differentiate childhood schizophrenia from autism (Kolvin, 1971). This body of work led to significant changes in the concept of childhood schizophrenia in DSM-III (APA, 1980).

In DSM-III, the term childhood schizophrenia was dropped as an official diagnostic category. Children with schizophrenia were diagnosed using the criteria developed for adults, albeit with some consideration of developmental factors in syndrome expression. Subsequent research has generally supported this strategy. While some investigators argued for a rather broad and inclusive diagnostic concept (e.g., Cantor et al., 1982), most have been persuaded that the much narrower diagnostic approach is, in fact, correct. With this narrower view, schizophrenia is observed in prepubertal children, although at very low rates. Rates of schizophrenia in individuals with autism also do not appear to be increased over rates in the general population (Volkmar & Cohen, 1991). The narrower and more stringent view of the diagnostic concept parallels, in many ways, concerns about the overdiagnosis of schizophrenia in adults (Cooper et al., 1972).

The DSM-III approach to the diagnosis of childhood schizophrenia was both supported and criticized. For example, Green et al. (1984) reported that the adult criteria for schizophrenia could be used in evaluating children. On the other hand, Volkmar et al. (1988) noted that it was sometimes difficult to establish clearly the required period of deterioration and the criteria for hallucinations and delusions were sometimes overly stringent. Some changes were made in DSM-III-R (APA, 1987), but more substantive changes were made in DSM-IV (APA, 1994).

In DSM-IV (as in DSM-III and III-R), the same criteria are used for childhood, adolescent, and adult forms of the disorder. These include characteristic psychotic symptoms, deficits in adaptive functioning, and duration of at least 6 months. The characteristic psychotic symptoms include delusions, hallucinations, disorganized speech, grossly disorganized or catatonic behavior, and negative symptoms such as flattened affect. Some consideration of age is made relative to social/occupational dysfunction. Signs of disturbance must be present for at least 6 months with at least 1 month during which active symptoms are present. Schizophrenia is not diagnosed in the presence of schizo-affective disorder or mood disorder with psychotic features or if the symptoms are directly due to substance abuse or a general medical condition. The accompanying text expands on differences in symptoms and issues in developmental diagnosis in children.

Unfortunately, tensions around these criteria still exist. Some features of schizophrenia, e.g., disorganized speech or behavior, are relatively frequent in children. In addition, the threshold for the number of characteristic psychotic symptoms has been reduced. These factors may result in overdiagnosis of schizophrenia in childhood. Conversely, adolescents with a history of substance abuse may be underdiagnosed. It appears that both false-positive and false-negative diagnoses are relatively common, and that a substantial group of psychotic children do not met criteria for any specific disorder (see McKenna et al., 1994). In ICD-10 (WHO, 1993), the approach to diagnosis of schizophrenia in children and adolescents is very similar, although Werry (1996) has noted that this system is even less developmentally oriented than DSM-IV.

Recent research suggests important continuities in the expression of schizophrenia in children, adolescents, and adults (Beitchman, 1985; Caplan et al., 1990a,c, 1993; Russell, 1992; Werry, 1992a,b). Deficits observed in children with schizophrenia include problems with illogical thinking and loosening of associations similar in many ways to the difficulties observed in adolescents and adults with the disorder. Since most core symptoms can be found in children, it is possible to apply what are, essentially, adult oriented criteria for the disorder. On the other hand, there are important developmental differences, both quantitative and qualitative, associated with the expression of the condition which have been increasingly appreciated. These differences, not surprisingly, are greatest for the youngest children (Werry, 1996). In very early onset schizophrenia (i.e., with onset under age 13), diagnostic difficulties are most frequently encountered. For example, the "negative" symptoms of schizophrenia may be less common in children (Garralda, 1985; Werry, 1996). Similarly, well-systematized delusions and particularly ones with more typical adult themes (e.g., sexual themes), are less frequent (Russell et al., 1989; Russell, 1992). Poverty of thinking and incoherence are apparently less likely to be encountered (Caplan et al., 1989, 1990a). Such differences are probably best explained by developmental factors (Caplan et al., 1989, 1990a,b; Thompson et al., 1990), but in any case suggest the need for careful consideration of developmental issues both in framing diagnostic criteria and evaluating children for schizophrenia. In this chapter developmental aspects of childhood schizophrenia are selectively reviewed relative to onset, clinical features, and course of the disorder. Finally, areas important for future research are summarized. While the present chapter is focused on childhood schizophrenia, it is important to note that developmental correlates of psychotic conditions exist throughout the life span (for a review, see Volkmar et al., 1994).

Clinical features of childhood onset schizophrenia

Hallucinations

Bleuler (1911/1951) defined hallucinations as "perceptions without corresponding stimuli from without." Slade and Bentall (1989, p. 23) define hallucination as any percept-like experience which (i) occurs in the absence of an appropriate stimulus, (ii) has the full force or impact of the corresponding actual (real) perception, and (iii) is not amenable to direct and voluntary control. In support of the latter view, hallucinations are relatively common in non-criminal populations, e.g., a substantial number of college students report having had at least brief hallucinatory experiences (Posey & Losch, 1983). Visual and non-threatening hallucinations are most frequently reported in non-clinical samples (Tien, 1991).

Hallucinations may be classified according to their complexity, the modality in which they occur (e.g., auditory or visual), the associated affective tone, and so forth (Asaad, 1990). Historically, these have been understood in two rather different ways. One approach views hallucinations as a psychopathologic symptom and focuses on the relationship of hallucinations to various forms of psychiatric disorder. The alternative approaches emphasize the continuities of normal mental imagery and hallucinations; this perspective emphasizes the similarities of hallucinatory phenomena to dreams and mental imagery, as well as to such common perceptual experiences such as hypnogogic imagery (see Bentall & Slade, 1985; Volkmar et al., 1994). Clearly, there are important individual differences in vulnerability to hallucinations, which may reflect

factors such as suggestibility which, in turn, have strong developmental correlates (Bentall, 1990); contextual and social factors are also important (Slade &
Bentall, 1989).

Developmental perspectives

Although the presence of hallucinations is difficult to establish in younger,
particularly preverbal, or non-verbal, children, they have been noted in
children between the ages of 3 and 4 (King & Noshpitz, 1991). In younger
children the presence of hallucinations may be difficult to establish, given
normative beliefs in fantasy figures and developing concepts of reality, e.g.,
hallucinations must be differentiated from such phenomena as imaginary
companions and dreams (Piaget, 1955).

Hallucinations and hallucinatory phenomena in children have only occasionally been studied, and the few reports available are limited in various ways,
e.g., by a lack of controls, little or no follow-up information, and very broad or
imprecise inclusion criteria (Despert, 1948; Egdell & Kolvin, 1972; Pilowsky &
Chambers, 1986; Rothstein, 1981). Essentially, no truly epidemiological data
are available. Transient, and more prognostically benign, hallucinations occur
in younger children, particularly in relation to anxiety or stress (Aug & Ables,
1971; Esman, 1962; Rothstein, 1981; Schreier & Libow, 1986; Wilking & Paoli,
1966). Such transient hallucinations tend to be primarily visual and/or tactile,
and occur in preschool children who are otherwise developing normally. Such
hallucinations may have an abrupt onset, often at night, and in some cases may
be related to a dream state, although they tend to persist for a period of several
days. Tactile hallucinations may include the sensation of insects crawling on
the child's skin, bed, or clothing; visual hallucinations may relate to threatening
animals or insects. Such hallucinations may be associated with some anxiety in
the child, who may then attempt to avoid sleep (Volkmar, 1996b).

Hallucinations in older, i.e., school age, children and adolescents tend to be
more persistent and are more likely to be associated with significant psychopathology (Del Beccaro et al., 1988; Russell et al., 1989; Volkmar et al., 1988).
Although it was once assumed that hallucinations were almost pathognomonic
of childhood schizophrenia, it is clear that they may be observed in bipolar and
other affective disorders (Ballenger et al., 1982; Carlson & Kashani, 1988), as
well as in conduct and personality disorders (Aug & Ables, 1971). As with
adults, childhood hallucinations can occur in the context of a wide variety of
organic syndromes, including progressive neuropathological processes, as well
as drug-related phenomena.

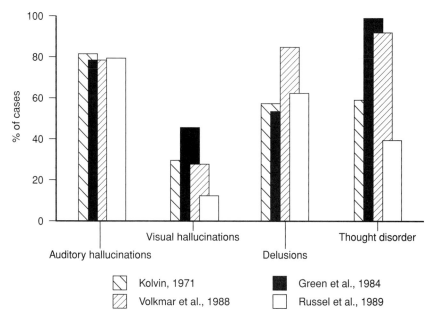

Fig. 4.1. Reported rates of auditory and visual hallucinations, delusions, and thought disorder in four series of cases of childhood schizophrenia. Data adapted from Green et al. (1984); Kolvin (1971); Russell et al. (1989); and Volkmar et al. (1988).

Hallucinations in childhood schizophrenia

In childhood schizophrenia auditory hallucinations are most consistently reported, in approximately 80% of cases (see Fig. 4.1). Auditory hallucinations may be similar to those observed in adults, e.g., with persecutory content of voices conversing or commenting about the child (Russell et al., 1989). Visual and somatic hallucinations are less frequently encountered. The frequency of visual hallucinations varies from one case series to another, from 13% to 46% (see Fig. 4.1). Particularly in younger children, hallucinations are more fluid and less complex than those usually observed in adults with the disorder. In childhood schizophrenia, hallucinations may reflect developmental concerns, e.g., the content may revolve around animals, toys, or monsters, rather than sexual or paranoid themes (Russell et al., 1989).

Delusions

A delusion is defined as a false belief, which remains firmly held even in the face of contradictory evidence and which is not held by other members of the culture (APA, 1987; Leon et al., 1989; Yager, 1989); delusions are grouped by their complexity, the degree to which they are systemized, their bizarreness, and whether they occur with or without pre-existing psychopathology (see Kendler et al., 1983). Delusions can also be classified according to their content (APA, 1987; Leon et al., 1989), e.g., whether they are persecutory delusions, delusions of reference or influence, religious, grandiose, and so forth. Delusions also may relate to thought broadcasting, thought insertion, and thought withdrawal. While delusions are pathognomonic of psychosis, not all individuals have delusions (Nicholi, 1978), and delusions may be associated with various psychotic conditions not limited to schizophrenia. Kraepelin (1907, 1921) made important distinctions between types of delusions, which continue to be embodied in many of the official diagnostic systems.

The organic basis for delusions is suggested by the observation of how commonly delusions are associated with disturbances which impact adversely on the central nervous system (for a review, see Cummings, 1985). Weinberger (1987) has proposed an interesting developmental model that involves a defect in the mesocortical dopaminergic system, occurring early during development, which leads to reduced prefrontal activation and eventually to positive symptomatology.

Developmental perspectives

The capacity for understanding reality and developing a shared view of reality with other members of the same culture has a strong developmental basis. Piaget (1955) has amply demonstrated marked developmental changes in children's understanding of reality over the course of development. Although some theorists have postulated that infants and very young children exhibit delusions (or hallucinations) as normal developmental phenomena, the available experimental data do not support this view. Rather, it appears that children's judgments about, and appreciation of, reality follow a steady developmental progression in which the child is, at first, totally dependent on external appearance but gradually comes to be able to appreciate such factors as conservation of mass and volume, discards animistic thinking, and develops hypotheses for predicting the behavior of the world and of others.

Young children have a tendency to blur the distinction between fantasy and reality and this, in combination with their inability to utilize logical reasoning fully, make it very difficult to demonstrate reliably delusions in children less than about 5 years of age. Developmental factors also impact on the ways in which delusions may be present at different developmental periods. The importance of developmental issues in the expression of delusional thinking has been repeatedly emphasized since the work of Kolvin (1971), which distinguished between early and late onset psychosis. Kolvin emphasized that allowance had to be made for both linguistic and cognitive factors, as well as for culturally congruent, normative beliefs, e.g., in fantasy figures. In children, delusions are less likely to be elaborate or richly detailed and are less likely to have a sexual component.

Delusions in childhood schizophrenia

Developmental factors also affect the manifestation of delusions in childhood schizophrenia. As compared to adolescent or adult schizophrenia, delusions are less frequent, particularly in children under 10 years of age. Only about 50% of cases may exhibit delusions (see Fig. 4.1). Delusional content may revolve around ideas of reference, somatic preoccupations, or grandiose or religious delusions or persecution (Russell et al., 1989). In school-age children, delusions are more likely to be less complex and non-systematized. They may center on disturbances in identity and may be hypochondriacal, persecutory, or grandiose; the latter appear even more frequently in adolescence (Beitchman, 1985; Cantor et al., 1982; Eggers, 1978; Garralda, 1985; Jordan & Prugh, 1971; Kolvin et al., 1971; Kydd & Werry, 1982; Russell et al., 1989; Volkmar et al., 1988). In younger children, delusions more typically revolve a round fantasy figures, animals, or family members (Arboleda & Holzman, 1985; Russell et al., 1989) and thus are more easily missed. The frequency of delusions begins to increase markedly in adolescence with the increase in schizophrenia. As with hallucinations, delusions in children may be seen in relation to organic states, as well as with bipolar disorder and psychotic depression (Volkmar et al., 1994).

Thought process disorder

The term "thought disorder" refers to a rather heterogeneous set of problems in the form, rather than content, of thought. Difficulties subsumed within this overarching construct vary widely (Andreasen & Grove, 1986; Butler & Braff, 1991). At one time, the term was used rather loosely either to refer to schizophrenia or to all the various symptoms of thought disturbance associated with schizophrenia. More recently, usage of the term has been restricted to the organization and presentation of thoughts (Holzman, 1986), i.e., in this view hallucinations and delusions are manifestations of psychotic thought content, rather than process. It is also the case that the more recent trend is to emphasize disorganized speech, rather than thought process difficulties, i.e., to focus on the more overtly observable manifestation of disordered thought process (Andreasen & Grove, 1986; Docherty et al., 1988; George & Neufield, 1985). Unfortunately inconsistency in terminology has complicated much of the available research on this condition in adults and in children. The recent development of assessment instruments has represented an important advance, e.g., Andreasen, 1979; Andreasen & Grove, 1982, 1986; Andreasen & Olsen 1982; Caplan et al., 1990a,b; 1992; Holzman, 1986).

Although there remains disagreement about the exact boundaries of thought disorder, there has been a consensus that it subsumes problems in the organization and expression of thought processes. Various terms have been used to describe aspects of these phenomena; unfortunately these are not always well defined and sometimes overlap each other. Loosening of associations is observed when the speaker's topic shifts are either totally unconnected or only very loosely connected; the speaker is not aware of his or her failure to connect the topics. When severe, the individual's speech may be incoherent. Circumstantial speech is characterized by long and elaborate statements in which relevant points of "connectedness" are maintained. In flight of ideas, the rapidly changing topics usually do have understandable points of connection; if severe, incoherence may then result. In derailment, thought processes are easily disrupted. In illogicality, basic violations in logical thought occur. Thought blocking is observed if the individual's speech is repeatedly interrupted; in this instance, the individual usually fails to recall the overarching goal of speech, but may be aware of having lost his or her train of thought. Thought process disorder may involve the use of neologisms (new, generally meaningless, words which may have a highly idiosyncratic meaning) or in clang associations, where word relationships reflect word sounds rather than meaning. The individual also may echo the speech of others (echolalia) or perseverate on some word or idea. Occasionally, speech is adequate in quantity but fails to convey much, if any, information (poverty of content). Features of thought process disorder may be based on either positive symptoms (e.g., clang associations) or negative ones (poverty of content of speech).

The concept of thought disorder has been central in the definition of schizophrenia historically (Bleuler, 1911/1951), but it is now clear that disturbed thought processes can be observed in various other disorders, such as manic episodes, drug intoxication, and dementia. In addition, cultural issues may complicate the interpretation of thought disorder (Volkmar et al., 1994). The use of a linguistic-communicative perspective has been emphasized by work with adults who have conditions such as aphasia. In such persons, various manifestations of difficulties in organization of thought process are observed (e.g., Faber et al., 1983). The advent of more precise diagnostic criteria and of reliable and valid assessment instruments has facilitated work in this area in both child and adult populations.

Developmental perspectives

Given the major changes in young children's conceptions of reality and their ability to communicate, it is not surprising that it is difficult to establish the presence of thought disorder in preschool children (Green et al., 1984; Russell et al., 1989; Volkmar et al., 1988). In normally developing children, loosening of associations is not typically observed after age 7, and illogical thinking decreases markedly at about the same time (Caplan et al., 1990a). During the early phase of childhood schizophrenia, the degree of thought disturbance sufficient to satisfy strict diagnostic criteria may not be met; rates of thought disorder vary from one case series to another (depending largely on definition) but generally are exhibited in more than half of cases.

Issues of assessment of thought disorder are most problematic in younger or developmentally delayed children (Caplan, 1994; Russell et al., 1989; Volkmar et al., 1988). The importance of developmental factors was emphasized by Despert (1948) but confusion about diagnostic concepts in the 1950s and 1960s resulted in the inability to interpret many publications dating from this period.

Thought disorder in childhood schizophrenia

With the publication of DSM-III (APA, 1980), diagnostic consistency improved and it became apparent that, by the time the child reaches middle childhood, problems in thought process are more like those observed in adolescents and adults (Bettes & Walker, 1987; Garralda, 1984). Earlier age of onset of child-hood schizophrenia is associated with higher levels of thought disorder as well as a worse prognosis (Werry, 1996). Children at risk for schizophrenia have exhibited greater levels of thought disturbance than normal controls (Johnson & Holzman, 1979) or depressed children (Tompson et al., 1990).

Several attempts have been made to develop more quantitative methods of assessing thought disturbance in children and adolescents following Johnson and Holzman's (1979) observation of the importance of developmental level in assessing thought disorder. Research has focused on clinical features (Arboleda & Holzman, 1985), on cognitive processes (Asarnow & Sherman, 1984), and communication (Caplan et al., 1992). Caplan et al. (1989, 1990a) developed the Kiddie Formal Thought Disorder Rating Scale (K-FTDS), which is based on Andreasen's Thought, Language, and Communication Scale (1979) in an in-direct interview (Caplan et al., 1989). The K-FTDS provides operational defini-tions of illogical thinking, incoherence, loosening of association, and poverty of speech content. Using this instrument, Caplan and colleagues (1989) reported that higher levels of illogical thinking and loose association strongly differenti-ated children with schizophrenia from normal controls, although not as strongly from those with schizotypal personality disorder (Caplan et al., 1989, 1990a,b).

The few studies available suggest some potential explanations for the nature of thought disturbance in childhood onset schizophrenia. For example, children with schizophrenia have been noted to have lower distractibility scores on the WISC-R (Asarnow & Ben-Meir, 1988) and deficits in visual information processing (Asarnow & Sherman, 1984). Indices of distractibility have also been related to a quantitative measure of loosening of associations (Caplan et al., 1990a). A few studies of information processing have noted potential developmental differences (Schneider & Asarnow, 1987). In both children and adults, measures of looseness of association and illogical thinking do relate strongly to the severity of thought process disorder.

The degree of communicative dysfunction in adults with schizophrenia is strongly related to the severity of associated thought disorder (Salzinger et al., 1964). Problems in the processing of verbal information and in the social uses of language (pragmatics) have also been reported (Harvey, 1983; Hoffman et al., 1986; Koh, 1978; Rochester & Martin, 1979). Caplan et al. (1992) reported deficits in the ability of children with schizophrenia to use cohesive devices.

As with hallucinations and delusions, disturbances in thought process are not necessarily specific to schizophrenia. Certain features of thought disorder, such as incoherence and poverty of content of speech, occurred at very low rates in childhood schizophrenia. In complex partial seizure disorder in childhood, illogical thinking may be present but usually is not associated with loose associations (Caplan et al., 1993). The latter diagnostic feature appears, in children, to be one of the more specific features of thought disturbance associated with schizophrenia.

Other features

Onset

One interesting, and relatively consistent, finding has been the observation that age at onset of childhood schizophrenia is a major prognostic feature. Children with very early onset schizophrenia tend to have the worst prognosis (Werry, 1996) and to have higher levels of apparent thought disorder (Caplan et al., 1990a). Distinctions between "early onset" and "very early onset" in childhood and adolescence have been suggested (Werry et al., 1994). Very early onset schizophrenia (i.e., before age 10) is extremely uncommon and associated with the worse prognosis whereas early onset childhood schizophrenia (i.e., after age 10 and before adolescence) is more common and associated with a somewhat better outcome. Although very young children are sometimes said to exhibit the disorder (e.g., Russell et al., 1989), it appears that this is extremely rare (Werry, 1996).

Numerous studies (Asarnow et al., 1989; Walker & Levine, 1990; Werry, 1992a) have confirmed that the earlier the age of onset the worse the outcome in various areas of the child's life. Premorbid difficulties appear more common in children with schizophrenia; this is less true in adolescents (Werry, 1996). It appears that individuals with early onset schizophrenia, particularly with very early onset schizophrenia, may have a higher genetic predisposition for the disorder (Hanson & Gottesman, 1976; Pulver et al., 1990; Werry, 1992a,b).

Several general patterns of onset in childhood have been identified (Volkmar, 1996a). Typically onset is more likely to be acute the older the age of the child (Werry, 1992a). It appears that, as with adult schizophrenia, males with the disorder have an earlier onset than females (Green et al., 1984). Developmental correlates of onset have not been clearly established, although it appears that, for a minority of cases, childhood schizophrenia develops in the context of a longstanding pattern of neurodevelopmental vulnerability (Werry, 1996). In younger children, the acute phase is more likely to be prolonged compared to that in older children (Asarnow et al., 1991; McClellan & Werry, 1991; Spencer et al., 1991; Werry et al., 1991a,b).

Outcome

The outcome of childhood schizophrenia, strictly defined, is relatively poor and probably much worse than for adolescent and adult onset schizophrenia. For example, in Bennett and Klein's follow-up (1966) of Potter's 1933 case series, only one case had a relatively good outcome. In Eggers (1978) 20-year follow-up of nearly 60 children with an onset of schizophrenia before age 14 about 50% had poor or moderately poor outcome with 20% apparently exhibiting remission. Although interpretation of these data is complicated by changes in diagnostic practice, in this series early onset in the context of premorbid difficulties was associated with the worst outcome. In their follow-up of a small group of children with schizophrenia, who were rediagnosed using DSM-III, Kydd and Werry (1982) reported that most continued to exhibit the disorder, while the remaining cases exhibited difficulties without meeting full criteria. Although the subsequent course of childhood schizophrenia is somewhat variable, it appears that the most typical course is one in which periodic acute exacerbations occur in the context of a steady deterioration in functioning. Some stabilization may, however, occur after many years (Werry, 1992b).

The explanation for the apparently much worse prognosis of childhood schizophrenia remains unclear but may relate to several factors. It is possible that childhood schizophrenia arises as a result of higher genetic loading, and that both earlier onset and worse outcome relate essentially to such loading. Alternatively, early onset of the condition may, of itself, impact negatively on subsequent development and thus intrinsically carry greater long term risk. Both factors may, of course, be operative, and it clearly is very difficult to tease out the effects of the illness *per se* from premorbid abnormalities, on the one hand, and the severely disruptive effects of an active psychotic process on subsequent development, on the other (Werry, 1992a).

As has been true for adults with schizophrenia, the advent of neuroleptic drug treatment in childhood schizophrenia has been particularly effective in relation to the "positive" symptoms of the disorder while the "negative" symptoms such as anhedonia are less responsive (McKenna et al., 1994). It remains unclear whether long-term drug treatment fundamentally impacts on outcome. It appears that prominent affective symptoms, acute onset, better premorbid adjustment, and well-differentiated symptomatology are associated with better outcome.

Cognitive factors and intelligence

While schizophrenia can occur at any level of cognitive ability several studies have suggested a relation between schizophrenia and lower levels of intellectual ability. This appears to be true in early onset schizophrenia (Werry, 1992a) and may be evidence of some earlier form of central nervous system damage (Werry et al., 1991b). In addition to overall differences in intellectual ability, several investigators have focused on specific psychological processes which may relate to pathophysiology in both adults and children (Asarnow et al., 1989, 1991; Goldstein, 1980). Attentional and other problems have been observed. Caplan and colleagues have also reported particular problems in language related to logical thinking and thought process (Caplan et al., 1989, 1990a). Problems in the ability to "plan forward" and change set (i.e., in executive functioning) have also been reported (Butler & Braff, 1991).

It is, of course, likely that any pre-existing difficulties in learning adversely impact the child's cognitive abilities and educational achievement. Various neurodevelopmental difficulties and minor neurological signs are apparently more frequent in early onset schizophrenia (Asarnow et al., 1989; Russell et al., 1989; Russell, 1992). Similar problems are sometimes seen in young adults with the disorder (Foerster et al., 1991; Walker & Levine, 1990).

As Werry (1996) suggests, there is some reason to suspect that there are at least two clinical phenotypes of schizophrenia. One form is apparently associated with a pattern of longstanding developmental abnormality in which the actual psychotic episode develops after some years of pre-existing abnormality, whereas in the other form the disorder develops in the context of previously normal development (Crow, 1980; Foerster et al., 1991; Lewis & Murray, 1987). Even in very early onset schizophrenia, at least one-fifth of cases apparently do not exhibit pre-existing abnormality prior to the onset of the condition (Werry, 1992a).

Developmental issues in differential diagnosis

Hallucinations and disorganized thinking can be observed in a range of conditions other than schizophrenia (Burke et al., 1989; Caplan et al., 1989, 1990b,c; Garralda, 1984; Rothstein, 1981; Werry, 1992b). Thus, in contrast to adults, these symptoms are less specific. The task of differential diagnosis in childhood can be difficult since disorders other than schizophrenia can be associated with psychosis, and since children with schizophrenia may exhibit other conditions and symptoms suggestive of other conditions. Disturbances in mood appear to be particularly common in childhood schizophrenia (Asarnow et al., 1991; Werry et al., 1991b). However, the presence of a prolonged mood disturbance and/or prominent affective symptoms associated with psychosis suggests the possibility that an affective or schizo-affective disorder is present (Eggers, 1989; Freeman et al., 1985). Hallucinations and delusions are common in bipolar disorder and may be taken to suggest the presence of schizophrenia (Werry et al., 1991a). Confusion may also arise around psychotic depression although, in that condition, the congruence of mood and psychotic features and the decreased frequency of delusions help to clarify the diagnosis (Volkmar, 1996b). Various disruptive behaviors suggestive of conduct or oppositional disorders may be observed particularly in the prodromal stage of the disorder (e.g., Russell, 1992; Werry, 1992a). The characteristic deterioration in multiple areas of functioning may also be taken to suggest the operation of some specific neuropathological process.

Occasionally, hallucinations occur as an isolated finding in younger children and, as noted previously, these tend to be prognostically rather benign. Also, on occasion, the ruminations of a child with severe obsessive compulsive disorder may present a diagnostic problem. In rare instances, the disorganized speech of a severely language disordered child might suggest schizophrenia although the history and absence of other symptoms of psychosis clarify the diagnostic picture. Transient psychotic phenomena can arise following trauma or in relation to dissociative states (Lewis, 1994; Lohr & Brimaher, 1995).

Childhood schizophrenia can co-occur with various other disorders including mental retardation, conduct disorder, specific developmental disorders and learning disability (McKenna et al., 1994). In the various developmental disorders, considerable caution should be used in making a diagnosis of schizophrenia, given the challenges that the presence of such conditions presents for assessment.

Somewhat paradoxically, it appears that much of the work in the 1950s and 1960s about childhood schizophrenia was really about autism. It appears that persons with autism seem not to be at increased risk for schizophrenia (Volkmar & Cohen, 1991); the risk for individuals with other pervasive developmental disorders, notably Asperger's syndrome, for schizophrenia may be increased (Klin & Volkmar, 1997).

Summary and directions for future research

Until children have reasonably sophisticated cognitive and linguistic abilities, it is extremely difficult to demonstrate psychotic processes. In younger, preschool children, possible signs of psychosis must be distinguished from sleep-related and developmental phenomena. Beliefs in fantasy figures, imaginary friends, and so forth are common at this time. Transient symptoms, such as hallucinations, may be observed in younger children in relation to stress and anxiety (Rothstein, 1981). The presence of thought disorder and delusional thinking is most difficult to establish in this age group (Caplan, 1994).

In middle childhood, psychotic phenomena are generally rather uncommon. Symptoms of psychosis are, however, more ominous during this period as they tend to persist and are frequently associated with serious disorders such as schizophrenia (Carlson & Kashani, 1988; Del Beccaro et al., 1988; Russell et al., 1989; Volkmar et al., 1988). Developmental issues and concerns color the content of hallucinations and delusions in this age period, e.g., they tend to evolve around familiar figures and aspects of identity and are not as complex or as systematized as in adults. The complexity of psychotic phenomena increases with developmental level (Garralda, 1985; Russell et al., 1989; Volkmar et al., 1988). In adolescence, the levels of psychosis increase markedly and clinical features are similar to those seen in adulthood. Substance abuse complicates the task of differential diagnosis as does the increased frequency of brief psychotic episodes associated with other conditions such as borderline personality disorder. The difficulties of some psychotic children appear to fall outside current syndrome boundaries (McKenna et al., 1994).

Although relatively rare in childhood, schizophrenia does occur and is a major concern because of its severity and duration. Current diagnostic approaches to childhood schizophrenia are, for the most part, based on work with adolescents and adults; developmental issues are considered only in passing. Differences in official diagnostic systems may continue to complicate conducting and interpreting research (Werry, 1996). Developmental effects on the expression of schizophrenia are observed in various features such as the form and content of delusions and hallucinations and in the nature of thought process disturbance. Early onset of the condition is uncommon but is associated with an even worse outcome; the meaning of this association remains unclear since the development of the syndrome usually has a profound impact on other aspects of the child's development.

REFERENCES

American Psychiatric Association (1980). *Diagnostic and Statistical Manual of Mental Disorders*, 3rd edn (DSM-III). Washington, DC: APA.

American Psychiatric Association (1987). *Diagnostic and Statistical Manual of Mental Disorders*, 3rd edn-Revised (DSM-III-R). Washington, DC: APA.

American Psychiatric Association (1994). *Diagnostic and Statistical Manual of Mental Disorders*, 4th edn (DSM-IV). Washington, DC: APA.

Andreasen, N.C. (1979). Thought, language, and communication disorders. I. Clinical assessment, definition of terms, and evaluation of their reliability. *Archives in General Psychiatry*, **36**, 1315–23.

Andreasen, N.C. & Olsen, S. (1982). Negative vs. positive schizophrenia: definition and validation. *Archives in General Psychiatry*, **39**, 789–94.

Andreasen, N.C. & Grove, W.M. (1986). Thought, language, and communication in schizophrenia: diagnosis and prognosis. *Schizophrenia Bulletin*, **12**, 346–59.

Arboleda, C. & Holzman, P.S. (1985). Thought disorder in children at risk for psychosis. *Archives in General Psychiatry*, **42**, 1004–13.

Asaad, G. (1990). *Hallucinations in Clinical Psychiatry: A Guide for Mental Health Professionals*. New York: Brunner/Mazel Publishers.

Asarnow, R.F. & Sherman, T. (1984). Studies of visual information processing in schizophrenic children. *Child Development*, **55**, 249–61.

Asarnow, J.R. & Ben-Meir, S. (1988). Children with schizophrenia spectrum and depressive disorders: a comparative study of premorbid adjustment, onset pattern, and severity of impairment. *Journal of Child Psychology and Psychiatry*, **29**, 477–89.

Asarnow, R.F., Asarnow, J.R., & Strandburg, R. (1989). Schizophrenia: a developmental perspective. *Rochester Symposium on Developmental Psychology*, ed. D. Cicchetti, pp. 189–220. New York: Cambridge University.

Asarnow, J.R., Bates, S., Tompson, M. et al. (1991). Depressive and schizophrenia spectrum disorders in childhood: a follow-up study. Paper presented to the annual meeting of the American Academy of Child and Adolescent Psychiatry, San Francisco.

Aug, R. & Ables, B. (1971). Hallucinations in nonpsychotic children. *Child Psychiatry and Human Development*, **1**, 153–67.

Ballenger, J.C., Reus, V.I., & Post, R.M. (1982). The "atypical" clinical picture of adolescent mania. *American Journal of Psychiatry*, **139**, 602–6.

Beitchman, J.H. (1985). Childhood schizophrenia: a review and comparison with adult-onset schizophrenia. *Psychiatric Clinics of North America*, **8**, 793–814.

Bender, L. (1947). Childhood schizophrenia: clinical study of one hundred schizophrenic children. *American Journal of Orthopsychiatry*, **17**, 40–55.

Bennett, S. & Klein, H.R. (1966). Childhood schizophrenia: thirty years later. *American Journal of Psychiatry*, **122**, 1121–4.

Bentall, R.P. (1990). The illusion of reality: a review and integration of psychological research on hallucinations. *Psychological Bulletin*, **107**, 82–95.

Bentall, R.P. & Slade, P.D. (1985). Reliability of a measure of disposition towards hallucination. *Personality and Individual Differences*, **6**, 527–9.

Bettes, B.A. & Walker, E. (1987). Positive and negative symptoms in psychotic and other psychiatrically disturbed children. *Journal of Child Psychology and Psychiatry*, **28**, 555–68.

Bleuler, E. (1911/1951). *Dementia Praecox, or the Group of Schizophrenia*. (Translated by J. Zinkin). New York: International Universities Press.

Burke, A.E., Crenshaw, D.A., Green, J., Schlosser, M.A., & Strocchia-Rivera, L. (1989). Influence of verbal ability on the expression of aggression in physically abused children. *Journal of the American Academy of Child and Adolescent Psychiatry*, **28**, 215–18.

Butler, R.W. & Braff, D.L. (1991). Delusions: a review and integration. *Schizophrenia Bulletin*, **17**, 633–47.

Cantor, S., Evans, J., Pearce, J., & Pezzot-Pearce, T. (1982). Childhood schizophrenia; present but not accounted for. *American Journal of Psychiatry*, **139**, 758–62.

Caplan, R. (1994). Thought disorder in childhood. *Journal of the American Academy of Child and Adolescent Psychiatry*, **33**, 605–15.

Caplan, R., Guthrie, D., Fish, B., Tanguay P.E., & David-Lando, G. (1989). The Kiddie Formal Thought Disorder Rating Scale (K-FTDS). Clinical assessment, reliability, and validity. *Journal of the American Academy of Child and Adolescent Psychiatry*, **28**, 208–16.

Caplan, R., Foy, J.G., Asarnow, R.F., & Sherman, T. (1990a). Information processing deficits of schizophrenic children with formal thought disorder. *Psychiatric Research*, **31**, 169–77.

Caplan, R., Foy, J.G., Sigman, M., & Perdue, S. (1990b). Conservation and formal thought disorder in schizophrenia and schizotypal children. *Developmental Psychopathology*, **2**, 183–90.

Caplan, R., Perdue, S., Tanguay, P.E., & Fish, B. (1990c). Formal thought disorder in childhood onset schizophenia and schizotypal personality disorder. *Journal of Child Psychology and Psychiatry*, **31**, 1103–14.

Caplan, R., Guthrie, D., & Foy, J.G. (1992). Communication deficits and formal thought disorder in schizophrenic children.

Caplan, R., Guthrie, D., Sheilds, D., Peacock, W.J., Vinters, H.V., & Yudovin, S. (1993). Communication deficits in children undergoing temporal lobectomy. *Journal of the American Academy of Child and Adolescent Psychiatry*, **32**, 604–11.

Carlson, G.A. & Kashani, J.H. (1988). Phenomenology of major depression from childhood through adulthood: analysis of three studies. *American Journal of Psychiatry*, **145**, 1222–5.

Cooper, H.E., Kendell, R.E., Gurland, B.J., Sharpe, L., Copeland, J.R.U. & Simon, R. (1972). *Psychiatric Diagnosis in New York and London* (Institute of Psychiatry, Maudlsey Monograph no. 20). London: Oxford University Press.

Creak, E.M. (1963). Childhood psychosis: a review of 100 cases. *British Journal of Psychiatry*, **109**, 84–9.

Crow, T.J. (1980). Molecular pathology of schizophrenia: more than one disease process? *British Medical Journal*, **20**, 66–8.

Cummings, J.L. (1985). Organic delusions: phenomenology, anatomical correlations, and review. *British Journal of Psychiatry*, **146**, 184–97.

Del Beccaro, M.A., Burke, P., & McCauley, E. (1988). Hallucinations in children: a follow-up study. *Journal of the American Academy of Child and Adolescent Psychiatry*, **27**, 462–5.

De Sanctis, S. (1906). Sopra alcune varieta della demenzi precoce. *Revista Sperimentale De Feniatria E. Di Medicina Legale*, **32**, 141–65.

Despert, L. (1948). Delusional and hallucinatory experiences in children. *American Journal of Psychiatry*, **1–4**, 528–37.

Docherty, D., Schnur, M., & Harvey, P.D. (1988). Reference performance and negative thought disorder: a follow-up study of manics and schizophrenics. *Journal of Abnormal Psychology*, **4**, 437–42.

Egdell, H.G. & Kolvin, I. (1972). Childhood hallucinations. *Journal of Child Psychology and Psychiatry*, **13**, 279–87.

Eggers, C. (1978). Course and prognosis of childhood schizophrenia. *Journal of Autism and Childood Schizophrenia*, **8**, 21–36.

Eggers, Ch. (1989). Schizo-affective psychoses in childhood: a follow-up study. *Journal of Autism and Developmental disorders*, **19**, 327–42.

Esman, A. (1962). Visual hallucinosis in young children. *Psychoanalytic Study of the Child*, **17**, 334–43.

Faber, R., Abrams, R., Tayor, M.A., Kasprison, A., Morris, C., & Weisc, R. (1983). Comparison of schizophrenic patients with formal thought disorder and neurogically impaired patients with aphasia. *American Journal of Psychiatry*, **140**, 1348–51.

Foerster, A., Lewis, S., Owen, M., & Murray, R. (1991). Pre-morbid adjustment and personality in psychosis: effects of sex and diagnosis. *British Journal of Psychiatry*, **158**, 171–6.

Freeman, L.N., Poznanski, E.O., Grossman, J.A., Buchsbaum, Y.Y., & Banegas, M.E. (1985). Psychotic and depressed children: a new entity. *Journal of the American Academy of Child Psychiatry*, **24**, 95–102.

Garralda, M.E. (1984). Hallucinations in children with conduct and emotional disorders: I. The clinical phenomena. *Psychological Medicine*, **14**, 589–96.

Garralda, M.E. (1985). Characteristics of the psychoses of late onset in children and adolescents: a comparative study of hallucinating children. *Journal of Adolescence*, **8**, 195–207.

George, L. & Neufeld, R.W.J. (1985). Cognition and symptomatology in schizophrenia. *Schizophrenia Bulletin*, **11**, 264–85.

Goldstein, M.J. (1980). The course of schizophrenic psychosis. In *Constancy and Change in Human Development*, ed. O. Brim & I. Kagan, pp. 325–58. Cambridge: Harvard University Press.

Green, W.H., Campbell, M., Hardesty, A.S., Grega, D.M., Padron-Gaylor, M., Shell, J., & Erlenmeyer-Kimling, L. (1984). A comparison of schizophrenic and autistic children. *Journal of the American Academy of Child and Adolescent Psychiatry*, **4**, 399–409.

Hanson, D.R. & Gottesman, I.I. (1976). The genetics, if any, of infantile autism and childhood schizophrenia. *Journal of Autism and Childhood Schizophrenia*, **6**, 209–34.

Harvey, P.D. (1983). Speech competence in manic and schizophrenic psychoses: the association between clinically rated thought disorder and performance. *Journal of Abnormal Psychology*, **92**, 8–77.

Hoffman, R.E., Stopek, S., & Andreasen, N.C. (1986). A comparative study of manic vs. schizophrenic speech disorganization. *Archives in General Psychiatry*, **43**, 831–8.

Holzman, P.S. (1986). Thought disorder in schizophrenia: editor's introduction. *Schizophrenia Bulletin*, **12**, 342–5.

Johnson, M.H. & Holzman, P.S. (1979). *Assessing Schizophrenic Thinking*, pp. 56–101. San Francisco: Jossey-Bass.

Jordan, K. & Prugh, D.G. (1971). Schizophreniform psychosis of childhood. *American Journal of Psychiatry*, **128**, 323–9.

Kanner, L. (1943). Autistic disturbances of affective contact. *Nervous Child*, **2**, 217–50.

Kendler, K.S., Glazer, W.M., & Morgenstern, H. (1983). Dimensions of delusional experience. *American Journal of Psychiatry*, **140**, 466–9.

King, R.A. & Noshpitz, J. (1991). *Pathways of Growth: Essentials of Child Psychiatry, Volume 2: Psychopathology*. New York: John Wiley.

Klin, A. & Volkmar, F.R. (1997). Asperger syndrome. In *Handbook of Autism and Pervasive Developmental Disorders*, ed. D.J. Cohen & F.R. Volkmar, 2nd edn, pp. 94–122. New York: John Wiley.

Koh, S.D. (1978). Remembering verbal materials by schizophrenic young adults. *Language and Cognition in Schizophrenia*, ed. S. Schwartz. Hillsdale: Lawrence Erlbaum Associates.

Kolvin, I. (1971). Studies in the childhood psychoses. I: Diagnostic criteria and classification. *British Journal of Psychiatry*, **118**, 381–4.

Kolvin, I., Ounsted, C., Humphrey, M., & McNay, A. (1971). Studies in the childhood psychoses, I: The phenomenology of childhood psychoses. *British Journal of Psychiatry*, **118**, 385–95.

Kraepelin, E. (1907). *Clinical Psychiatry: A Textbook for Students and Physicians* (Translated by A.R. Diefendorf). New York: McMillan.

Kraepelin, E. (1921). *Manic-Depressive Insanity and Paranoia* (Translated by R.M. Barclay). Edinburgh: E. & S. Livingstone.

Kydd, R.R. & Werry, J.S. (1982). Schizophrenia in children under 16 years. *Journal of Autism and Developmental Disorders*, **12**, 343–57.

Leon, R.L., Bowden, C.L., & Faber, R.A. (1989). The psychiatric interview, history, and mental status examination. *Comprehensive Textbook of Psychiatry*, 5th edn, ed. H.I. Kaplan & B.J. Sadock, pp. 449–62. Baltimore, MD: Williams & Wilkins.

Lewis, M. (1994). Borderline disorders in childhood. *Child and Adolescent Psychiatry Clinics of North America*, **3**, 31–42.

Lewis, S.W. & Murray, R.M. (1987). Obstetric complications, neurodevelopmental deviance, and risk of schizophrenia. Munich Genetic Discussion International Symposium (1986, Berlin, Federal Republic of Germany). *Journal of Psychiatric Research*, **21**, 413–21.

Lohr, D. & Brimaher, B. (1995). Psychotic disorders. *Child and Adolescent Psychiatry Clinics of North America*, **4**, 237–54.

McClellan, J.M. & Werry, J.S. (1991). Schizophrenia. *Psychiatric Clinics of North America*, **15**, 131–48.

McKenna, K., Gorton, C.T., Lenane, M., Kayes, D., Fahey, K., & Rapoport, J.L. (1994). Looking for childhood-onset schizophrenia: the first 71 cases screened. *Journal of the American Academy of Child and Adolescent Psychiatry*, **33**, 636–44.

Nicholi, A.M. (1978). History and mental status. In *The Harvard Guide to Modern Psychiatry*, ed. A.M. Nicholi, pp. 25–40. Cambridge, MA: Belknap Press.

Piaget, J. (1955). *The Child's Construction of Reality*. London: Routledge and Kegan Paul.

Pilowsky, D. & Chambers, W. (1986). *Hallucinations in Children*. Washington, DC: American Psychiatric Press.

Posey, T.B. & Losch, M.E. (1983). Auditory hallucinations of hearing voices in 375 normal subjects. *Imagination, Cognition, and Personality*, **2**, 99–113.

Potter, H.W. (1933). Schizophrenia in children. *American Journal of Psychiatry*, **12**, 1253–70.

Pulver, A.E., Brown, C.H., Wolyntec, P. et al. (1990). Schizophrenia: age at onset, gender and familial risk. *Archives in Psychiatric Scandinavia*, **82**, 344–51.

Rochester, S.R. & Martin, J.R. (1979). *Crazy Talk: A Study of the Discourse of Schizophrenic Speakers*. New York: Plenum Press.

Rothstein, A. (1981). Hallucinatory phenomena in childhood: a critique of the literature. *Journal of the American Academy of Child Psychiatry*, **20**, 623–35.

Russell, A.T. (1992). Schizophrenia. In *Assessment and Diagosis of Child and Adolescent Psychiatric Disorders: Current Issues and Procedures*, ed. S.R. Hooper & G.W. Hynd. Hillsdale, NJ: Lawrence Ehrlbaum.

Russell, A.T., Bott, L., & Sammons, C. (1989). The phenomenology of schizophrenia occurring in childhood. *Journal of the American Academy of Child and Adolescent Psychiatry*, **28**, 399–407.

Rutter, M. (1972). Childhood schizophrenia reconsidered. *Journal of Autism and Childhood Schizophrenia*, **2**, 315–37.

Salzinger, K., Portnoy, S., & Feldman, R.S. (1964). Verbal behavior of schizophrenic and normal subjects. *Annals of the New York Academy of Sciences*, **105**, 845–60.

Schneider, S.G. & Asarnow, R.F. (1987). A comparison of cognitive/neuropsychological impairments of nonautistic and schizophrenic children. *Journal of Abnormal Child Psychology*, **15**, 29–36.

Schreier, H.A. & Libow, J.A. (1986). Acute phobic hallucinations in very young children. *Journal of the American Academy of Child Psychiatry*, **25**, 574–8.

Slade, P.D. & Bentall, R.P. (1989). *Sensory Deception: A Scientific Analysis of Hallucination.* Baltimore, MD: Johns Hopkins University Press.

Spencer, E.K., Mecker, W., Kafantaris, V. et al. (1991). Symptom duration in schizophrenic children: DSM-III-R compared with ICD-10 criteria. Paper presented at the annual meeting of the American Academy of Child and Adolescent Psychiatry, San Francisco, 1991.

Tien, A.Y. (1991). Distributions of hallucinations in the population. *Social Psychiatry and Psychiatric Epidemiology*, **26**, 287–92.

Tompson, M.C., Asarnow, J.R., Goldstein, M.J., & Mikowitz, D.J. (1990). Thought disorder and communication problems in children with schizophrenia spectrum and depressive disorders and their parents. *Journal of Clinical Child Psychology*, **19**, 159–68.

Volkmar, F.R. (1996a). Childhood schizophrenia. *Child and Adolescent Psychiatry*, 2nd edn, ed. M. Lewis, pp. 629–35. Baltimore: Williams & Wilkins.

Volkmar, F.R. (1996b). Childhood and adolescent psychosis: a review of the past 10 years. *Journal of the American Academy of Child and Adolescent Psychiatry*, **35**, 843–51.

Volkmar, F.R. & Cohen, D.J. (1991). Comorbid association of autism and schizophrenia. *American Journal of Psychiatry*, **148**, 1705–7.

Volkmar, F.R., Cohen, D.J., Hoshino, Y., Rende, R.D., & Paul, R. (1988). Phenomenology and classification of the childhood psychoses. *Psychological Medicine*, **18**, 191–201.

Volkmar, F.R., Becker, D.F, King, R.A. & McGlashan, T.H. (1995). Psychotic Processes. In *Handbook of Developmental Psychopathology*, ed. D. Cicchetti & D. Cohen, vol. 1, pp. 512–34. New York: John Wiley.

Walker, E. & Levine, R.J. (1990). Prediction of adult-onset schizophrenia from childhood home movies of the patient. *American Journal of Psychiatry*, **147**, 1052–6.

Weinberger, D.R. (1987). Implications of normal brain development for the pathogenesis of schizophrenia. *Archives of General Psychiatry*, **44**, 660–9.

Werry, J.S. (1992a). Child and early adolescent schizophrenia: a review in the light of DSM-III-R. *Journal of Autism and Developmental Disorders*, **22**, 610–14.

Werry, J.S. (1992b). Child psychiatric disorders: Are they classifiable? *British Journal of Psychiatry*, **161**, 472–80.

Werry, J.S. (1996). Childhood schizophrenia. In *Psychoses and Pervasive Developmental Disorders in Childhood and Adolescence*, ed. F. Volkmar. Washington, DC: American Psychiatric Press.

Werry, J.S., Andrews, L.K., & McClellan, J.M. (1991a). Do mood symptoms differentiate misdiagnosed early onset bipolar disorder from schizophrenia? Paper presented to the NIMH Workshop on Early Onset Schizophrenia, Bethesda.

Werry, J.S., McClellan, J.M., & Chard, L. (1991b). Childhood and adolescent schizophrenia, bipolar and schizoaffective disorders: a clinical and outcome study. *Journal of the American Academy of Child and Adolescent Psychiatry*, **30**, 457–65.

Werry, J.S., McClellan, J.M., Andrews, L.K., & Ham, M. (1994). Clinical features and outcome in child and adolescent schizophrenia. *Schizophrenia Bulletin*, **20**(4), 619–30.

Wilking, V. & Paoli, C. (1966). The hallucinatory experience. *Journal of the American Academy of Child and Adolescent Psychiatry*, **5**, 431–40.

World Health Organization (1993). *International Classification of Diseases: Diagnostic Criteria for Research* (ICD-10), 10th edn. Geneva: WHO.

Yager, J. (1989). Clinical manifestations of psychiatric disorders. In *Comprehensive Textbook of Psychiatry*, 5th edn, ed. H.I. Kaplan & B.J. Sadock, pp. 553–82. Baltimore, MD: Williams & Wilkins.

5

Diagnosis and differential diagnosis

Chris Hollis

Introduction

The diagnostic construct of schizophrenia as applied to children assumes the principle of "developmental homotypy". This view asserts that psycho-pathological disorders have similar presentations at different stages of development and it is implicit in the DSM-IV (APA, 1994) and ICD-10 (WHO, 1993) diagnostic criteria for schizophrenia. In producing a common diagnostic construct across the age range, less emphasis is given to the principle of "developmental heterotypy," which asserts that the symptoms, or manifestations, of psychopathological disorders can vary with age.

The importance of the effect of developmental heterotypy in childhood and adolescence is illustrated by the example of Wilson's disease (hepatolenticular degeneration). In prepubertal children, Wilson's disease presents predominantly with hepatic symptoms, while in adolescence the symptom picture changes to one of a neurological syndrome – with extrapyramidal (parkinsonian) features. If the later onset symptom pattern alone was used to define the condition, then most prepubertal cases would be missed. In addition, the lack of specificity of the neurological symptoms would also make it impossible to distinguish "true" cases from those resulting from mimicking syndromes such as antipsychotic-induced parkinsonism. However, because the underlying pathogenesis of Wilson's disease is known and confirmatory diagnostic tests are available, it has been possible to show that quite different clinical presentations at different ages are manifestations of the same underlying disorder.

In contrast to Wilson's disease, it has been very difficult to establish the true extent of developmental variability of schizophrenic symptoms because the disorder is defined by its manifestations and there is no "gold standard" to validate clinical diagnosis. Phenomenological comparisons between childhood and adult-onset cases using the same diagnostic criteria contain an inherent circularity which could mask true developmental differences. There are two main risks of ignoring developmental heterotypy in the diagnosis of child and adolescent onset schizophrenia. First, phenotypes which lie outside the diagnostic cutoffs, but share a common pathogenesis, cannot be given a diagnosis of schizophrenia. Developmental variability would mean that a greater proportion of "true" cases of schizophrenia would lie outside the boundaries of DSM-IV and ICD-10 in childhood than in adult life. Secondly, the symptoms of specific developmental disorders affecting language and social relatedness in childhood may mimic the "adult" diagnostic criteria for schizophrenia. This could result in a greater number of schizophrenic "phenocopies" occurring in childhood than in adult life.

At this point, some readers may object to the idea that the phenotype of schizophrenia may extend in children and adolescents beyond the diagnostic boundaries set by DSM-IV and ICD-10. After all, why do you need to invoke the possibility of developmental variants when the "full" syndrome can be recognized in children? However, if we accept the assumption that the symptoms of schizophrenia are manifestations of an underlying brain disorder, then the principles of developmental heterotypy should apply equally to schizophrenia as they do in the example of Wilson's disease. However, unlike Wilson's disease, schizophrenia lacks an independent diagnostic test, and until one is available (e.g., molecular genetic markers), individual clinical diagnoses must be validated by longitudinal clinical course. It is a mistake to assume that clinical diagnosis using DSM or ICD criteria represents a "gold standard" in itself and is free of diagnostic error other than that due to problems of reliability.

In this chapter, a central theme will be the idea that the clinical diagnosis of schizophrenia is always a probabilistic exercise associated with the risk of both "true" cases being missed and "false" cases being inappropriately diagnosed. While this is true at any age, there are specific diagnostic challenges in childhood. First, developmental variability in symptoms can blur the distinction between "true" cases and in "non-cases" – reducing diagnostic accuracy. Secondly, the relative rarity of schizophrenia in children and adolescents compared to adults increases the risk of diagnostic error. A theme running through this chapter is the recognition that the usefulness of diagnostic criteria varies according to the needs of the user and the characteristics of those diagnosed. Hence, clinicians and researchers have different needs when using a diagnostic instrument, and therefore are likely to want to use different cutoffs or diagnostic boundaries.

The chapter is organized in the following sections. First, we review the historical development of the construct of schizophrenia as applied to both adults and children. Secondly, we present some of the basic tools of clinical epidemiology which can help to quantify diagnostic certainty in children and adolescents. The aim is that the reader can critically appraise the usefulness of diagnostic instruments and can assess the likely effects of changing diagnostic cutoffs for schizophrenia. Thirdly, we compare DSM-IV and ICD-10 diagnostic criteria and examine the implications for their different diagnostic thresholds when applied to children and adolescents. Fourthly, we consider the use of assessment instruments, in particular the potential for using symptom rating scales to improve diagnostic accuracy. Fifthly, the evidence for the validity of adult diagnostic criteria in children and adolescents is reviewed. Sixthly, we discuss the issue of developmental variability and the specific problem of assessing psychotic symptoms in children. Seventhly, we review the process of differential diagnosis, and in the final section discuss the potential for prevention and early diagnosis. Throughout the chapter, we reiterate the theme that an understanding of developmental variability and clinical epidemiology are essential tools if "adult" diagnostic criteria for schizophrenia are to be applied to children and adolescents.

Historical background: an evolving diagnostic construct

The onset of schizophrenia in childhood was noted in the descriptions of the illness by both Kraepelin (1919) and Bleuler (1911). Kraepelin (1919) found that 3.5% of cases of dementia praecox had onsets before the age of 10 years, with a further 2.7% of cases developing between 10 to 15 years. He also remarked that these cases frequently had an insidious onset. In 1906, De Sanctis described a group of young children who exhibited catatonia, stereotypies, negativism, mannerisms, echolalia and emotional blunting (De Sanctis, 1906). De Sanctis viewed this condition as an early onset from of Kraepelin's dementia praecox, and coined the term "dementia praecoccissima."

Shifting diagnostic fashions and boundaries

Without the benefit of confirmatory diagnostic tests, the boundaries of schizophrenia have expanded and contracted during the twentieth century. Kraepelin's (1919) description of "dementia praecox" was of an illness with an insidious deterioration of personality and coping abilities. Kraepelin believed that dementia praecox was characterized by a deteriorating course which differentiated it from manic depressive illness. Bleuler's concept (1911) of schizophrenia focused on a constellation of psychological deficits including thought disorder, social withdrawal and affective flattening. He believed that these symptoms were "primary" deficits, and that symptoms such as hallucinations and delusions were of "secondary" importance and consequences of a breakdown in more fundamental psychological processes. Bleuler's primary symptoms correspond broadly to the current concepts of "disorganized" and "negative" symptom dimensions.

However, Bleuler's concept proved difficult to define precisely – and this led, in the USA, to the application of looser diagnostic criteria and resultant higher prevalence rates for schizophrenia than in the UK (Cooper et al., 1972). Reliable diagnostic criteria to determine the "true" prevalence were needed, a process which was accelerated by the successful use of lithium in manic depressive illness and the need to differentiate the two disorders.

The "first-rank" symptoms of Schneider (1974) formed a reliable set of symptoms for this purpose. These symptoms are now described as "positive" symptoms and they formed the basis of standardized interviews such as the present state examination (PSE), and diagnostic systems including ICD-9. The problem with first rank criteria is that they define a group of patients in whom the onset of the illness is often abrupt, the course benign and family history weighted towards affective illness rather than schizophrenia (Pope & Lipinski, 1978; Kendell et al., 1979). The publication of DSM-III criteria in 1980 sought to remedy this situation by excluding episodes with a continuous disturbance of less than 6 months. DSM-III also broadened Schneiderian symptoms by including all hallucinations and delusions as long as they lasted for a week.

The paradox of the shift from Bleurerian to Schneiderian concepts was that a gain in reliability was accompanied by a loss of sensitivity and diagnostic validity. Schneiderian criteria exclude those patients whose illness is characterized by insidious social withdrawal, cognitive impairment and disorganized language and behavior – and who never experience overt positive symptoms. However, it is these "negative" symptoms, and not Schneiderian "positive" symptoms, which are associated with increased family risk for psychosis (Van os et al., 1997), premorbid and structural brain abnormalities (Weinberger et al., 1980), cognitive impairments (Johnstone & Frith, 1996) and poorer clinical outcome (Van os et al., 1996).

The concept of schizophrenia in children and adolescents

The history of the concept of schizophrenia in childhood has reflected a shifting dominance between the principles of developmental homotypy and developmental heterotypy. In child psychiatric practice, following the contribution of Kraepelin and De Sanctis, until the early 1930s, schizophrenia in children and adults was seen as essentially the same disorder with a broadly similar presentation. However, in the 1930s, coinciding with the emergence of child psychiatry as a separate discipline, a "unitary" view of childhood psychoses was proposed which included present-day concepts of autism, schizophrenia, schizotypal and borderline personality disorder (Potter, 1933; Fish & Rivito, 1979). This broad definition of schizophrenia dominated research and clinical practice from the 1940s to the 1970s, and was endorsed by DSM-II and ICD-8, which grouped all childhood-onset psychoses, including autism, under the category of "childhood schizophrenia." The "unitary" view of childhood psychoses began to be challenged in the 1970s, following the landmark studies of Kolvin (1971) and Rutter (1972), who demonstrated that autism and childhood onset schizophrenia could be distinguished in terms of age at onset, phenomenology and family history. This led to the differentiation of adult-type schizophrenia with childhood onset from autism and other psychoses. The use of adult criteria for schizophrenia in cases with childhood onset was endorsed in DSM-III and ICD 9 and has been maintained in DSM-IV and ICD-10.

Recent conceptual developments

Neurodevelopmental models

In the last 10 years the concept of schizophrenia as a neurodevelopmental disorder has replaced earlier notions that schizophrenia was a progressive, degenerative condition (Murray & Lewis, 1987; Weinberger, 1987). The model proposes that the biological origins of schizophrenia lie in fetal neurodevelopment. It is argued that the manifestation of this early developmental "lesion" can subsequently be traced in premorbid developmental, behavioural and cognitive impairments. Later, as a result of normal brain development in adolescence, e.g., synaptic pruning and myelination of frontolimbic connections (Purves & Lichtmen, 1980), the putative neuropathology is finally expressed as classic psychotic symptoms.

Although there is a lively debate about whether premorbid schizophrenic impairments are best understood as precursors or more non-specific risk factors (Hollis & Taylor, 1997) – the neurodevelopmental model has considerable heuristic value and has raised new and important questions about the diagnosis and timing of onset in schizophrenia. First, it may be mistaken to think of schizophrenia having a single onset coinciding with the manifestation of positive psychotic symptoms. Rather, there may be a sequence of onsets, starting with a "biological onset" in fetal life, followed by a "preclinical onset" with the development of premorbid behavioral changes during childhood, and finally a "clinical-onset" coinciding with the emergence of positive and negative psychotic symptoms, typically in late adolescence and early adult life.

Secondly, the model embodies the principle of developmental variability in symptoms (developmental heterotypy) – with premorbid impairments conceptualized as age-specific manifestations of underlying neuropathology.

Symptom dimensions and associated neurocognitive mechanisms

The second major development in the last decade has been research linking schizophrenic symptoms to underlying neurocognitive processes. There is a long history of subtyping in schizophrenia – in fact, the categories of hebephrenia, catatonia and paranoia predate the description of schizophrenia. However, this recent exercise has had a different purpose, namely to group psychotic symptoms (rather than patients) according to altered function in specific brain regions. Liddle (1987) used factor analysis of standardized symptom assessments to identify three symptom dimensions in adult schizophrenic patients: psychomotor poverty (flattened affect, withdrawal), disorganization (thought disorder, inappropriate behavior) and reality distortion (hallucinations and delusions). Liddle et al. (1992) showed that these three symptom dimensions were correlated with altered functional brain activity in the frontolateral (psychomotor poverty), fronto-orbital (disorganization) and temporal (reality distortion) cortical regions.

The only published factor analysis of schizophrenic symptoms in child and adolescent patients produced a two, rather than a three, factor solution (Maziade et al., 1996). In their study, the "positive" dimension included hallucinations, delusions, bizarre behaviour and thought disorder, while the "negative" dimension included affective blunting, alogia, apathy and anhedonia.

This approach of identifying symptom dimensions has a number of exciting implications: first, it may be possible to trace the developmental continuities and neural substrate of different symptom dimensions. For example, there is evidence that psychomotor poverty and disorganization are associated with premorbid developmental impairments and functional abnormalities of the frontal lobes, while reality distortion is not (Baum & Walker, 1995). This link may reflect underlying continuity in brain development linking frontal lobe maturation, premorbid developmental impairments and psychomotor poverty/disorganization. Secondly, it may be more useful when studying the etiological risk factors and predictors of outcome of psychotic disorders to use symptom dimensions rather than categorical diagnostic constructs (Van os et al., 1996). There seems good reason to believe that mutiple-gene influences in psychiatric disorders result in continuous dimensions rather than categorical disorders (Plomin et al., 1994).

Principles of clinical epidemiology: tools to estimate the usefulness of diagnostic criteria

Accuracy of diagnosis is acknowledged to be crucial. But, what factors influence accuracy, how can it be estimated and improved? To answer these questions we need to apply the principles of clinical epidemiology to assessment and diagnosis (Sackett et al., 1991; Verhulst & Koot, 1992). First, we consider the issue of "false-negative" and "false-positive" diagnoses. Secondly, we consider a number of indices of diagnostic accuracy and illustrate the estimation of diagnostic accuracy with a worked example. Finally, we consider the differing needs of clinicians and researchers and how this may influence their choice of diagnostic cutoffs.

The main argument used by proponents of developmental homotypy is that schizophrenia can be recognized in children as young as 7 years of age using "adult" criteria (Green et al., 1984; Russell et al., 1989; Werry, 1992). As we have already discussed, there is a circularity in this argument which ignores the possibility that developmental variability in symptoms may result in an unidentified population of "true" cases, which lie outside these diagnostic criteria. These missed cases can be considered as "false-negatives." In addition, an unknown proportion of positive diagnoses will be phenocopies. We will call these inappropriately diagnosed cases "false-positives."

When evaluating the usefulness of DSM-IV and ICD-10 criteria we need to know how good these criteria are at discriminating "true" cases of schizophrenia from a population of children and adolescents with psychotic symptoms. In order to answer this question, we need to apply the concepts of sensitivity (the proportion of "true" cases correctly identified) and the specificity (the proportion of those without the disorder correctly identified) to the diagnostic criteria. While the sensitivity and specificity of the diagnostic criteria need to be considered at any age, the effect of developmental variability on sensitivity and specificity is a key issue for the diagnosis of schizophrenia in childhood.

A useful index is the positive predictive value (PPV). This is the proportion of positively diagnosed cases who, in fact, turn out to have the disorder (confirmed by a "gold standard" test – or in the case of schizophrenia, by clinical course). An advantage of the PPV is that it can be easily interpreted. As we have already discussed, diagnostic sensitivity may be reduced by developmental variability of symptoms (i.e., more "true" cases fall outside the cutoff). Diagnostic specificity will also be reduced if other competing presentations become more common at a younger age. However, unlike sensitivity and specificity, the PPV of a diagnosis will always be reduced if the prevalence of the target disorder decreases. For example, if our criteria for the diagnosis of schizophrenia have sensitivity and specificity of 95%, but the prevalence (or "pretest probability") of the disorder drops from 1% in adults to 0.1% in early adolescence, then the PPV of a diagnosis of schizophrenia would fall from 16% in adults to only 2% in early adolescence (PPV is also known as the "post-test probability"). Hence, the rarity of childhood onset schizophrenia and the difficulty in differentiating psychotic symptoms from normal cognitive immaturity in children or the symptoms of other disorders (low "signal" to "noise" ratio) will reduce the likelihood of making an accurate diagnosis.

In summary, the concepts of sensitivity, specificity and positive predictive value help us to quantify diagnostic uncertainty. We can then assess different diagnostic cutoffs in terms of the relative costs and benefits resulting from adopting either strict criteria (fewer falsely diagnosed cases vs. more missed cases) or looser criteria (fewer missed cases vs. more falsely diagnosed cases).

Table 5.1 provides a worked example of these principles based on a follow-up study of adolescent onset psychotics by Werry et al. (1991). There were 60 cases with index DSM-IIIR diagnoses of schizophrenia ($n = 34$), schizophreniform psychosis ($n = 13$), schizoaffective psychosis ($n = 1$), bipolar disorder ($n = 9$) and psychotic depression ($n = 3$). At follow-up, 30 subjects were given a diagnosis of schizophrenia, 23 of bipolar disorder (12 schizophrenic at index diagnosis) and 6 schizoaffective (all schizophrenic at index diagnosis). Therefore, of the original 34 index cases of schizophrenia, at follow-up 16 still had schizophrenia, 12 had bipolar disorder and 6 had schizoaffective disorder. We can see that the initial DSM-III-R diagnosis of schizophrenia has a sensitivity of 53% and a specificity of 40%. The PPV is 47% (i.e., not very good!).

The final index presented here is the likelihood ratio (LR), which gives the odds of a positive diagnosis occurring in a "true" case as opposed to a subject without the disorder. The likelihood ratio has the advantage that it is not affected by the prevalence of the disorder within a particular sample The likelihood ratio for the initial DSM-III-R diagnosis is 0.88:1, or expressed as a probability, there is a 47% chance that someone with a DSM-III-R diagnosis of schizophrenia will actually have schizophrenia validated by follow-up, if the prediagnosis odds of schizophrenia in the sample are 1:1 (as they would be in this sample of psychotic adolescents). If the results of this study were taken to their logical conclusion, it would be quicker and just as accurate to base the diagnosis of schizophrenia on tossing a coin! It is not surprising that an astute clinician might look at these results and chose to adopt a "wait and see" approach to the diagnosis of schizophrenia in the adolescent psychotic patient.

Table 5.1. Calculating sensitivity, specificity, positive predictive value and likelihood ratios for the diagnosis of schizophrenia

Definitions

		"Gold standard" diagnosis		
		Yes	No	
Clinical diagnosis	Yes	a	b	a + b
	No	c	d	c + d
		a + c	b + b	a + b + c + d

Sensitivity = a/a + c (True positive rate)
Specificity = d/b + d (True negative rate)
Positive predictive value = a/a + b
False-positive rate = 1 − specificity
   = b/b + d
Likelihood ratio   = Sensitivity/1 − specificity

Worked Example: Data from Werry et al. (1991)

		Follow-up diagnosis of schizophrenia		
		Yes	No	
Initial diagnosis of schizophrenia	Yes	16	18	34
	No	14	12	26
		30	30	60

Sensitivity = 16/30 = 53%
Specificity = 12/30 = 40%
Positive predictive value = 16/34
   = 47%
Likelihood ratio   = 0.53/(1 − 0.6):1
   = 0.88:1

It is important to remember that clinicians and researchers tend to require different things from the diagnostic process. For clinicians, a useful diagnosis is one which reliably identifies patients who may benefit from a specific treatment and/or are likely to follow a defined clinical course. That is to say, it should provide a good guide to treatment and prognosis. Until recently, the poor benefit-to-risk ratio of traditional antipsychotics, the apparent instability of early diagnosis and possible fears of premature diagnostic labeling – all contributed to an understandable skepticism among clinicians about the value of making an early diagnosis of schizophrenia. However, the arrival of a new generation of "atypical" antipsychotic drugs with improved benefit to risk ratios (Remschmidt et al., 1994), has forced clinicians to reconsider the need for accurate early detection and diagnosis of schizophrenia in young people.

Compared to clinicians, researchers are likely to have different requirements from the diagnostic process. In general, "false-negatives" are not a concern in research. Instead, the aim is to improve reliability and increase homogeneity in samples by excluding phenocopies or "false-positives." The result is that researchers tend to advocate strict, operationally defined criteria. Clinicians may feel that this approach unhelpfully excludes the bulk of "subthreshold" or borderline cases for which they need diagnostic guidance. Diagnostic sensitivity could be improved by broadening criteria to include borderline conditions such as "simple" schizophrenia or schizotypal disorder. However, the risk is that broader criteria could lead to poorer reliability and more "false-positives." Whether or not this matters depends on whether it is more important not to miss "true" cases or conversely, whether it is more important not to inappropriately label cases who have other conditions or who are simply "normal variants."

In summary, it is necessary to understand how the sensitivity and specificity of diagnostic criteria for schizophrenia are affected by developmental and epidemiological factors. For example, the overlap between symptoms such as thought disorder and immature language in young children can significantly reduce the diagnostic specificity of this symptom. The very low prevalence of schizophrenia in prepubertal children also reduces the positive predictive value of a clinical diagnosis of schizophrenia. In both circumstances, the probability of an accurate diagnosis is reduced even if the diagnostic criteria are being applied with precision.

Diagnostic criteria: DSM-IV and ICD-10

The publication of DSM-IV in 1994 (APA, 1994), ICD-10 (clinical guidelines) in 1992 (WHO, 1992) and ICD-10 (research criteria) in 1993 (WHO, 1993) aimed to achieve greater convergence between the DSM and ICD classification systems. However, a number of differences remain, which are likely to affect the relative sensitivity and specificity of these criteria when applied to children and adolescents. The aim is to provide a guide to the important differences between DSM-IV and ICD-10, and the relevance of these differences to diagnosis in children and adolescents. In order to apply the diagnoses, the reader must consult the DSM-IV and ICD-10 manuals, hence the full criteria are not provided here. We start first by considering the changes from DSM-III-R to DSM-IV.

Changes from DSM-III-R to DSM-IV

DSM-IV replaced DSM-III-R which was published in 1987 (APA, 1987). The DSM-IV criteria for schizophrenia incorporate a number of small, but significant, changes from DSM-III-R:

(i)   The criterion for the duration of psychotic symptoms in the active phase was increased from 1 week to 1 month.

(ii)   The symptom of "grossly disorganized behavior" has been added in addition to the symptom of catatonic behavior.

(iii) The list of characteristic symptoms (criterion A in DSM-IV) refers to the broader categories of "disorganized speech" and "negative symptoms" rather than the specific symptoms described in DSM-III-R.

The division of the characteristic symptoms (DSM-IV criterion A) reflects the influence of recent research into symptom dimensions. Hence, the "psychotic dimension" comprises delusions or hallucinations, "disorganization dimension" consists of a description of disorganized speech and behavior, and a "negative dimension" is reflected by the inclusion of negative symptoms. However, the continuing influence of Schneider's "first rank" symptoms can be seen in the fact that, while psychotic symptoms are normally required from at least two categories (e.g., hallucinations and negative symptoms) – only one "first rank" symptom is required for the diagnosis.

Comparison between DSM-IV and ICD-10

ICD-10 was published in 1992, and research diagnostic criteria published in 1993. For the first time, the ICD system provided detailed operational criteria. The major differences between the diagnostic criteria for schizophrenia in DSM-IV and ICD-10 are as follows:

(i)   Both ICD-10 and DSM-IV require a minimum duration of 1 month for active psychotic symptoms. However, ICD-10 excludes "prodromal" and "residual" symptoms from its criteria for schizophrenia because it states that they are non-specific and cannot be reliably defined. Hence, ICD-10 requires a shorter overall duration of symptoms (1 month of active symptoms) compared with 6 months in DSM-IV (combined duration of active and residual/prodromal symptoms).

(ii)   ICD-10 does not have an equivalent category to "schizophreniform disorder (DSM-IV295.4)". Cases which fall into this DSM-IV category would be classified as having schizophrenia in ICD-10.

(iii) The schizophrenic subtypes in the two systems are broadly comparable and share the same labels except the DSM-IV "disorganized type" (295.1) which is equivalent to ICD-10 "hebephrenic schizophrenia" (F20.1). An important difference in ICD-10 is the inclusion of the category of "simple schizophrenia" (F20.6) which is characterized by insidious onset of social withdrawal, oddities of conduct and deteriorating social performance over a period of at least 1 year without active psychotic symptoms. There is no equivalent category in DSM-IV.

(iv)   ICD-10 places "schizotypal disorder" (F21) in the broad group of "schizophrenia and other psychotic disorders," while in DSM-IV, "schizotypal personality disorder" (301.22) is placed in the section of personality disorders.

Implications of differences between DSM-IV and ICD-10

At first sight, DSM-IV would appear to set more stringent criteria for diagnosis with a 6-month minimum for overall symptom duration compared to 1 month in ICD-10. Certainly, all cases classified as having schizophreniform disorder in DSM-IV would be diagnosed as schizophrenia in ICD-10. Hence, the concept of schizophrenia in ICD-10 includes some psychoses excluded from DSM-IV, which have a more acute onset and rapid offset and probably a more favorable outcome. However, the inclusion of simple schizophrenia in ICD-10 may have the converse effect of identifying a group excluded from DSM-IV, which has a particularly insidious onset of withdrawal and social deterioration associated with very poor outcome. This type of presentation may be more common in some child and adolescent-onset psychoses (Volkmar et al., 1988) when positive psychotic symptoms can be absent or fragmentary and negative symptoms difficult to disentangle from premorbid impairments. Finally, ICD-10 defines hallucinations and delusions with greater stringency than DSM-IV. For example, simple persecutory delusions would be accepted by DSM-IV but not by ICD-10. This higher threshold for positive symptoms set by ICD-10 may be important in younger children where it is particularly difficult to differentiate positive symptoms from normal age-related phenomena.

In summary, ICD-10 appears to define a rather broader phenotype than DSM-IV, which includes both a greater variability of presentation and potential outcome. The exception is the more stringent definition of positive symptoms in ICD-10. Any gain in sensitivity in ICD-10 is likely to be accompanied by a loss of specificity. The effect of this difference on clinical course is difficult to predict. It is possible that ICD-10 criteria would result in greater variability of outcome, while comparisons of mean outcome scores would show little difference between the two systems. Diagnostic studies which apply a range of diagnostic criteria to the same subjects (polydiagnostic studies) could compare the effects of using ICD-10 and DSM-IV cutoffs in children and adolescents. The use of the OPCRIT (OPerational CRITeria in psychotic illness) diagnostic algorithm in adult onset psychoses has proved to be a very useful way of comparing the effect of different diagnostic cutoffs within the same adult-onset subjects (McGuffin et al., 1991). The results of current research using OPCRIT in child and adolescent-onset psychoses to compare the positive predictive values and likelihood ratios of different diagnostic cutoffs is awaited with interest.

Assessment: the pursuit of reliability

A basic requirement of any clinical diagnosis is that it should be reliable and reproducible. Only when reliability is achieved is it meaningful to go on to test the validity of the diagnosis. The introduction of DSM-III in 1980, went a long way towards improving reliability by publishing explicit operational criteria for use in clinical practice and research. However, the existence of standard diagnostic criteria will not improve reliability if two clinicians or researchers ask the same patient different questions and receive different information. For example, if one interviewer asks a child in great detail about hallucinations, while another focuses on mood disturbance, information bias may lead to different diagnostic criteria being met. The answer is to use a standard procedure for eliciting clinical information, which ensures a systematic coverage of symptoms.

A range of instruments now exists for use with children and adolescents with suspected psychotic disorders (see Table 5.2). In general, these instruments have been adapted for use in younger subjects after first being developed for use with adults. They fall into two main categories. First, diagnostic interviews with the aim of arriving at a categorical DSM or ICD diagnosis. Secondly, symptom rating scales which have the aim of assessing particular aspects, or consequences, of psychopathology on a continuous scale (e.g., positive symptoms, thought disorder or functional impairment). Apart from the scales measuring thought disorder, all the schedules described here draw information from the parent, the child and other sources such as teachers. This is an obvious difference from adult schedules, which usually rely on the patient as the sole informant.

Table 5.2. A selection of assessment instruments for evaluating schizophrenic symptoms in children and adolescents

Clinical interviews	Description	Informant	Age range
K-SADS-E Schedule for Affective Disorder and Schizophrenia for School-Age Children Epidemiological version (Ovaschel & Puig-Antich, 1987)	Semistructured diagnostic interview designed to assess past and current DSM-III and DSM-III-R disorders	Parent Child	6–17
ICDS Interview for Childhood Disorders and Schizophrenia (Russell et al., 1989)	Semistructured interview	Parent Child	6–18
CAPA The Child and Adolescent Psychiatric Assessment (Angold et al., 1995)	Semistructured interview. Focus on past 3 months. Includes severity ratings	Parent Child	8–18
DICA Diagnostic Interview for Children and Adolescents (Herjanic & Reich, 1982)	Highly structured interview designed to assess DSM-III and III-R diagnoses. Available in computerized version	Parent Child	6–17
NIMH DISC The NIMH Diagnostic Interview Schedule for Children (NIMH, 1992)	Highly structured interview designed to give DSM-III and III-R diagnoses. Available in computerized version	Parent Child	9–17
Rating scales KIDDIE-PANSS Positive and Negative Syndrome Scale for Children and Adolescents (Fields et al., 1994)	Rating scale for positive and negative symptoms and other symptoms	Interviewer rating Parent/Child	6–16
CPRS Children's Psychiatric Rating Scale (Fish, 1985)	Symptoms ratings based on severity/degree of abnormality. Good coverage of schizophrenic symptoms	Interviewer rating child	Up to 15
C-GAS Children's Global Assessment Scale (Shaffer et al., 1983)	A rating of the severity of functional impairment on 0–100 scale	Rating based on review of all available sources	4–16
Thought disorder scales K-FTDS Kiddie-Formal Thought Disorder Story Game and Kiddie Formal Thought Disorder Scale (Caplan et al., 1989)	Procedures for eliciting and scoring speech samples	Child	5–13
TDI Thought Disorder Index (Arboleda & Holzman, 1985)	Codes thought disorder from speech samples	Child	5–16

Adapted from Asarnow (1994).

The use of standardized assessments are now almost mandatory in research studies. The reason is clear; if one researcher describes a finding in a group of "schizophrenic" adolescents, an attempt to replicate this finding by another research team can only be made if they use exactly the same diagnostic procedures. In the past, the failure to do this has led to a plethora of incompatible findings in the research literature. Whether standardized assessments should become routine in clinical practice is a moot point. As we mentioned earlier, the clinician uses the diagnostic process in a rather different way from the researcher. While the researcher primarily wants to classify the subjects into homogeneous groups to investigate biological or psychosocial correlates of the disorder, the clinician uses diagnosis as a guide to individual case management. As a result, the clinician may legitimately want to keep a degree of flexibility in their assessment to gather information which goes beyond that required for classification.

Assessment instruments are described under two headings, diagnostic interview schedules and rating scales. Only a brief overview will be provided here. For more details on the content, reliability and validity of each instrument the reader should refer to the references given in Table 5.2.

Diagnostic interview schedules

A selection of the most commonly used instruments are set out in Table 5.2. They fall into two main groups. First, the semistructured interviews which include the K-SADS-E, the ICDS and the CAPA. These are investigator-based interviews, which assume a high level of training and give considerable responsibility to the interviewer to decide whether an item has been answered satisfactorily, or whether further probes are required to elicit more information. The second group are the highly structured interviews such as the DICA and the NIMH-DISC. These are respondent-based interviews which place the responsibility on the subject, rather than the interviewer, to make certain questions are understood before moving on to the next item. As a logical extension, these highly structured schedules have now been developed in a self-administration and computerized format.

Rating scales

While the aim of diagnostic interviews is to place subjects within a diagnostic category, rating scales provide a continuous measure of psychotic symptoms or global functioning. This information can add significantly to a categorical diagnosis by providing a measure of symptom variability within diagnostic groups and as well as symptom change within subjects over time. For example, this information can be used to study predictors of outcome, or treatment response in individual patients.

There are three main types of rating scales available: first, general psychotic symptom scales such as the K-PANSS and the Children's Psychiatric Rating Scale (CPRS). These cover a broad range of positive and negative psychotic symptoms. Secondly, the global rating scales such as the Children's Global Assessment Scale (C-GAS). These scales provide an overall measure of severity of disturbance. Thirdly, the thought disorder scales which include the Kiddie Formal Though Disorder Story Game and The Thought Disorder Index. These scales have been developed specifically for the purpose of rating thought disorder in children.

A relatively unexplored possibility is the use of rating scales for diagnostic purposes. The advantage of continuous measures is that ROC (Receiver/ Response Operating Characteristic) curves can be drawn (Verhulst & Koot, 1992). Using ROC curves, it is possible to devise multiple cutoffs on a rating scale in order to discriminate much more accurately between true cases and non-cases. For example, cutoffs on the K-PANSS could be investigated which either maximize or minimize the likelihood ratio of detecting "true" cases of schizophrenia in childhood and adolescence validated by follow-up.

Diagnostic validity

Without a classical "gold standard" against which to compare clinical diagnosis, diagnostic validity can be measured in two ways. First, at the group level, the correlates of child and adolescent onset schizophrenia can be compared to the correlates of adult onset schizophrenia. For example, if similar patterns are found in premorbid impairment, family history or structural brain abnormalities then this would provide evidence for the continuity between schizophrenia in childhood and adult life. The second method, which is applicable to individual cases, is to validate childhood diagnoses using longitudinal course and outcome.

A more powerful test of childhood to adult continuities is to test whether child and adolescent-onset cases fit a model which proposes a continuum of liability to schizophrenia with an inverse relationship between age at onset and the "dose" of risk factors (Childs & Scriber, 1986). This model predicts that childhood onset cases should lie at an extreme end of a continuum of liability for schizophrenia. Hence, the "dose" of risk factors should be greatest in very early onset cases and they should have a poorer outcome compared to adult onset cases. The importance of this "model fitting" approach is that continuity of the diagnostic construct would be supported by quantitative etiological and phenotypic differences in children and adolescents when compared with adults. This can be contrasted to the more traditional approach of inferring continuity between childhood and adult onset cases by demonstrating similarity, or lack of difference, in terms of correlates and outcome.

Overall, child and adolescent onset schizophrenia appears to resemble adult onset schizophrenia when compared in terms of premorbid adjustment (Asarnow & Ben-Meir, 1988), structural brain changes (Frazier et al., 1996), neuropsychological performance (Asarnow et al., 1994b), attention and information processing deficits (Strandberg et al., 1994), eye tracking (Iacono & Koenig, 1983) and psychophysiological measures (Gordon et al., 1994). Of course, all these comparisons are indirect (comparisons made between rather than within studies) and none of these associations is in themselves specific to schizophrenia.

An important test of the validity of the diagnosis of schizophrenia in childhood is to examine the continuity of the disorder over time. Furthermore, the model of age at onset and liability to schizophrenia would predict that childhood onset cases would have a particularly poor outcome. Unfortunately, there have been relatively few follow-up studies of child and adolescent onset schizophrenia and several have been restricted to only adolescent onset cases.

Werry et al.(1991) followed 60 psychotic patients (mean age at index admission 13.9 years) over a period ranging from 1 to 16 years. They found a striking lack of diagnostic continuity, with a positive predictive value of only 47% for the diagnosis of schizophrenia (see the section on "Clinical epidemiology and diagnosis" for a detailed discussion). The outcome of the group diagnosed as schizophrenic at follow-up was very poor, with an average general adaptive functioning (GAF) score of 40, and a mortality rate of 15%. Out of those initially diagnosed as schizophrenic, diagnostic continuity was predicted by insidious onset, poor premorbid function, and the absence of prominent affective symptoms. Positive psychotic symptoms did not differentiate between schizophrenic cases and those with a psychotic mood disorder. Werry et al. (1991) restricted their analysis of outcome to cases where the diagnosis was validated at follow-up, clearly, a method which contains an inherent circularity. Schmidt et al.(1995) compared the outcome of adolescent onset and adult onset patients from the same catchment area using the disability assessment scale (DAS). They found that the adolescent onset patients had significantly greater impairments in self-care and social competence. Overall, the evidence available suggests that schizophrenia with onset in early adolescence tends to run a chronic course with a very poor outcome. This resembles the finding of poor outcome in schizophrenia with an adult onset under 25 years of age (Murray et al., 1988).

If there is an age-related continuum of liability for schizophrenia, we would expect an even worst outcome in preadolescent onset cases. We are aware of only two follow-up studies of this age group. Eggers (1978) reported on a follow-up of 57 patients aged 7–13 years with a diagnosis of "childhood schizophrenia" made before the introduction of DSM-III and ICD-9 criteria in childhood. Although his results suggest a somewhat better prognosis, with 50% showing some form of improvement, the lack of operational diagnostic criteria make these findings difficult to interpret. Asarnow et al. (1994a) reported a recent follow-up study of childhood onset schizophrenia using DSM-III-R criteria (age range at onset 6–11.3 years). They found diagnostic continuity in 61% of index schizophrenic cases over a 2–7 year follow-up period, with 56% showing improvement in functioning, and the remainder minimal improvement or a deteriorating course. Somewhat surprisingly, 28% of the sample were classified as having a good outcome, based on a global adjustment scale (GAS) score of 60 or over. The variability of outcome in this young onset sample suggests the possibility of considerable etiological heterogeneity in schizophrenia with onsets below the age of 11 or 12 years. Variability in outcome may also result from the inclusion of phenocopies such as the group of children labeled by Gordon et al. (1994) "multidimensionally impaired" (see "Differential diagnosis" for a more detailed description of this category).

In summary, does childhood onset schizophrenia lie on a continuum with adult schizophrenia? Using a definition of childhood onset schizophrenia based on phenotypic resemblance with adult schizophrenia, there appears to be evidence of continuity of psychophysiological and neuropsychological measures, premorbid impairments and structural brain abnormalities, and clinical course. The variability in outcome of childhood onset schizophrenia is broadly similar to that seen in young adults and does not suggest that childhood onset cases have any greater etiological homogeneity. Overall, the findings support the view of diagnostic continuity with some age dependent variations in presentation. Fitting the correlates of child and adolescent onset cases against age-dependent models (e.g., increasing familial risk with younger age of onset) is a more powerful test of childhood to adult continuities than simple comparisons between childhood onset and adult onset cases. Finally, there is rather greater uncertainty about the validity of the diagnosis of schizophrenia in preadolescent children. It appears that both developmental and epidemiological factors reduce diagnostic accuracy quite markedly in this age group, and this increases the likelihood of false-positive diagnoses.

Developmental variability: symptoms and associated features

Both the DSM and ICD systems (DSM-IV and ICD-10) use a polythetic criteria set for schizophrenia, which means that diagnosis is based on a subset of items from a longer list. This allows for some degree of variability of symptomatology within the overall diagnostic boundaries. In this section we will consider how the pattern of premorbid and psychotic symptoms differs between childhood onset and adult onset schizophrenia.

Premorbid abnormalities

Premorbid developmental impairments appear to be particularly prevalent in prepubertal or childhood onset schizophrenia. Watkins et al. (1988) found that 70% of children with onsets of schizophrenia under the age of 10 had significant language and motor impairments in infancy. Over one-third of children had a history of autistic symptoms and 17% met criteria for either autism or childhood onset pervasive developmental disorder prior to the onset of schizophrenia. Hollis (1995) dichotomized childhood onset schizophrenics into onsets of 7–13 years and 14–17 years and found that developmental impairments, in particular language impairments, were more common in the younger (7–13 years) onset group. In this study, approximately 20% of the younger onset group would have been diagnosed as having atypical or childhood onset pervasive developmental disorder (PDD) prior to their psychosis. While there is no evidence to suggest that autism and schizophrenia are etiologically related disorders, these studies do indicate that autistic symptoms are associated with an earlier onset of schizophrenia in children. Alaghband-Rad et al. (1995) examined premorbid functioning in the National Institutes of Mental Health (NIMH) study of childhood onset schizophrenia. They found that 36% of their cases had a premorbid history of at least one PDD feature and 13% had full autism. Although Kolvin (1971) found it relatively straightforward to distinguish autism with onset less than 36 months from late childhood onset schizophrenia, there were a small number of children between the ages of 7 to 11 years where the diagnostic distinction between late onset autism and childhood onset schizophrenia proved to be very difficult.

Developmental variability in psychotic symptoms

There have been surprisingly few direct comparisons between clinical features in childhood and adult onset schizophrenia. Werry et al. (1994) reported that their sample of adolescent onset schizophrenics was characterized by fewer well-formed systematized delusions, fewer auditory hallucinations, and more undifferentiated subtypes when compared to the published rates for adult schizophrenia. In a study of the age at onset of DSM-III-R schizophrenia subtypes, Beratis et al. (1994) found that, in a sample of first episode schizophrenics, the disorganized subtype (ICD-10 hebephrenic) had a mean age at onset of 16.7 years (s.d. 2.5), compared with 22.9 years (s.d. 5.5) for the undifferentiated subtype and 29.9 years (s.d. 9.4) for the paranoid subtype. While all subtypes can occur in childhood, there appears to be a relative predominance of disorganised and undifferentiated cases and fewer paranoid cases, when compared to adult samples. Galdos and Van os (1995) found that Schneiderian "first-rank" symptoms were more common in older psychotic adolescents compared with younger psychotic adolescents. Yang et al. (1995) dichotomized adolescent onset patients into onset before and after 15 years of age. When assessed as adults, the younger onset group had lower performance IQ scores and more prominent negative symptoms. Recent studies also support Kraepelin's observation that most cases of childhood onset schizophrenia present with a slow, insidious onset (Asarnow & Ben-Meir, 1988; Green et al., 1992). Russell (1994) described the results of two studies of childhood onset schizophrenia with onsets before the age of 12 (Russell et al., 1989; Green et al., 1992). The most striking finding was the frequency of insidious onsets (acute onset in only 14%) with non-specific psychiatric symptoms emerging, on average, 2–3 years before the emergence of psychotic symptoms. In summary, when compared with adult onset schizophrenics, childhood onset cases are characterized by greater premorbid impairments, a more insidious onset, more negative and disorganized symptoms, and fewer systematised or persecutory delusions.

The influence of age and cognition on symptom assessment

Positive symptoms

Age-specific factors will restrict the possibility of making a phenomenological diagnosis in very young children. For example, distinguishing true delusions and hallucinations from childhood fantasies can present diagnostic dilemmas. Similarly, the interpretation of thought disorder will be affected by the level of the child's language and cognitive development.

Garralda (1984) in a child psychiatric clinic sample found no reports of hallucinations in children under 7 years of age. Bettes and Walker (1987), in a population-based survey of psychiatric symptoms in children aged 5 to 18 years, found a positive linear association between positive symptoms (including hallucinations) and age. Interestingly, after controlling for age, positive symptoms were associated with higher IQ. This supports the view that the expression of positive symptoms is associated with increasing cognitive development.

While it cannot be certain that hallucinations do not occur in younger children, they are likely to have difficulty in discriminating "inner speech or thoughts" from other subjective phenomena like hallucinations. This may be related to developmental issues in the localization of hallucinations in space. Bender (1970) emphasized the shift from an internal to an external location of voices with age. Garralda (1984) found that auditory hallucinations were located predominantly in internal space before age of 13, and in external space in older children. In studies of preadolescent onset schizophrenia using DSM-III criteria auditory hallucinations are described in about 80% of cases (Green et al., 1992; Russell et al., 1989). Russell (1994) provides examples of psychotic symptoms including command hallucinations: "shut up," "smash your mom" and "help your mom with dinner." These examples illustrate the problematic issue of differentiating genuine psychopathological phenomena from normal experiences of childhood.

Thought disorder/disorganisation of speech and language

Arboleda and Holzman (1985) using the Thought Disorder Index (TDI) and Caplan et al. (1989) using the Kiddie-Formal Thought Disorder (K-FTDS) story game have shown that the symptoms of thought disorder, such as illogical thinking and lose associations, are more common in younger children. These findings indicate the difficultly in distinguishing between developmentally normal patterns of immature speech and language and clinically significant thought disorder in young children. The distinction is even more difficult to make between psychotic children and those with a developmental language disorder who present with symptoms of incoherence, poverty of speech and derailment. Because developmental language disorders are more commonly found in psychiatrically disturbed children than in adults, it is likely that the DSM-IV criterion of "disorganized speech" will have less specificity for schizophrenia when applied to children compared with adults.

Negative symptoms

While positive symptoms are associated with increasing cognitive maturity, negative symptoms appear to be more common in younger children and those with poorer cognitive abilities. Bettes and Walker (1987) found an association between negative symptoms and lower IQ and younger age at presentation. Because their study did not relate symptoms to diagnostic groups, it is difficult to know what type of disorders (i.e., psychosis or pervasive and other developmental disorders) accounted for a peak of negative symptoms in children in the 5 to 6 years age range. As with thought disorder, it is very difficult to discriminate between negative psychotic symptoms and the symptoms of flat or inappropriate affect and language impairment found in a range of developmental disorders.

Are there continuities between premorbid developmental impairments and psychotic symptoms?

An obvious question to ask is whether the difficulties described in distinguishing developmental impairments and negative symptoms arise because both are manifestations of the same underlying neurodevelopmental process. Baum and Walker (1995) explored the specific relationship between premorbid childhood impairments (parental reported CBCL scores) and symptom dimensions ("reality distortion," "disorganization" and "psychomotor poverty") of schizophrenia in adult life. They found a positive relationship between childhood "withdrawal" and the "negative-type" dimensions of psychomotor poverty and disorganization. They found no association between childhood behaviors and the "positive" dimension of reality distortion. These findings provide some support for Carpenter et al.'s (1988) contention that primary negative symptoms show developmental continuity with premorbid impairments, and that this neurodevelopmental process is at least partly independent of the processes subserving positive symptoms.

From a diagnostic perspective, continuity between premorbid and psychotic symptoms would make it almost impossible to reliably define the "onset" of the disorder. The tendency for insidious onset in child and adolescent schizophrenia is well recognized, and the difficulty in reliably timing the onset has led many research studies to define "onset" as the point when positive symptoms are first noted. The risk of this approach in clinical practice is that diagnosis may be deferred in cases where negative symptoms precede the onset of positive symptoms.

Differential diagnosis

Differential diagnosis refers to the hypothetico-deductive process of generating and then excluding possible diagnoses that could account for a particular clinical presentation. In essence, this process involves estimating the prior probability of a range of potential diagnoses and then using clinical information to either increase or decrease the probability of each potential diagnosis until a point is reached when they can either be excluded or definitely accepted. If a symptom is specific to a particular diagnosis, its presence will "rule-in" the

Table 5.3. NIMH study of childhood-onset schizophrenia: diagnoses for the first 98
subjects assessed by research interviews (up to 8/94)

Diagnosis	n
Schizophrenia	28
Multidimensionally impaired	21
Bipolar disorder	11
Major depression	8
Asperger's syndrome/pervasive developmental disorder NOS	7
Schizotypal personality disorder	4
ADHD/conduct disorder/oppositional defiant disorder	7
Dissociative disorder NOS/PTSD	4
Obsessive compulsive disorder	2
Schizoaffective disorder	2
Organic psychosis	3
Tourette's syndrome	1

From Gordon et al. (1994).

diagnosis and "rule-out" all others. Conversely, if a symptom is a very sensitive marker of a diagnosis, then its absence will rule the diagnosis out. Of course, in psychiatry most symptoms have only moderate specificity and sensitivity, hence, comorbid or multiple diagnostic formulations are common.

A dilemma arises when psychotic children fail to fit into conventional DSM and ICD diagnostic categories. Should these cases be considered as having separate diagnoses, or are they developmental variants of schizophrenia? This question can only be resolved by careful longitudinal follow-up of these psychotic children. The results of the NIMH study of childhood onset schizophrenia (Gordon et al., 1994) have been valuable in describing the range of diagnoses which followed a initial broad screen for cases with "probable" symptoms of childhood onset schizophrenia. The diagnoses of the first 98 subjects assessed at NIMH (up to August 1994) are presented in Table 5.3.

Jacobson and Rapoport (1998) provide a more recent update on the NIMH study with results for 160 children who have been invited to NIMH for a research assessment following a positive case record screening for schizophrenia. Up to December 1996, 36 subjects (22.5% of the screen positive sample) were given a DSM-III-R diagnosis of schizophrenia. These cases were characterized by prominent positive and negative symptoms, and insidious onset with a prodrome which included deteriorating school performance, social withdrawal and disorganized behavior. In the premorbid course, specific developmental disabilities and transient early symptoms of autism were common.

In about 20% of the screened cases, the diagnosis was affective disorder with psychotic features. However, an even larger subgroup of about 30% failed to fit any known diagnostic category and were labeled by the study team as "multi-dimensionally impaired" (MDI) (McKenna et al., 1994). These children had brief, transient psychotic symptoms, excessive age inappropriate fantasy or magical thinking which was not clearly delusional, emotional lability, poor interpersonal skills without social withdrawal, and multiple deficits in information processing including memory and visuospatial skills. Compared to schizophrenic children, the most striking difference in the MDI group was a far lower rate of negative symptoms and less marked social impairment.

The MDI children have symptoms that cross a number of diagnostic boundaries including schizoptypal personality and affective disorder but fail to meet these criteria in full. Towbin et al. (1993) described a similar syndrome characterized by "disturbances in affect modulation, social relatedness and thinking" which they labeled "Multiple complex developmental disorder" (MCDD). Compared to the MDI syndrome, the construct of MCDD appears closer to the pervasive developmental disorder spectrum.

Is there continuity between the MDI syndrome and schizophrenia?

A preliminary 2-year follow-up of 19 MDI patients shows that most do not progress within this period to full schizophrenic presentations, and so this does not seem to represent a prodromal state (Jacobson & Rapoport, 1998). However, there is a higher rate of schizophrenia spectrum disorders in their first-degree relatives, and there are also similarities in brain abnormalities between MDI and age-matched schizophrenic subjects. This evidence suggests that MDI subjects may lie on a schizophrenic spectrum and represent a broader developmental phenotype. Hopefully, further follow-up and neurobiological and genetic studies at NIMH will help to clarify the nosological status of MDI children.

Perhaps the most remarkable feature of the NIMH study is that only about 5% of cases (36 out of over 700) referred with a clinical diagnosis of schizophrenia with onset before age 12 actually had a validated diagnosis of schizophrenia. Why was the positive predictive value (PPV) of clinical diagnoses so low and false positives so common? Earlier in "Clinical epidemiology and diagnosis," we learned that, if the pretest probability or prevalence of the disorder is very low, then even with good sensitivity and specificity of diagnostic criteria the PPV will be low. Given the extreme rarity of schizophrenia before the age of 12 in child psychiatric practice (an incidence of perhaps 50–100 times less than adult onset schizophrenia), it is not surprising that the PPV of diagnosis would be so low from a nationally referred sample from non-specialist centers. Furthermore, we have argued that developmental factors reduce the sensitivity and specificity of "adult" diagnostic criteria in preadolescent children. Hence, in this age group it would seem more appropriate for non-specialist centers to simply register children as screen positive for psychosis/complex developmental disorder, and leave the final diagnostic discrimination to specialist centers, who can collect samples where the prevalence of schizophrenia is say, 20% vs. 0.1% in non-specialist clinics. In these settings, the risk of diagnostic errors is likely to be much smaller.

The differential diagnosis of psychotic symptoms in children and adolescents

A list of differential diagnoses with their clinical characteristics and differentiating features will be presented here. First, in order to demonstrate the process of differential diagnosis we present a brief case example.

An 11-year-old girl reports hearing "voices." What are the diagnostic hypotheses? It would be easy to generate a very long list, so the challenge is to reduce this list by estimating the prior likelihood of the diagnoses and then obtaining extra information which can help to "rule-in" or "rule-out" each condition. First, it is important to remember that non-psychotic conditions such as conduct and emotional disorders exist as well as rarer non-psychotic developmental disorders such as Asperger's syndrome and receptive language disorders. On the other hand, symptoms lasting over a month are more specific to schizophrenic, affective, and organic psychoses. Hence, a history of persistent hallucinations would help to discriminate between non-psychotic and psychotic disorders. However, it is still difficult to differentiate between schizophrenic, affective and organic psychoses on the basis of positive symptoms alone. Drug-induced psychoses are the most common organic cause and they should be confirmed though a positive drug history and urine testing. Other organic disorders are far rarer, and should only be considered in the presence of confirmatory neurological signs or with a history of a loss of cognitive skills. It is particularly important to enquire about the onset pattern, and the presence of negative symptoms as these features provide better discrimination between schizophrenic and affective psychoses than does the presence or absence of positive symptoms.

Differential diagnoses

Conduct and emotional disorders

Hallucinations have been described in conduct and emotional disorders (Garralda, 1984) particularly at times of stress. However, positive symptoms are usually transient and fragmentary and negative symptoms (e.g., avolition, social withdrawal) are very unusual. The problem of misdiagnosis usually arises when undue emphasis is placed on symptoms such as pseudo-hallucinations, persecutory ideas and ideas of reference.

Affective psychoses (psychotic depression and bipolar disorder)

There has been considerable debate about whether a valid distinction can be drawn between schizophrenia and affective psychoses in children and adolescents. In a follow-up study of adolescent-onset psychoses, Werry et al. (1991) found that, at follow-up, over 50% of the bipolar cases had initial diagnoses of schizophrenia. Positive symptoms occur in bipolar disorder and affective psychoses and distinctions such as mood congruency can be difficult to apply. Negative-type symptoms also occur in depression; however, it should be possible to distinguish between affective flatness associated with despair and depression and the "blunted" or incongruous emotional expression commonly seen in schizophrenia. Onset pattern and premorbid functioning may also be helpful distinguishing features. In schizophrenia, the usual presentation follows an insidious onset with poor premorbid functioning. In affective psychoses, the onset of psychotic symptoms is often rapid with relatively good premorbid social and scholastic functioning. However, whether these constructs describe two extreme ends of a continuum, or two discrete diagnostic entities is still subject to debate.

Asperger's syndrome and the autistic spectrum

Positive symptoms may develop in Asperger's syndrome and autistic spectrum disorders (atypical-PDD) in adolescence. DSM-IV does not exclude a diagnosis of schizophrenia in cases of PDD/autism so long as prominent delusions or hallucinations are present for a month. This avoids the misclassification of cases with transient psychotic symptoms. In childhood onset schizophrenia, there is usually a history of deteriorating social and scholastic functioning arising in late childhood or early adolescence. In Asperger's syndrome and atypical PDD, social and cognitive impairments are more longstanding and progressive deterioration of functioning prior to onset is less marked. However, the distinction becomes increasingly difficult in the youngest onset schizophrenic cases.

Alaghband Rad et al. (1995) found that 36% of their NIMH sample of childhood onset schizophrenics had at least one feature of PDD, and 13% met full criteria for infantile autism. The question remains as to whether these cases are best viewed as autistic "phenocopies" or display genuine comorbidity.

Organic brain conditions

The traditional "functional / organic" dichotomy used to classify psychoses has become relatively meaningless as our knowledge of the neuropathological basis of schizophrenia has grown over the last 20 years. A range of acute and chronic organic states can give rise to psychotic symptoms and may be confused with schizophrenia. By far the most common are drug-induced psychoses. Much rarer causes are temporal lobe epilepsy and the neuro-degenerative disorders.

Drug-induced psychoses

The high incidence of drug-induced psychoses places them at the top of any differential diagnosis list of organic psychotic conditions. A vast array of substances may be implicated, some known and well described and others unknown. The best known substances include cocaine, amphetamines, and hallucinogens. Psychotic symptoms may also occur with the withdrawal of alcohol, sedatives, hypnotics and anxiolytics. Cocaine and amphetamine psy-choses may include the following symptoms: persecutory delusions, perceptual distortions, and vivid hallucinations in any modality, most classically visual and tactile hallucination of insects crawling under the skin (formication).

A substance abuse history may be elicited from the history and confirmed by finding urinary metabolites. Confirmation of schizophrenia can only be made if the psychotic symptoms persist for at least a month following drug withdrawal. However, this distinction can sometimes be difficult because drug-induced psychotic symptoms can sometimes persist for weeks following withdrawal.

Temporal lobe epilepsy

The association between epilepsy and psychosis has produced a lengthy and rather bewildering literature. Part of the problem lies in the confusing terminol-ogy used to describe a range of epileptic states, all of which can be associated with behavioral and perceptual disturbances. The term "psychomotor seizure" is used to refer to any epileptic discharge which is associated with a behavioral or experiential manifestation. While this most commonly involves discharges from the temporal lobes, in about 20% of cases other brain regions are implicated.

The most common origin of epileptic psychotic phenomena are lesions of the left temporal lobe. The seizures are sometimes described as "twilight states" or "psychomotor status" and commonly last several hours but may continue for up to a week. Consciousness is always impaired and patients seem retarded, absent minded and tend to perseverate. Automatisms may be seen such as lip smacking or picking at cloths. Hallucinations are usually visual and may be vivid in content; however, memory for the episodes may be incomplete or fragmentary. These episodes are accompanied by EEG disturbance, most commonly with a focus in the medial temporal lobes. The differentiation of this group of seizures from schizophrenia is based on the presence of clouding of consciousness, their brief and episodic nature, with partial amnesia for the episodes. Twenty-four-hour EEG recording with event monitoring may be needed to establish the association between the temporal lobe discharge and the psychotic and behavioral symptoms.

Neuro-degenerative disorders

In neurological textbooks, one can often find cautionary tales of neuro-degenerative disorders which psychiatrists failed to diagnose. While the prevalence of these conditions is very low, it is certainly worth bearing in mind that a variety of brain disorders can produce psychotic symptoms prior to the development of obvious physical signs.

These very rare disorders include juvenile metachromatic leukodystrophy, adrenoleukodystrophy, Wilson's disease and Huntington's chorea. A detailed description of these disorders is beyond the scope of this chapter; however some general diagnostic points can be made. First, all these conditions are associated with movement disorders, particularly gait disturbance. Clearly, a full neurological examination is mandatory in the assessment of all psychotic patients. In addition, it is important to attempt to distinguish between primary and secondary (antipsychotic-related) movement disorder. Secondly, these conditions are characterized by a progressive loss of cognitive skills. This is in contrast to the more relative decline seen in schizophrenia and other developmental disorders, where a loss of previously learned skill is unusual.

Prevention and detection of "at risk" or prodromal states

There is great intuitive appeal in the idea of early diagnosis and prevention of child and adolescent-onset schizophrenia. The aim would be to identify and treat "high-risk" or preschizophrenic children before they developed the full

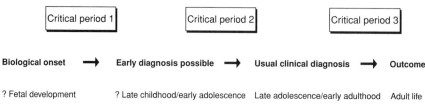

Fig. 5.1. Possible critical periods for detection and early intervention in schizophrenia.

clinical presentation of schizophrenia. However, the important question to ask is whether such a strategy would be possible or effective?

The strategy of early detection of disorders is based on the assumption that there exists a critical period for intervention before the full clinical presentation of the disorder (see Fig. 5.1). A critical period is defined as a time before which therapy is easier to apply or is more effective than when applied afterwards. There are a number of different points in the development of a disorder when critical periods may occur. Early detection will only be useful if there is a critical period after the point when early diagnosis is possible but before clinical diagnosis is usually possible (Critical Period 2). If the critical period comes before the point at which early detection is possible (Critical Period 1), then it will not make any difference at what stage you intervene after this. If the critical period does not arise until after the full clinical presentation (Critical Period 3), then early detection and intervention will not be effective.

The neurodevelopmental model of schizophrenia provides the best theoretical underpinning to the idea of a developmental progression of disease illustrated in Fig. 5.1. According to this model, the biological onset occurs during fetal neurodevelopment, and the putative neuropathology would remain relatively silent in early childhood, manifest perhaps as mild developmental delays and non-specific behavioral problems. The developmental progression of symptoms suggests that, in later childhood, social and cognitive difficulties become more apparent, and the emergence of negative symptoms may mark the beginnings of a schizophrenic prodrome. Most of the data we have on "preschizophrenic" symptoms comes from genetic "high-risk" studies following children of schizophrenic parents (Asarnow, 1988; Fish et al., 1992) and birth cohort studies, using childhood records to examine the antecedents of schizophrenia in a representative population (Jones et al., 1994; Done et al., 1994). While these studies have identified premorbid features such as language delay, social impairments and attentional problems, which are more common in preschizophrenic children, none of these features has the necessary sensitivity and specificity to be useful in clinical screening (Yung & McGrory, 1996). A further problem is that the low prevalence of schizophrenia means that, even if we were able to identify early symptoms with high sensitivity and specificity, their positive predicative value would still be unacceptably low. For example, if only 15% of screen positive cases went on to develop schizophrenia, then the dangers of inappropriately labeling and treating false-positives would have to be balanced against any potential gain of early treatment for the correctly identified cases. In summary, there seems little evidence at present to suggest that identification and treatment of preschizophrenic children would be worthwhile or effective.

For most clinicians, the question of early diagnosis relates to the period *after* the development of psychotic symptoms not before. The important question here is whether there is a critical period for intervention soon after the emergence of psychotic symptoms (Critical Period 3)? It has been suggested that psychotic symptoms may have a toxic effect on the brain, a mechanism analogous to the "kindling" effect of seizures (Wyatt, 1995). Evidence has also been cited that outcome in first-episode schizophrenics is worse for those with a longer duration of untreated psychosis before first presentation (Loebel et al., 1992). Although these findings are of interest, they do not provide direct support for a critical period either before or after the emergence of psychotic symptoms. What is really needed is a randomized controlled trial of "early intervention" in first-onset child and adolescent schizophrenic patients. For example, the components of an "early-intervention" package could include new atypical antipsychotics and psychoeducation started within 6 months of the onset of psychotic symptoms. The control group would have access to the same package, but only after 18–24 months of conventional management.

Much depends on establishing the positive predictive value (PPV) of DSM-IV and ICD-10 diagnostic criteria in first episode psychoses in children and adolescents. If the PPV of early diagnosis is sufficiently high, then clinicians may feel more confident in initiating treatment with new atypical antipsychotics and providing diagnosis specific psychoeducation. However, if the PPV is only 50%, then clinicians may well be justified in waiting and allowing the natural course of the illness to emerge and then make a diagnosis with greater certainty. This strategy would reduce the risk of inappropriately labeling and treating non-schizophrenic psychoses. As we have mentioned earlier, this is a crucial issue in preadolescent children where there is considerable overlap between the phenomenology of normal developmental variation and psychotic symptoms.

In conclusion, it will be important to resolve whether premorbid impairments are precursors or risk factors for later schizophrenia. If they are precursors, they may be legitimate targets for early diagnosis – if they are simply non-specific risk factors, then diagnosis may be premature – and a "high-risk" status may be more appropriate. Despite considerable intuitive appeal, early intervention to prevent psychosis in "high-risk" children and adolescents would seem to have more risks than benefits. The target symptoms for screening simply do not have sufficient predictive value, given their low sensitivity and specificity and the low prevalence of the disorder. Early intervention for first-episode psychoses in children and adolescents is more likely to be of value; however, randomized controlled trials are needed. More research is required on the predictive value of early diagnosis, particularly in prepubertal children.

Conclusions

Perhaps the most important conceptual development over the last 20 years has been the realization that schizophrenia in children and adolescents lies on a continuum with schizophrenia in adults. Hence, it was appropriate that the separate category of "childhood schizophrenia" was removed from DSM-III. However, because the definition of schizophrenia is symptom based, diagnostic criteria using prototypic adult manifestations of the disorder will miss some of the developmental variability in symptoms seen in children and adolescents. While adult criteria will identify cases of schizophrenia in childhood, developmental variability means that they will have less sensitivity and specificity than when applied to adults. This could result in missed diagnoses, particularly as presentations with an insidious onset and predominant negative-type symptoms are more common in childhood. The converse problem is lack of specificity of psychotic symptoms in childhood due to the overlap with developmental disorders and delay (e.g., the difficulty in distinguishing psychotic thought disorder from developmental language disorders) and the symptom overlap with other psychotic disorders (e.g., affective psychoses in adolescence).

Clearly, the diagnosis of schizophrenia carries uncertainty at all ages, but this is even greater in childhood due to developmental variation in symptomatology and reduced prevalence. As the sensitivity and specificity of diagnostic cutoffs vary with age, it is important that clinicians and researchers understand the degree of uncertainty inherent in the diagnostic process and the need for diagnostic validation. The development of more effective, diagnosis-specific treatments such as the atypical antipsychotics will force clinicians to demand more accurate diagnostic measures. Further refinement of diagnostic cutoffs, possibly using psychotic symptom rating scales is needed to improve the accuracy of early diagnosis.

At present, there is insufficient evidence to suggest that prodromal or "at-risk" states have sufficient specificity to justify early detection and treatment programmes. However, we are just beginning to gather evidence to validate phenotypic variants of childhood onset schizophrenia. The use of neurobiological and genetic markers is already facilitating an exploration of the status of various phenotypic variants of childhood onset schizophrenia, including those children designated as "multidimensionally impaired." Future studies will need to include a broad range of children with "atypical" developmental psychoses, as they are at least as common as children meeting full schizophrenic criteria, yet it is unclear whether or not they are part of the schizophrenia spectrum. Longitudinal diagnostic validation of a group of broadly defined psychotic children would also help to identify the extent of phenotypic variation in childhood onset schizophrenia and overcome the circularity inherent in the use of unmodified "adult" diagnostic criteria for schizophrenia in children.

REFERENCES

Alaghband-Rad, J., McKenna, K., Gordon, C., Albus, K., Hamburger, S., Rumsey, J., Frazier, J., Lenane, M., & Rapoport, J. (1995). Childhood-onset schizophrenia: the severity of premorbid course. *Journal of the American Academy of Child and Adolescent Psychiatry*, **34**, 1273–83.

American Psychiatric Association (1987). *Diagnostic and Statistical Manual of Mental Disorders*, 3rd edn-Revised (DSM-III-R). Washington, DC: APA.

American Psychiatric Association (1994). *Diagnostic and Statistical Manual of Mental Disorders*, 4th edn (DSM-IV). Washington, DC: APA.

Angold, A., Prendergast, M., Cox, A., Harrington, R., Simonoff, E., & Rutter, M. (1995) . The Child and Adolescent Psychiatric Assessment (CAPA). *Psychological Medicine*, **25**, 739–53.

Arboleda, C. & Holzman, P. (1985). Thought disorder in children at risk for psychosis. *Archives of General Psychiatry*, **42**, 1004–13.

Asarnow, J.R. (1988). Children at risk for schizophrenia: converging lines of evidence. *Schizophrenia Bulletin*, **14**, 613–31.

Asarnow, J.R. (1994). Childhood-onset schizophrenia. *Journal of Child Psychology and Psychiatry*, **35**, 1345–71.

Asarnow, J.R. & Ben-Meir, S. (1988). Children with schizophrenia spectrum and depressive disorders: a comparative study of premorbid adjustment, onset pattern and severity of impairment. *Journal of Child Psychology and Psychiatry*, **29**, 477–88.

Asarnow, J.R., Thompson, M.C., & Goldstein, M.J. (1994a). Childhood-onset schizophrenia: a follow-up study. *Schizophrenia Bulletin*, **20**, 599–617.

Asarnow, R., Asamen, J., Granholm, E., Sherman, T., Watkins, J.M., & William, M.E. (1994b). Cognitive/neuropsychological studies of children with schizophrenic disorder. *Schizophrenia Bulletin*, **20**, 647–69.

Baum, B.M. & Walker, E.F. (1995). Childhood behavioural precursors of adult symptom dimensions in schizophrenia. *Schizophrenia Reserch*, **16**, 111–20.

Bender, L. (1970). The maturational process and hallucinations in children. In *Origins and Mechanisms of Hallucinations*, ed. W. Keup, pp. 95–102. New York: Plenum Press.

Beratis, S., Gabriel, J., & Hoidas, S. (1994). Age at onset in subtypes of schizophrenic disorders. *Schizophrenia Bulletin*, **20**, 287–96.

Bettes, B. & Walker, E. (1987). Positive and negative symptoms in psychotic and other psychiatrically disturbed children. *Journal of Child Psychology and Psychiatry*, **28**, 555–68.

Bleuler, E. (1911). *Dementia praecox oder die Gruppe der Schizophrenien*. In *Handbuch der Psychiatrie*, special part, fasc. 4, ed. G. Aschaffenburg. Vienna: Deuticke.

Caplan, R., Guthrie, D., Tanguay, P., Fish, B., & David-Lando, G. (1989). The Kiddie Formal Thought Disorder Scale (K-FTDS): clinical assessment, reliability and validity. *Journal of the American Academy of Child Psychiatry*, **28**, 408–16.

Carpenter, W., Heinrichs, D., & Wagman, A. (1988). Deficit and non-deficit forms of schizophrenia: the concept. *American Journal of Psychiatry*, **145**, 578–83.

Childs, B. & Scriber, C. (1986). Age at onset and cause of disease. *Perspectives in Biology and Medicine*, **29**, 437–60.

Cooper, J., Kendell, R., Gurland, B., Sharp, L., Copland, J., & Simon, R. (1972). *Psychiatric Diagnosis in New York and London*. London: Oxford University Press.

De Sanctis, S. (1906). On some varieties of dementia praecox. In *Rivista Sperimentale de Freniatria e Medicina Legale delle Alienazioni Mentale*, ed. J.G. Howell, pp. 141–65 [translated by M.L. Osbourn]. New York: Brunner Mazel.

Done, J.D., Crow, T.J., Johnstone, E.C., & Sacker, A. (1994). Childhood antecedents of schizophrenia and affective illness: social adjustment at ages 7 and 11. *British Medical Journal*, **309**, 699–703.

Eggers, C. (1978). Course and prognosis in childhood schizophrenia. *Journal of Autism and Childhood Schizophrenia*, **8**, 21–36.

Fields, J., Grochowski, S., Linenmayer, J., Kay, S., Grosz, D., Hyman, R., & Alexander, G. (1994). Assessing positive and negative symptoms in children and adolescents. *American Journal of Psychiatry*, **151**, 249–53.

Fish, B. (1985). Children's Psychiatric Rating Scale. *Psychopharmacological Bulletin*, **21**, 753–65.

Fish, B. & Rivito, E.R. (1979). Psychoses of childhood. In *Basic Handbook of Child Psychiatry: Vol. 2*, ed. J.D. Noshpitz, pp. 249–304. New York: Basic Books.

Fish, B., Marcus. J., Hans, S.L., Auerbach, J.C., & Perdue, S. (1992). Infants at risk for schizophrenia: sequelae of a genetic neurointegrative defect. *Archives of General Psychiatry*, **49**, 221–35.

Frazier, J., Giedd, J, Hamberger, S., Albus, K., Kaysen, D., Vaituzis, A., Rajapakse, J., Lenane, M.,

McKenna, K., Jacobson, L., Gordon, C., Breier, A., & Rapoport J. (1996). Brain anatomic magnetic resonance imaging in childhood-onset schizophrenia. *Archives of General Psychiatry*, **53**, 617–24.

Galdos, P. & Van os, J. (1995). Gender, psychopathology, and development: from puberty to early adulthood. *Schizophrenia Research*, **14**, 105–12.

Garralda, M. (1984). Hallucinations in children with conduct and emotional disorders; I. The clinical phenomena. *Psychological Medicine*, **14**, 589–96.

Gordon, C.T., Frazier, J.A., McKenna, K. Giedd, J., Zametkin, A., Zahn, T, Hommer, D, Hong, W., Kaysen, D., Albus, K.E., & Rapoport, J.L. (1994). Childhood-onset schizophrenia: a NIMH study in progress. *Schizophrenia Bulletin*, **20**, 697–712.

Green, W., Campbell, M., Hardesty, A., Grega, D., Padron-Gayol, M., Shell, J., & Erlenmeyer-Kimling, L. (1984). A comparison of schizophrenic and autistic children. *Journal of the American Academy of Child Psychiatry*, **23**, 399–409.

Green, W., Padron-Gayol, M., Hardesty, A., & Bassiri, M. (1992). Schizophrenia with childhood onset: a phenomenological study of 38 cases. *Journal of the American Academy of Child and Adolescent Psychiatry*, **35**, 968–76.

Herjanic, B. & Reich, W. (1982). Development of a structured psychiatric interview for children: agreement between child and parent on individual symptoms. *Journal of Abnormal Child Psychology*, **10**, 307–24.

Hollis, C. (1995). Child and adolescent (juvenile onset) schizophrenia: a case control study of premorbid developmental impairments. *British Journal of Psychiatry*, **166**, 489–95.

Hollis, C. & Taylor, E. (1997). Schizophrenia: a critique from the developmental psychopathology perspective. In *Neurodevelopment and Adult Psychopathology*, ed. M. Keshervan & R. Murray. Cambridge: Cambridge University Press.

Iacono, W.G. & Koenig, W.G.R. (1983). Features that distinguish smooth pursuit eye tracking performance in schizophrenic, affective disordered and normal individuals. *Journal of Abnormal Psychology*, **92**, 29–41.

Jacobsen, L. & Rapoport, J. (1998). Childhood onset schizophrenia: implications of clinical and neurobiological research. *Journal of Child Psychology and Psychiatry*, **39**, 101–13.

Johnstone, E. & Frith, C. (1996). Validation of three dimensions of schizophrenic symptoms in a large unselected sample of patients. *Psychological Medicine*, **26**, 667–79.

Jones, P., Rogers, B., Murray, R., & Marmot, M. (1994). Child development risk factors for adult schizophrenia in the British 1946 birth cohort. *Lancet*, **344**, 1398–1402.

Kendell, R., Brockington, I., & Leff, J. (1979). Prognostic implications of six different definitions of schizophrenia. *Archives of General Psychiatry*, **36**, 25–31.

Kolvin, I. (1971). Studies in the childhood psychoses: I. Diagnostic criteria and classification. *British Journal of Psychiatry*, **118**, 381–4.

Kraepelin, E. (1919). *Dementia Praecox* (Translated by R. Barclay). Edinburgh, UK: Livingstone.

Liddle, P. (1987). The symtoms of chronic schizophrenia: a re-examination of the positive–negative dichotomy. *British Journal of Psychiatry*, **151**, 145–51.

Liddle, P.F., Friston, K.J., Frith, C.D., Hirsch, S.R., Jones, T., & Frackowiak, R.S.J. (1992). Patterns of cerebral blood flow in schizophrenia. *British Journal of Psychiatry*, **160**, 179–86.

Loebel, A., Lieberman, J., Alvir, J., Mayerhoff, D., Geisler, S., & Szymanski, S. (1992). Duration of psychosis and outcome of first episode schizophrenia. *American Journal of Psychiatry*, **149**, 1183–8.

McGuffin, P., Farmer, A., & Harvey, I. (1991). A polydiagnostic application of diagnostic criteria in psychotic illness: development and relaibility of the OPCRIT system. *Archives of General Psychiatry*, **41**, 541–5.

McKenna, K., Gordon, C.,Lenane, M., Kaysen, D., Fahey, K., & Rapoport, J. (1994). Looking for childhood onset schizophrenia: the first 71 cases screened. *Journal of the American Academy of Child and Adolescent Psychiatry*, **33**, 636–44.

Maziade, M., Bouchard, S., Gingras, N., Charron, L., Cardinal, A., Roy, M-A., Gauthier, B., Tremblay, G., Cote, S., Fournier, C., Boutin, P., Hamel, M., Merette, C., & Martinez, M. (1996). Long term stability of diagnosis and symptom dimensions in a systematic sample of patients with onset of schizophrenia in childhood and early adolescence. II. Positive/negative distinction and childhood predictors of adult outcome. *British Journal of Psychiatry*, **169**, 371–8.

Murray, R.M. & Lewis, S.W. (1987). Is schizophrenia a neurodevelopmental disorder? *British Medical Journal*, **295**, 681–2.

Murray, R.M., Lewis, S.W., Owen, M.J., & Foerster, A. (1988). The neurodevelopmental origins of demential praecox. In *Schizophrenia: The Major Issues*, ed. P. McGuffin & P. Bebbington, pp. 90–107. London: Heinemann.

National Institute of Mental Health (NIMH) (1992). *The NIMH Diagnostic Interview Schedule for Children*. Rockville, MD: National Institute of Mental Health.

Orvaschel, H. & Puig-Antich, J. (1987). Schedule for affective disorders and schizophrenia for school-age children: epidemiological version. Unpublished manuscript. Medical College of Pennsylvania, Eastern Pennsylvania Psychiatric Institute.

Plomin, R, Owen, M., & McGuffin, P. (1994). The genetic basis of complex human behaviours. *Science*, **264**, 1733–9.

Pope, H. & Lipinski, J. (1978). Differential diagnosis of schizophrenic and manic-depressive illness. *Archives of General Psychiatry*, **25**, 811–36.

Potter, H.W. (1933). Schizophrenia in children. *American Journal of Psychiatry*, **12**, 1253–70.

Purves, D.L. & Lichtmen, J.W. (1980). Elimination of synapses in the developing nervous system. *Science*, **210**, 153–7.

Remschmidt, H., Schulz, E., & Martin, M. (1994). An open trial of clozapine in thirty-six adolescents with schizophrenia. *Journal of Child and Adolescent Psychopharmacology*, **4**, 31–41.

Russell, A.T. (1994). The clinical presentation of childhood-onset schizophrenia. *Schizophrenia Bulletin*, **20**, 631–46.

Russell, A.T., Bott, L., & Sammons, C. (1989). The phenomena of schizophrenia occurring in childhood. *Journal of the American Academy of Child and Adolescenct Psychiatry*, **28**, 399–407.

Rutter, M. (1972). Childhood schizophrenia reconsidered. *Journal of Autism and Childhood Schizophrenia*, **2**, 315–407.

Sackett, D., Hayes, R., Guyatt, G., & Tugwell, P. (1991). *Clinical Epidemiology: A Basic Science for Clinical Medicine*. Boston: Little Brown.

Schmidt, M., Blanz, B., Dippe, A., Koppe, T., & Lay, B. (1995). Course of patients diagnoses as having schizophrenia during first episode occurring under age 18 years. *European Archives of Psychiatry and Clinical Neuroscience*, **245**, 93–100.

Schneider, K. (1974). Primary and secondary symptoms in schizophrenia (Translated by H. Marshall from *Fortschr. Neurol. Psychiat. 1957*, **25**, 487–90). In ed. S. Hirsch & M. Shepard, *Themes and Variations in European Psychiatry*, pp. 40–4. Bristol: John Wright.

Shaffer, D., Gould, M., Brasic, J., Ambrosini, P., Fisher, P., Bird, B., & Aluwahlia S. (1983). A Children's Global Assessment Scale (CGAS). *Archives of General Psychiatry*, **40**, 1228–31.

Strandberg, R.J., Marsh, J.T., Brown, W.S., Asarnow, R.F., & Guthrie, D. (1994). Information processing deficits accross childhood and adult onset schizophrenia. *Schizophrenia Bulletin*, **20**, 685–96.

Towbin, K., Dykens, E., Pearson, G., & Cohen, D. (1993). Conceptualising "borderline syndrome of childhood" and "childhood schizophrenia" as a developmental disorder. *Journal of the American Academy of Child and Adolescenct Psychiatry*, **32**, 775–82.

Van os, J., Fahy, T., Jones, P., Harvey, I., Sham, P., Lewis, S., Bebbington, P., Toone, B., Williams, M., & Murray, R. (1996). Psychopathological syndromes in the functional psychoses: associations with course and outcome. *Psychological Medicine*, **26**, 161–76.

Van os, J., Marcelis, M., Sham, P., Jones, P., Gilvarry, K., & Murray, R. (1997). Psychopathological syndromes and familial morbid risk of psychosis. *British Journal of Psychiatry*, **170**, 241–6.

Verhulst, F. & Koot, H. (1992). Assessment and diagnosis. In *Child Psychiatric Epidemiology: Concepts, Methods and Findings*, pp. 42–96. Newbury Park, CA: Sage Publications.

Volkmar, F., Cohen, D., Hoshino, Y, Rende, R., & Rhea, P. (1988). Phenomenology and classification of the childhood psychoses. *Psychological Medicine*, **18**, 191–201.

Watkins, J.M., Asarnow, R.F., & Tanguay, P. (1988). Symptom development in childhood onset schizophrenia. *Journal of Child Psychology and Psychiatry*, **29**, 865–978.

Weinberger, D.R. (1987). Implications of normal brain development for the pathogenesis of schizophrenia. *Archives of General Psychiatry*, **44**, 660–9.

Weinberger, D.R., Cannon-Spoor, E., Potkin, S.G., & Wyatt, R. (1980). Poor premorbid adjustment and CT scan abnormalities in chronic schizophrenia. *American Journal of Psychiatry*, **137**, 1410–13.

Werry, J.S. (1992). Child and adolescent (early onset) schizophrenia. A review in light of DSM-IIIR. *Journal of Autism and Developmental Disorders*, **22**, 601–24.

Werry, J.S., McClellan, J.M., & Chard, L. (1991). Childhood and adolescent schizophrenia, bipolar and schizoaffective disorders: a clinical and outcome study. *Journal of the American Academy of Child and Adolescent Psychiatry*, **30**, 457–65.

Werry, J., McClellan, J., Andrews, L., & Ham, M. (1994). Clinical features and outcome of child and adolescent schizophrenia. *Schizophrenia Bulletin*, **20**, 619–30.

World Health Organization (1992). *The ICD-10 Classification of Mental and Behavioral Disorders. Clinical Descriptions and Diagnostic Guidelines*. Geneva: WHO.

World Health Organization (1993). *The ICD-10 Classification of Mental and Behavioral Disorders. Diagnostic Criteria for Research*. Geneva: WHO.

Wyatt, R.J. (1995). Early intervention in schizophrenia: can the course of the illness be altered? *Biological Psychiatry*, **38**, 1–3.

Yang, P.-C., Liu, C.-Y., Chiang, S.-Q., Chen, J.-Y., & Lin, T.-S. (1995). Comparisons of adult manifestations of schizophrenia with onset before and after 15 years of age. *Acta Psychiatrica Scandinavica*, **91**, 209–12.

Yung, A. & McGrory, P. (1996). The prodromal phase of first episode psychosis: past and current conceptualisations. *Schizophrenia Bulletin*, **22**, 353–71.

6

Genetic aspects

Jane Scourfield and Peter McGuffin

Introduction

Beliefs about the nature and etiology of schizophrenia have been influenced by the changing political and social climates of the twentieth century. In the early decades of the century there was a general consensus that schizophrenia was hereditary, but the excesses of the eugenics movement in the 1930s and 1940s, together with the popularity of psychoanalytic theory in North America, and the growth of the antipsychiatry movement in the 1960s resulted in psychiatric genetics becoming decidedly unfashionable (Stromgren, 1994). Despite this, the observation that schizophrenia clusters in families has not been seriously disputed and the past quarter of a century has seen a marked return of interest in the genetic factors involved in schizophrenia. Twin and adoption studies, as described below, provide support for genetic contributions and there is a general consensus nowadays that schizophrenia, although a heterogeneous disorder, has a substantial genetic component to its etiology.

Most genetic research to date concerns adult subjects with schizophrenia, and there is a relative dearth of information regarding the genetics of the childhood onset disorder. This chapter will therefore draw on evidence from adults as well as from the small amount of literature pertaining specifically to children.

Defining the phenotype

Any genetic research requires first that a clearly defined phenotype be agreed upon. With many psychiatric disorders this has not been the case, but it is especially true of childhood onset schizophrenia which has been subject to considerable disagreement regarding its diagnostic boundaries. Until the 1970s childhood psychoses were grouped together according to the theory of "equality of schizophrenias," that is, that there is a single psychosis of childhood

(Kolvin, 1971). This grouping included infantile autism and a broad set of disorders with severe impairments of early onset, many of which would be diagnosed as having questionable or no psychotic symptoms today. This approach was reflected in DSM-II and ICD-8, which grouped all psychotic disorders under the broad category of "childhood schizophrenia."

Although there was some debate during the 1960s regarding the boundaries of childhood schizophrenia (Tsiantis et al., 1986) the first systematic study was that of Kolvin in 1971. This work confirmed earlier reports that early and late childhood psychoses are fundamentally different in age of onset, symptomatology, family history, evidence of cerebral dysfunction and social circumstances (Kolvin, 1971). This led to the recognition of infantile autism as a discrete diagnostic entity, which was incorporated as such in DSM-III (American Psychiatric Association, 1980) and ICD-9 (World Health Organization, 1978). These diagnostic systems included a separate category of infantile autism, and adopted the current practice of using the same criteria to diagnose schizophrenia in children and adults.

Markers of vulnerability and childhood precursors

Although it is generally accepted that the signs and symptoms of overt schizophrenia in children are the same as those in adults, there has been much interest in "preschizophrenic" markers in childhood. Fish (1977) argued that "soft" neurological signs may be a childhood manifestation of a genetic susceptibility to schizophrenia. Other workers have also investigated this question, by following "high risk" offspring of schizophrenic parents. This has revealed an increased incidence of neurosensory and neuromotor deficits in the children of schizophrenic mothers (Erlenmeyer-Kimling & Cornblatt, 1984); marked autonomic reaction to stress (Mednick et al., 1974); and complicated births (Parmas et al., 1982). An investigation supported by the NIMH using a clinical sample has found impaired smooth pursuit eye movements and high baseline autonomic activity with slow habituation and adaptation in a group of children diagnosed with childhood onset schizophrenia (Gordon et al., 1994a). Two recent investigations into behavioral precursors of schizophrenia have analyzed data from prospective population-based cohort studies, following all individuals born in the UK during a 1-week period in 1946 and 1958, respectively. Done et al. (1994) using data from the 1958 cohort, showed that preschizophrenic boys were more likely to be rated as overactive than boys who later developed affective psychosis, neurosis or no psychiatric illness. Preschizophrenic girls were more likely to be rated as withdrawn. Jones et al. (1994), using data from the 1946 cohort, found later attainment of developmental milestones in schizophrenic cases than in normal controls, a preference for solitary play aged 4–6, and higher self- and teacher-ratings of anxiety. This analysis found no association between antisocial behavior and later schizophrenia. Both reports are based on data from standardized rating scales and diagnostic tools and are methodologically robust.

Although the findings to date are interesting, no biological marker has emerged as a reliable diagnostic aid in schizophrenia, either in adults or children, so the boundaries of schizophrenia continue to be defined using detailed descriptions of psychopathology generated using standardized interview techniques.

Genetic epidemiology

Family studies

Study of the aggregation of diseases/traits within families is a central theme in genetic epidemiology. If familial aggregation is found, the next step is to distinguish whether environmental, cultural and/or genetic factors are contributing. Family studies compare the frequency of schizophrenia in the relatives of cases with the frequency in a group of controls drawn from the general population. It is estimated that the lifetime morbid risk for schizophrenia in the worldwide population is about 1%, and family studies have shown that the relatives of schizophrenics are at significantly increased risk of the disorder, the risk increasing with the genetic closeness of the relationship. The highest risks are seen in identical twins of schizophrenics (48%) and in the offspring of two schizophrenic parents (46%). The results of 40 family studies are illustrated in Fig. 6.1 which shows average lifetime risks according to genetic relatedness (Gottesman, 1991).

An earlier onset of schizophrenia might result from an increased genetic load or a more potent environmental insult, and would therefore be expected to result in increased familiality. This has, indeed, been observed in schizophrenic males with onset of psychosis before 17 (Pulver et al., 1990). Also, a large Swedish family study of schizophrenia showed that earlier age of onset in the proband was associated with an increased risk of schizophrenia in the relatives (Sham et al., 1994). However, the small number of family studies of childhood schizophrenia have so far not demonstrated higher rates of disorder among relatives than is found for adult probands. Results of the early studies (Kallman & Roth, 1956; Kolvin et al., 1971a,b) are difficult to interpret because of a lack of standardized diagnoses and the one recent study (Gordon et al., 1994a) has only published preliminary results so far and a larger sample size is needed.

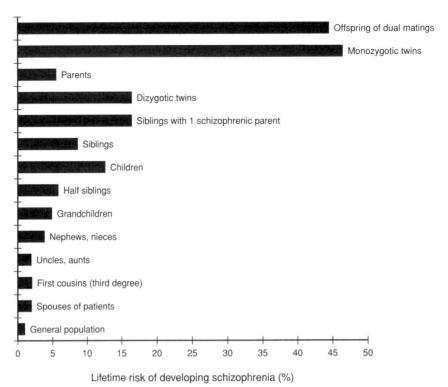

Fig. 6.1. Average risks for developing schizophrenia, compiled from European studies 1920–87 (from Gottesman, 1991). Irving I. Gottesman © 1991. Used with permission of W.H. Freeman and Company.

Most of the family studies cited above are based on relatives of adult schizophrenic subjects. Few family studies to date have dealt specifically with relatives of probands with childhood onset schizophrenia but two early studies warrant discussion; those of Kolvin et al. (1971a) and Kallman and Roth (1956). The methods used were possibly not as rigorous as is the current norm and did not include standardized diagnosis. Therefore, the findings need to be interpreted cautiously (Werry, 1992). Kolvin (1971) divided childhood psychosis into "Infantile Psychosis" (IP) with onset before age 3, and "Late onset psychosis" (LOP) with onset after age 5 and adult first rank symptoms. Using hospital records, cases of schizophrenia among the parents of psychotic children were traced. In the LOP group, 6 of 64 parents (9.4%) had schizophrenia, a rate which is considerably higher than the expected population rate of 1%. Only one parent in the IP group had schizoaffective disorder. Of the 68 siblings of the IP children, none presented with schizophrenia, whilst one out of 56 siblings of the LOP group had an adult type of schizophrenia. Kolvin concluded that LOP of childhood resembles adult schizophrenia at least in its familial aspects.

Kallman and Roth (1956) found rates of schizophrenia of 8.8% (12.5% age corrected) among the parents of their sample of childhood schizophrenics, and of 12.2% among siblings. The results of both studies reveal higher rates of schizophrenia among parents than are seen in the parents of adult schizophrenics, as illustrated in Fig. 6.1. A more recent study (Gordon et al., 1994a) using structured interviews and best estimate diagnostic methods have reported preliminary results of an overall rate of 13% for non-affective psychotic illness among the first degree relatives of subjects with childhood-onset schizophrenia. This rate is comparable to that found among relatives of adult schizophrenics, although the results await confirmation in a larger sample. To date, then, there is not consistent support for an increased risk to relatives of childhood-onset as opposed to adult-onset schizophrenics, although the results of early studies point to increased illness in parents. This would be consistent with the notion that early onset of schizophrenia reflects greater severity and that risk to relatives increases as severity increases. However, methodological shortcomings of these early studies prevent confident conclusions and more data are needed.

The aggregation of schizophrenia in families, an observation which is a prerequisite for further genetic studies, may of course be due to factors other than genetic transmission. For example, it has been suggested that some forms of parental behavior are "schizophrenogenic" (Alanen, 1958). Familiality of schizophrenia has also been attributed to abnormal communication styles in parents (Bateson et al., 1956; Wynne & Singer, 1963) or transmission of viruses (Mednick et al., 1988). In order to clarify whether the aggregation is due to shared genes, shared environment, or both, it is necessary to examine data from adoption and twin studies.

Adoption studies

Adoption studies allow the separation of the effects of genes and family environment. There are three commonly used methods:

The adoptee study

Offspring of parents with the disorder of interest who were adopted away are compared with control adoptees with normal biological parents.

The adoptee's family study

Adopted subjects with the disorder of interest are ascertained and rates of the disorder in their biological and adoptive relatives are compared.

The cross-fostering study

Adoptees whose biological parents have the disorder of interest, but who grew up with unaffected adoptive parents, are studied and their rates of disorder compared with adoptees whose biological parents are normal but who grew up with affected adoptive parents.

Although adoption studies allow the separation of genes from environment, they are not without drawbacks. The placement of adoptees is not random and agencies tend to look for what are considered well-matched families. Also, studies have tended to find higher rates of psychopathology among adoptees than in the general population. However, with these reservations in mind, it is still possible to say that adoption studies have confirmed a genetic contribution to the etiology of schizophrenia. All studies to date have used adult probands with schizophrenia (we are not aware of any adoption studies in childhood schizophrenia) and are summarized in Table 6.1.

The earliest study by Heston (1966) examined 47 adoptees who had been separated from their schizophrenic mothers within 3 days of birth. Five of the subjects developed schizophrenia compared with none of 50 control adoptees. These results were confirmed by two later adoptee studies (Rosenthal et al., 1968; Tienari, 1991). It can be seen from the table that the evidence from adoption studies is compelling, with consistently higher rates of schizophrenia among biological relatives compared with adoptive relatives or controls.

Twin studies

Monozygotic twins share 100% of their genes whereas dizygotic twins share on average 50%, as do ordinary siblings. By examining the concordance rate for schizophrenia in MZ and DZ twins, it is possible to estimate the extent to which the disorder has a genetic component. If genes are playing a significant role, then the concordance rate among MZ pairs should be significantly higher than among DZ pairs.

The main assumption of twin studies is that MZ and DZ pairs have equally shared environments. This assumption has been criticized on the grounds that MZ twins share a unique environment because they are identical and therefore are treated more similarly by parents and friends. There is indeed some evidence that MZ twins share childhood environments to a greater extent than DZ twins. However, support for the assumption of equal environmental sharing comes from MZ twins who have been reared apart. Such twins are rare and data is only available for adults with schizophrenia but shows a concordance rate of 58%, which is slightly higher than that seen in twins raised together (Gottesman & Shields, 1982).

Table 6.1. Adoption studies

Study	Type of study	Diagnosis	Genetic relatives of a schizophrenic	Not genetically related to a schizophrenic
Heston (1966)	Adoptee	Schizophrenia	10.6% of 47 adoptees who had a schizophrenic biological mother	0% of 50 control adoptees
Rosenthal et al. (1968)	Adoptee	Schizophrenia spectrum disorder	18.8% of 69 children of schizophrenics raised by normals	10.1% of 79 control adoptees
Wender et al. (1974)	Cross-fostering	Schizophrenic spectrum disorder	18.8% of 69 children of schizophrenics raised by normals	10.7% of 28 children of controls raised by future schizophrenics
Kety (1983); Kety et al. (1994)	Adoptee's family: national sample (47 chronic schizophrenic adoptees)	Chronic and latent (DSM-III) schizophrenics	15.8% of 279 biological relatives of adopted-away schizophrenics	1.8% of 228 adoptive relatives of schizophrenics and relatives of control adoptees
Kendler & Gruenberg (1984); Kendler et al. (1994)	Reassessment of Kety's data (31 adoptees with spectrum disorder)	DSM-III schizophrenia plus schizotypal personality disorder plus RDC schizoaffective disorder, mainly schizophrenic	14.4% of 209 biological relatives of adopted-away schizophrenics (23% in first-degree relatives, 9.9% in second-degree relatives)	3% of 229 adoptive relatives of schizophrenics and relatives of control adoptees
Tienari (1991)	Adoptee	Any form of psychosis	9% of 138 adoptees who had a schizophrenic biological parent	1.2% of 171 control adoptees

From McGuffin et al. (1994). Reprinted with permission of Royal College of Psychiatrists.

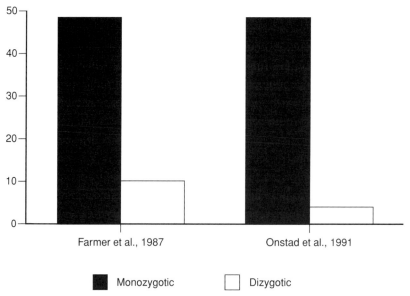

Fig. 6.2. Twin concordance for DSM III/DSM IIIR schizophrenia.

As with family and adoption studies, an important criticism of the early twin studies is their lack of standardized diagnostic practices. Two recent studies using operational diagnostic criteria (Farmer et al., 1987; Onstad et al., 1991) are illustrated in Fig. 6.2. Both found concordance rates for MZ twins to be almost 50% and for DZ to be considerably less at 5–10%, supporting the results of earlier work.

Another criticism of twin studies is ascertainment bias. Reports of concordance among clinical samples tend to be biased towards concordance and MZ pairs because these are the most memorable and tend to be recruited. This will have the tendency to inflate the genetic effect. Such biases are overcome by using systematically ascertained samples such as twin registers. Data from studies using European twin registers have been summarized by Gottesman and Shields (1982), and show a MZ concordance of 46% compared with a DZ concordance of 14%. This large ratio of MZ:DZ concordances supports a role for genes in schizophrenia but illustrates that the disorder is not entirely genetic since, if this were true, we would expect the concordance between MZ twins to be 100%.

There has been one twin study of childhood schizophrenia which warrants discussion. Kallman and Roth (1956) recruited a sample of 52 twins and 50 singletons under age 15 from admissions to a hospital in the State of New York.

Diagnoses were made by a single clinician. Pairwise concordance rates for monozygotic and dizygotic twins were 70.6% and 17.1%, respectively, rates which are comparable to those found in adults, although the MZ concordance rate is slightly higher, possibly a result of the clinical sampling frame which, as mentioned above, can inflate the genetic effect. There was also an unexpectedly large proportion of same sex DZ pairs (same sex and opposite sex DZ pairs are expected with equal frequency), which might have been due to the mistaken identification of MZ pairs as DZ. This would have increased DZ and lowered MZ concordances (Hanson & Gottesman,1976). Additionally, the composition of the sample in this study is rather surprising, with a statewide longitudinal sampling strategy producing only 50 singletons compared with 52 pairs of twins, which is very unlike the general population ratio of approximately 1 set of twins for every 100 singletons born (Hanson & Gottesman, 1976).

Type of inheritance

Various genetic mechanisms have been offered as explanations of the similarity between relatives in liability to schizophrenia. The most simple is that of a single major gene. However, even allowing for incomplete penetrance, single locus inheritance is not consistent with the observed segregation patterns and can be shown statistically to be incompatible with the available data (McGue et al., 1985).

Alternative modes of inheritance may involve many genes of small effect, with (multifactorial) or without an environmental effect. A mixed model involving a major locus with a multifactorial background is another possibility. The complex inheritance of schizophrenia has made genetic marker studies difficult, but progress is now being made.

Molecular genetics

Genetic markers

While family, twin and adoption studies provide convincing evidence that schizophrenia clusters in families, this is only indirect support for a genetic mode of transmission. Studies using genetic markers provide a more direct approach to identifying and locating genes and therefore to understanding the molecular basis of the disease. A genetic marker is any characteristic which can be reliably measured, has simple Mendelian transmission and exists in two or more allelic forms with at least a 1% frequency in the population. Very many markers are now available from reference genetic linkage maps, such as the Généthon human linkage map (Dib et al., 1996), and have resulted in a great increase in feasibility of linkage studies in complex disorders.

Linkage studies

This approach employs the use of genetic markers in families which contain several members with the disease of interest. Linkage occurs when a genetic marker and the disease are found to occur together more frequently than would be expected by chance. The marker and disease gene are then said to be "linked" and can be assumed to lie close together on the chromosome. Genes which are in close proximity to each other will recombine less frequently than expected during meiosis and therefore do not follow Mendel's law of independent assortment.

The frequency of recombination is measured by the recombination fraction (Θ) which can vary from 0 (tight linkage) to 0.5 (independent assortment). It is estimated using the lod (log of the odds) score method where the lod score is calculated for a range of possible values of Θ between 0 and 0.5 and the peak lod score is taken as the maximum likelihood estimate of the recombination fraction. Within certain limits, this is proportional to the distance between the marker and the disease locus. By convention, for simple Mendelian traits, a lod score of 3 or more is taken as acceptable evidence that linkage is present, while a lod score of -2 or less excludes linkage. A lod score of 3 corresponds to odds on linkage of 1000:1, whereas a score of -2 corresponds to odds of 100:1 against (Morton, 1955; Ott, 1991).

Complex modes of inheritance, genetic heterogeneity and unclear phenotypic boundaries are all problems which complicate linkage studies. There is also still considerable debate regarding what can legitimately be included in the adult schizophrenia spectrum as well as in the spectrum of childhood onset disorder. The literature regarding linkage and schizophrenia is so far based on adult data only. Early studies looked at classical markers such as HLA types (Turner, 1979) and, whilst initial results looked encouraging, these were not replicated by other workers (McGuffin, 1989). More recently, attention has focused on chromosome 11 following two reports of albinism and schizophrenia cosegregating (Baron, 1976; Clarke & Buckley, 1989). The dopamine D_2 receptor gene is located near the albinism gene on chromosome 11, prompting much interest in this region; however no positive linkage results have emerged (Moises et al., 1991; Gill et al., 1993).

Reports of an unbalanced translocation of the long arm of chromosome 5 in a pair of relatives affected by schizophrenia (Bassett et al., 1988) prompted linkage studies of this region, and much excitement was generated when positive linkage was reported in five Icelandic and British pedigrees (Sherrington et al., 1988). However, subsequent studies in families from Sweden, Scotland, North America, Ireland and Wales (Kennedy et al., 1989; St. Clair et al., 1989; Detera-Wadleigh et al., 1989; Diehl & Kendler, 1989; McGuffin et al., 1990) have failed to replicate these results.

Schizophrenic siblings are more frequently of the same gender and this observation has led to speculation that a gene for schizophrenia may be located in the pseudoautosomal region of the X chromosome (Crow, 1988). However, early support for this hypothesis (Collinge et al., 1991) has not been replicated by other groups (Asherson et al., 1992).

Linkage analyses based on adult data have therefore, so far, been inconclusive. A recent report by Gordon et al. (1994b) described a balanced translocation between chromosomes 1 and 7 in a boy with childhood onset schizophrenia. The breakpoints were at p22 on chromosome 1 and q22 on chromosome 7. The report is interesting, given a previous case of chromosomal rearrangement involving chromosomes 1, 7, and 21 in a 6-year-old autistic boy where the break point on chromosome 1 was also 1p22 (Lopreiato & Wulfsberg, 1992). A small number of case reports have described early autistic symptoms followed by development of schizophrenia in adolescence and early adulthood. Whilst the full syndromes of autism and schizophrenia appear to be distinct, as Gordon et al. (1994b) suggest, it is possible that a subgroup of childhood schizophrenics and autistics share a similar genetic abnormality. This observation makes the break points of chromosomes 1 and 7 likely sites for further linkage studies.

Association studies

While linkage studies can detect genes of major effect, genes of small effect may go unnoticed. Such genes may be detectable using association studies which investigate whether a particular marker is more common in a sample of unrelated schizophrenics than in a control sample. Although potentially comparable with linkage studies, association studies have the drawback of being "shortsighted." That is, the marker and the susceptibility locus have to be very close together, resulting in the phenomenon called linkage disequilibrium. In practice, this means that association is only likely to be detected for recombination fractions of 0.01 or less. Alternatively, association may be detectable if the marker itself confers susceptibility to the disorder.

Early studies in schizophrenics investigated possible associations with classical markers such as ABO blood groups and the HLA system. Recent results do not support an association with ABO blood groups, but are more supportive of an association between schizophrenia and HLA A9, although the effect is small (McGuffin & Sturt, 1986). An association study using a large European sample

(Williams et al., 1996) has found an increase of allele 2 of a polymorphism in the 5-hydroxytryptamine type 2a-receptor gene among schizophrenics, suggesting that this allele confers increased susceptibility to schizophrenia.

A recent association study from Canada (Maziade et al., 1997) is the only one we are aware of which includes data from a sample of childhood onset schizophrenics. This group tested for an allelic association between schizophrenia and a marker at the dopamine D_3 receptor locus in a sample from Eastern Quebec. The sample was divided into cases with onset before and after the age of 17, and was compared with controls. Positive association was found only among the adult-onset group and not among those with childhood-onset, supporting the authors' hypothesis that extreme age of onset may identify a homogeneous subgroup of schizophrenia. The finding of an association between D_3 and adult schizophrenia had earlier been reported by groups in Wales and France, with homozygosity at this locus approximately doubling the risk of schizophrenia (Crocq et al., 1992; Mant et al., 1994).

Limitations of association studies

As with linkage studies, association studies are limited by the quality of definition of the phenotype in question. A second problem is that of stratification effects; this refers to a phenomenon whereby there has been a recent admixture of populations with different frequencies of both disease and marker alleles. This can result in apparent marker-disease association without any causal relationship existing between them. Additionally, statistical allowance must be made for the use of multiple markers in association studies and the probability level needs to be corrected for multiple tests. A further limitation of these studies is that unlike with linkage, it is so far not feasible to carry out systematic genome searches because of the need for very large numbers of markers. This is because of the fact that, in order for linkage disequilibrium to exist, markers and disease susceptibility loci have to be very close so that a minimum of 2000 evenly spaced markers would be needed to scan the genome. One solution to this difficulty is the recently developed technique of sample pooling in which DNA from all patients and all controls can be combined to form two pools. The initial genotyping is performed on the pools and positive results then confirmed by conventional individual genotyping (Daniels et al., 1996).

Conclusions

Evidence from adult data provides compelling support for an important genetic component in the etiology of schizophrenia. The evidence regarding childhood onset schizophrenia is sparse and conclusions are difficult to draw. The small amount of epidemiological data supports an increased risk to relatives of childhood schizophrenics compared with general population rates, but not over and above that found among relatives of adult schizophrenics. The exception to this is among parents of childhood schizophrenics, who have almost double the rates of illness seen in parents of adult schizophrenics. This provides some support for the notion that childhood-onset schizophrenia represents a greater genetic loading. One could speculate that schizophrenia is like breast cancer with very early-onset cases appearing to have Mendelian genetic transmission, while later onset cases are multifactorial in their etiology. However, the only studies available do not meet modern standards for diagnostic rigor, so interpretation can only be made cautiously. There is a need for methodologically rigorous genetic epidemiological studies in this area, in order to point the way forward for future molecular genetic searches.

REFERENCES

Alanen, Y.O. (1958). The mothers of schizophrenic patients. *Acta Psychiatrica Scandinavica*, suppl. 124.

American Psychiatric Association (1980). *Diagnostic and Statistical Manual of Mental Disorders*, 3rd edn. Washington DC: APA.

Asherson, P., Parfitt, E., Sargeant, M., Tidmarsh, S., Buckland, P., Taylor, C., Clements, A., Gill, M., McGuffin, P., & Owen, M. (1992). No evidence for a pseudoautosomal locus for schizophrenia. Linkage analysis of multiply affected families. *British Journal of Psychiatry*, **161**, 63–8.

Baron, M. (1976). Albinism and schizophreniform psychosis. *American Journal of Psychiatry*, **133**, 1070–3.

Bassett, A.S., McGillivray, B.C., Jones, B.D., & Pantzar, J.T. (1988). Partial trisomy chromosome 5 cosegregating with schizophrenia. *The Lancet*, i(8589), 799–801.

Bateson, G., Jackson, D.D., Hayley, J., & Weakland, J.H. (1956). Towards a theory of schizophrenia. *Behavioral Science*, **1**, 251–64.

Clarke, D.J. & Buckley, M.E. (1989). Familial association of albinism and schizophrenia. *British Journal of Psychiatry*, **155**, 551–3.

Collinge, J., DeLisi, L.E., Boccio, A., Johnstone, E.C. Lane, A., Larkin, C., Leach, M., Lofthouse, R., Owen, F., Poulter, M. et al. (1991). Evidence for a pseudo-autosomal locus for schizophrenia using the methods of affected sibling pairs. *British Journal of Psychiatry*, **158**, 624–9.

Crocq, M.A., Mant, R., Asherson, P., Williams, J. Hode, Y., Mayerova, A., Collier, D. Lannfelt, L., Sokoloff, P., Schwartz, J.C., et al. (1992). Association between schizophrenia and homozygosity at the dopamine D3 receptor gene. *Journal of Medical Genetics*, **29**, 858–60.

Crow, T.J. (1988). Sex chromosomes and psychosis. *British Journal of Psychiatry*, **153**, 675–83.

Daniels, J., McGuffin, P. & Owen, M. (1996). Molecular genetic research on IQ: can it be done?

Should it be done? *Journal of Biosocial Science*, **28**, 491–507.

Detera-Wadleigh, S.D., Goldin, L.R., Sherrington, R., Encio, I. de Miguel, C. Berrettini, W., Gurling, H., & Gershon, E.S. (1989). Exclusion of linkage to 5q11–13 in families with schizophrenia and other psychiatric disorders. *Nature*, **339**, 331–93.

Dib, C., Faure, S., Fizames, C., Samson, D., Drouot, N., Vignal, A., Millasseau, P., Marc, S., Hazan, J., Seboun, E., Lathrop, M., Gyapay, G., Morissette, J., & Weissenbach, J. (1996). A comprehensive genetic map of the human genome based on 5,264 microsatelllites. *Nature*, **380**(6570), 152–4.

Diehl, S.R. & Kendler, K.S. (1989). Strategies for linkage studies of schizophrenia: Pedigrees, DNA markers and statistical analyses. *Schizophrenia Bulletin*, **15**, 403–19.

Done, J.D., Crow, T.J., Johnstone, E.C., & Sacker, A. (1994). Childhood antecedents of schizophrenia and affective illness: social adjustment at ages 7 and 11. *British Medical Journal*, **309**, 699–703.

Erlenmeyer-Kimling, L. & Cornblatt, B. (1984). Biobehavioural risk factors in children of schizophrenic parents. *Journal of Autism and Developmental Disorders*, **14**, 357–73.

Farmer, A.E., McGuffin, P. & Gottesman, I.I. (1987). Twin concordance and DSM III schizophrenia: scrutinizing the valildity of the definition. *Archives of General Psychiatry*, **44**, 634–40.

Fish, B. (1977). Neurobiologic antecedents of schizophrenia in children. *Archives of General Psychiatry*, **34**, 1297–313.

Gill, M., McGuffin, P., Parfitt, E., Mant, R. Asherson, P., Collier, D., Vallada, H., Powell, J., Shaikh, S., Taylor, C. et al. (1993). A linkage study of schizophrenia with DNA markers from the long arm of chromosome 11. *Psychological Medicine*, **23**(1), 27–44.

Gordon, C.T., Frazier, J.A., McKenna, K., Giedd J. Zametkin, A., Zahn, T., Hommer, D., Hong, W., Kaysen, D., Albus, K.E. et. al. (1994a). Childhood-onset schizophrenia: an NIMH study in progress. *Schizophrenia Bulletin*, **20**, 697–712.

Gordon, C.T., Krasnewich, D., White, B., Lenane, M., & Rappoport, J.L. (1994b). Translocation involving chromosomes 1 and 7 in a boy with childhood-onset schizophrenia. *Journal of Autism and Developmental Disorders*, **24**(4), 537–45.

Gottesman, I.I. (1991). *Schizophrenia Genesis: The Origins of Madness*. New York: W.H. Freeman.

Gottesman, I.I. & Shields, J. (1982). Schizophrenia, the epigenetic puzzle. Cambridge: Cambridge University Press.

Hanson, D.R. & Gottesman, I.I. (1976). The Genetics, if any, of infantile autism and childhood schizophrenia. *Journal of Autism and Childhood Schizophrenia*, **6**(3), 209–34.

Heston, L.L. (1966). Psychiatric disorders in foster home reared children of schizophrenic mothers. *British Journal of Psychiatry*, **112**, 819–25.

Jones, P., Rodgers, B., Murray, M., & Marmot, M. (1994). Child developmental risk factors for adult schizophrenia in the British 1946 birth cohort. *The Lancet*, **344**, 1398–402.

Kallman, F.J. & Roth, B. (1956). Genetic aspects of preadolescent schizophrenia. *American Journal of Psychiatry*, **112**, 599–606.

Kendler, K.S. & Gruenberg, A.M. (1984). An independent analysis of the Danish adoption study of schizophrenia VI. The patterns of psychiatric illness as defined by DSM III in adoptees and relatives. *Archives of General Psychiatry*, **41**, 555–64.

Kendler, K.S., Gruenberg, A.M., & Kinney, D.K. (1994). Independent diagnoses of adoptees and relatives as defined by DSM-III in the provincial and national samples of the Danish adoption study of schizophrenia. *Archives of General Psychiatry*, **51**(6), 456–68.

Kennedy, J.L., Giuffra, L.A., Moises, H.W., Wetterberg, L., Sjogren, B., Cavalli-Sforza, L.L., Pakstis, A.J., Kidd, J.R., & Kidd, K.K. (1989). Molecular genetic studies in schizophrenia. *Schizophrenia Bulletin*, **15**, 383–91.

Kety, S.S. (1983). Mental illness in the biological and adoptive relatives of schizophrenic adoptees, findings relevant to genetic and environmental factors in etiology. *American Journal of Psychiatry*, **140**, 720–7.

Kety, S.S., Wender, P.H., Jacobsen, B., Ingraham, L.J. Jansson, L., Faber, B., & Kinney, D.K. (1994). Mental illness in the biological and adoptive relatives of schizophrenic adoptees. Replication of the Copenhagen study in the rest of Denmark. *Archives of General Psychiatry*, **51**(6), 442–55.

Kolvin, I. (1971). Studies in the childhood psychoses. *British Journal of Psychiatry*, **118**, 381–4.

Kolvin, I., Ounsted,C., Humphrey, M., & McVay, A. (1971a). The phenomenology of childhood psychoses. *British Journal of Psychiatry*, **118**, 385–95.

Kolvin, I., Ounsted, C., Richardson, L.M., & Garside, R.F. (1971b). The family and social background in childhood psychoses. *British Journal of Psychiatry*, **118**, 396–402.

Lopreiato, J.O. & Wulfsberg, E.A. (1992). A complex chromosome rearrangement in a boy with autism. *Journal of Developmental and Behavioral Pediatrics*, **13**, 281–3.

Mant, R., Williams, J., Asherson, P. Parfitt, E., McGuffin, P., & Owen, M.J. (1994). The relationship between homozygosity at the dopamine D3 receptor gene and schizophrenia. *American Journal of Medical Genetics (Neuropsychiatric Genetics)*, **54**, 21–6.

Maziade, M., Martinez, M., Rodrigue, C., Gauthier, B., Tremblay, G., Fournier, C., Bissonnette, L., Simard, C., Roy, M.A., Rouillard, E., & Merette, C. (1997). Childhood-early adolescence onset and adult onset schizophrenia. Heterogeneity at the dopamine D3 receptor gene. *British Journal of Psychiatry*, **170**, 27–30.

McGue, M., Gottesman, I.I., & Rao, D.C. (1985). Resolving genetic models for the transmission of schizophrenia. *Genetic Epidemiology*, **2**, 99–110.

McGuffin, P. (1989). Genetic markers: an overview and future perspectives. In *A Genetic Perspective for Schizophrenia and Related Disorders*, ed. E. Smeraldi & L. Belloni. Milan: Edi-Ermes.

McGuffin, P. & Sturt, E. (1986). Genetic markers in schizophrenia. *Human Heredity*, **16**, 461–5.

McGuffin, P., Sargeant, M., Hetti, G., Tidmarsh, S., Whatley, S., & Marchbanks, R.M. (1990). Exclusion of a schizophrenia susceptibility gene from the chromosome 5q11–q13 region. New data and reanalysis of previous reports. *American Journal of Human Genetics*, **47**, 524–35.

McGuffin, P., Owen, M.J., O'Donovan, M.C., Thapar, A., & Gottesman, I.I. (1994). *Psychiatric Genetics*. College Seminars Series. London: Royal College of Psychiatrists.

Mednick, S.A., Schulsinger, F., Higgins, J., & Bell, B. (1974). *Genetics, Environment and Psychopathology*. New York: American Elsevier.

Mednick, S.A., Machon, R.A., Huttunen, M.D., & Bonett, D. (1988). Adult schizophrenia following prenatal exposure to an influenza epidemic. *Archives of General Psychiatry*, **45**, 189–92.

Moises, H.W., Gelernter, J., Giuffra, L., Zarcone, V.P. Wetterberg, L., Civelli, O., Kidd, K.K., Cavalli-Sforza, L.L., Grandy, D.K., Kennedy, J.L. et al. (1991). No linkage between D2 dopamine receptor region and schizophrenia. *Archives of General Psychiatry*, **48**, 643–7.

Morton, N.E. (1955). Sequential tests for the detection of linkage. *American Journal of Human Genetics*, **7**, 227–318.

Onstad, S., Skre, I., Torgersen, S., & Kringlen, E. (1991). Twin concordance for DSM-IIIR schizophrenia. *Acta Psychiatrica Scandinavica*, **83**, 395–401.

Ott, J. (1991). *Analysis of Human Genetic Linkage*. Baltimore: Johns Hopkins University Press.

Parmas, J., Schulsinger, F., Teasdale, T., Schulsinger, H., Felbman, P., & Mednick, S. (1982). Perinatal complications and clinical outcome within the schizophrenia spectrum. *British Journal of Psychiatry*, **140**, 416–20.

Pulver, A., Brown, C.H., Wolnyiec, P., McGrath, J., Tam, D., Adler, L., Carpenter, W.T., & Childs, B. (1990). Schizophrenia: age at onset, gender, and familial risk. *Acta Psychiatrica Scandinavica*, **82**, 344–51.

Rosenthal, D., Wender, P., Kety, S.S., Schulsinger, F., Welner, J., & Østergaard, L. (1968). Schizophrenics' offspring reared in adoptive homes. In *The Transmission of Schizophrenia*, ed. D. Rosenthal & S.S. Kety. Oxford: Pergamon Press.

Sham, P.C., MacLean, C.J., & Kendler, K.S. (1994). A typological model of schizophrenia based on age at onset, sex and familial morbidity. *Acta Psychiatrica Scandinavica*, **89**, 135–41.

Sherrington, R., Brynjolfsson, J., Petursson, H., Potter, M., Potter, M., Dudleston, K., Barraclough, B., Wasmuth, J., Dobbs, M., & Gurling, H. (1988). Localization of a susceptibility locus for schizophrenia on chromosome 5. *Nature*, **336**, 164–7.

St. Clair, D., Blackwood, D., Muir, W., Baillie, D., Hubbard, A., Wright, A., & Evans, H.J. (1989). No linkage of chromosome 5q11–q13 markers to schizophrenia in Scottish families. *Nature*, **339**, 305–9.

Stromgren, E. (1994). Recent history of European psychiatry – ideas, developments and personalities: the annual Eliot Slater lecture. *American Journal of Medical Genetics*, **54**, 405–10.

Tienari, F. (1991). Gene–environment interaction in adoptive families. In *Search for the Causes of Schizophrenia*, vol. 2, ed. H. Häfner & W.F. Gattaz, pp. 126–143. Heidelberg: Springer.

Tsiantis, J., Macri, I., & Maratos, O. (1986). Schizophrenia in children: a review of European research. *Schizophrenia Bulletin*, **12**, 101–19.

Turner, W.H. (1979). Genetic markers for schizotaxia. *Biological Psychiatry*, **14**, 177–206.

Wender, P.H., Rosenthal, D., Kety, S.S., Schulsinger, F., & Welner, J. (1974). Crossfostering. A research strategy for clarifying the role of genetic and experimental factors in the etiology of schizophrenia. *Archives of General Psychiatry*, **30**, 121–8.

Werry, J.S. (1992). Child and adolescent (early onset) schizophrenia: a review in light of DSMIIIR. *Journal of Autism and Developmental Disorders*, **22**, 601–24.

Williams, J., Spurlock, G., McGuffin, P., Mallet, J., Nothen, M.M., Gill, M., Aschauer, H., Nylander, P.O., Macciardi, F., & Owen, M.J. (1996). Association between schizophrenia and T102C polymorphism of the 5-hydroxytryptamine type 2a-receptor gene. *The Lancet*, **347**, 1294–6.

World Health Organization (1978). *International Classification of Diseases* (9th Revision) of Mental and Behavioural Disorders. Geneva: WHO.

Wynne, L.C. & Singer, M.T. (1963). Thought disorder and family relations of schizophrenics II. Classification of forms of thinking. *Archives of General Psychiatry*, **9**, 191–8.

7

Neurobehavioral perspective

Robert F. Asarnow and Canan Karatekin

Introduction

Schizophrenia provides a compelling challenge to neurobehavioral approaches to understanding mental disease. The neurobehavioral approach attempts to identify the central nervous system (CNS) substrates of a variety of psychiatric/behavioral disorders. There is an underlying CNS dysfunction in most schizophrenic individuals. However, the nature of this CNS dysfunction is not well understood. Genetic factors have been implicated in the etiology of schizophrenia (Gottesman & Shields, 1982). The efficacy of neuroleptic drugs in reducing positive symptoms of schizophrenia suggests that, in some schizophrenic patients, there may be a "neurochemical" lesion involving (at least indirectly) certain aspects of the dopamine system. Anatomical changes have been demonstrated in schizophrenic patients with both computer tomography and magnetic resonance imaging (MRI). One of the most replicated findings in schizophrenia research is that the third and fourth ventricles are enlarged in many schizophrenic patients (Nasrallah, 1990). Histological studies of the fine structure of schizophrenic brains have detected subtle cytoarchitectural anomalies, including loss or disarray of hippocampal tissue (Kovelman & Scheibel, 1986). Positron emission tomography studies indicate relative hypometabolism in a variety of brain structures, including the frontal lobes (Buchsbaum et al., 1990). There is clearly no dearth of putative CNS abnormalities in schizophrenic patients. The number and sheer diversity of these abnormalities have resulted in a situation where, while there is general agreement that many schizophrenic individuals have some form of CNS dysfunction, the specific nature of that dysfunction has yet to be detailed. Thus, the major challenge to a neurobehavioral approach to schizophrenia is to elucidate the nature of the CNS impairments underlying this disorder.

The data presented in this chapter can inform neurobehavioral models of schizophrenia, which attempt to understand the complex pathways from CNS dysfunction to the symptoms of the disorder. Many of these data are the products of the ongoing family genetic study of schizophrenic children we are conducting at the University of California, Los Angeles (UCLA), while some of the data come from the work of other investigators. The working assumption of our study is that schizophrenia is a disorder involving impaired CNS functioning. We further believe that there is a genetic basis for this CNS disturbance in many of the patients. We are studying schizophrenic children because of prior research (for review see Asarnow & Asarnow, 1994; Fish & Ritvo, 1979) suggesting that, compared to schizophrenic adults, they have a more homogeneous, familial, and severe form of schizophrenia in which the CNS dysfunction is more readily discernible.

This chapter summarizes three complementary sets of data that help elucidate the nature of neurobehavioral impairments in schizophrenia. The first set of data comes from studies that retrospectively characterize the development and course of neurobehavioral impairments in schizophrenic children. These studies reveal that there are certain neurobehavioral impairments in these children prior to the onset of psychotic symptoms. The second set of data comes from a series of cross-sectional studies examining cognitive/ neuropsychological functioning using behavioral and psychophysiological methods. These studies attempt to delimit the cognitive processes that are impaired in schizophrenic children. Thirdly, we summarize studies designed to identify aspects of brain structure and function underlying the neurobehavioral impairments found in schizophrenic children. Finally, we attempt to integrate cross-sectional and longitudinal analyses of the nature and evolution of neuro-behavioral impairments in schizophrenic children within a neurodevelopmental framework.

The children included in the studies reviewed here had an onset of schizophrenic psychosis prior to 13 years of age (there is some overlap among the subjects included in the various UCLA studies). Only children who obtained DSM-III (American Psychiatric Association, 1980) or DSM-III-R (APA, 1987) diagnoses of schizophrenia were included in these studies.

Precursors of psychotic symptoms in schizophrenic children

To identify the precursors of psychotic symptoms in schizophrenic children, we employed a follow-back design similar to that used in studies of adult schizophrenia (Watt & Lubensky, 1976), and examined early records of a group of children who subsequently developed schizophrenia (Watkins et al., 1988). The design provided a means of rating behavior and the presence of psychiatric symptoms using multiple, contemporaneous accounts of each child's behavior, medical status, and school performance in each age range.

A symptom rating database was developed by obtaining copies of records from all hospitals, clinics, schools, mental health professionals, physicians, and other relevant professionals seen by the children prior to their referral to UCLA. Two rating scales were used to characterize the children: a DSM-III Symptom Rating Scale and the Achenbach Child Behavior Checklist (CBCL; Achenbach & Edelbrock, 1983). The DSM-III Symptom Rating Scale was used to rate each symptom of schizophrenia, schizotypal personality disorder, pervasive developmental disorder, and infantile autism included in DSM-III. The CBCL provided broad coverage of behavioral problems, associated with a wide variety of childhood psychiatric disturbances, that were not covered by the Symptom Rating Scale. Symptoms were rated at four age ranges: 0 to 30 months, 31 months to 5 years 11 months, 6 years to 8 years 11 months, and 9 years to 11 years 11 months.

The majority of the schizophrenic children had significant developmental delays beginning in infancy. No language prior to 30 months or gross deficits in language development were reported in 72% of the children. However, the frequency of language deficits decreased gradually across the four age ranges. Problems in motor development were also noted in the records, including delays in reaching milestones and poor coordination in 72% and hypotonia in 28% of the children. Fig. 7.1 summarizes the neurobehavioral impairments most frequently observed in each of the four age ranges.

There appeared to be two somewhat different patterns of symptom development prior to the onset of psychotic symptoms in these children. The children with the most severe language problems had a number of autistic-like symptoms, including peculiar speech, pervasive lack of social responsiveness, and self-mutilation. The other children tended to have less severe language problems and no autistic-like symptoms.

The children with the more severe language problems and autistic-like symptoms generally manifested schizophrenic psychotic symptoms during the 6- to 8-year range, one age range earlier than the remaining children. During this age range, schizophrenic symptoms in 71% of this subgroup consisted primarily of incoherence, loosening of associations, and other symptoms of formal thought disorder (FTD), and flat or inappropriate affect. Only two children showed diagnostically significant delusions or hallucinations during this period. By the 9- to 11-year age range, however, 71% of the children had developed diagnostically significant delusions and hallucinations in addition to FTD and flat or inappropriate affect. Differences in symptomatology between

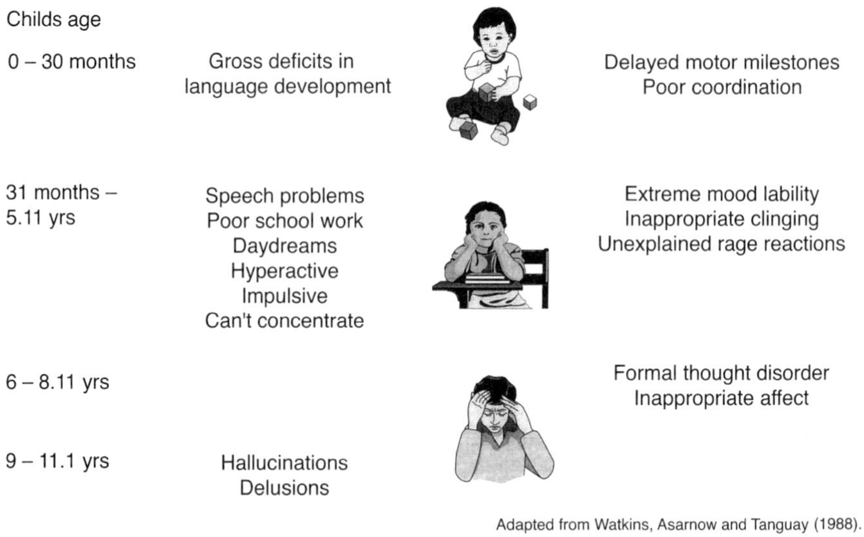

Childs age

0 – 30 months   Gross deficits in   Delayed motor milestones
                 language development   Poor coordination

31 months –   Speech problems   Extreme mood lability
5.11 yrs   Poor school work   Inappropriate clinging
                 Daydreams   Unexplained rage reactions
                 Hyperactive
                 Impulsive
                 Can't concentrate

6 – 8.11 yrs   Formal thought disorder
                                                            Inappropriate affect

9 – 11.1 yrs   Hallucinations
                 Delusions

Adapted from Watkins, Asarnow and Tanguay (1988).

Fig. 7.1. Sequence of symptom development in childhood-onset schizophrenia.

children with and without autistic-like symptoms faded with age as rates of hallucinations and delusions increased in both groups during the 9- to 11-year age range.

The other group, schizophrenic children *without* autistic-like symptoms, showed a relatively chronic gradual worsening of symptoms. While less disturbed during infancy than children with autistic-like symptoms, the majority of these children also had significant developmental delays beginning in infancy. Most of the children without early histories of autistic-like symptoms first manifested schizophrenic psychotic symptoms during the 9- to 11-year age range. However, during the age range immediately preceding the onset of psychotic symptoms, 82% of the children were rated as *both* socially impaired and presented with at least one of the following potential prodromata of schizophrenia identified in prior research: excessive anxiety and panic, constricted or inappropriate affect, magical thinking, suspiciousness, undue social anxiety and hypersensitivity to criticism. Interestingly, given data suggesting that depressive symptoms in adult schizophrenic patients are associated with more positive outcomes, schizophrenic children *without* autistic-like symptoms showed higher rates of depressive symptoms on the CBCL at the time of the onset of the schizophrenic episode than children *with* autistic-like symptoms.

Prior to the onset of psychotic symptoms, symptoms associated with the Hyperactive factor of the CBCL were observed in over 50% of the children in both groups. The items on this factor include: "hyperactive", "speech problems", "clumsy", "acts too young for age", "poor school work", "daydreams", "can't concentrate", "impulsive", and "confused".

These data indicate that there was a gradual, developmental unfolding of a broad spectrum of symptoms affecting social, cognitive, sensory, and motor functioning in these schizophrenic children. The symptoms usually began in infancy, many years before the appearance of schizophrenic symptoms. Overall, there were far more severe symptoms and far greater social impairment prior to the onset of schizophrenia in these children than is seen in the childhood histories of adult-onset schizophrenics.

Additional support for the view that impairments can be identified in schizophrenic children prior to the onset of the first schizophrenic episode is provided by follow-back analyses conducted by J.R. Asarnow and colleagues (Asarnow & Ben-Meir, 1988; Asarnow et al., 1994b). Using a sample of schizophrenic children who had been psychiatric inpatients (a small subset of whom were also in the Watkins et al. (1988) sample), J.R. Asarnow and colleagues (1994a) found that schizophrenic children were most likely to present with insidious, as opposed to acute, onset. Only 1 of the 21 schizophrenic children (5%) in their sample presented with an acute onset. When compared to a group of child psychiatric inpatients with major depression, schizophrenic children showed significantly poorer overall premorbid adjustment, as well as significantly poorer premorbid functioning in peer relationships, scholastic performance, school adaptation, and interests. However, schizophrenic children showed variability in the level of their premorbid adjustment, with the subgroup of children with depressive symptoms tending to show higher levels of premorbid adjustment.

Convergent findings have emerged from studies of childhood-onset schizophrenia at the National Institutes of Mental Health (NIMH). Parental reports at initial assessment and review of early records of the schizophrenic children studied by the NIMH group revealed that 60% of the subjects met criteria for previous developmental disorders of language and/or speech, and that 34% had shown early transient symptoms of pervasive developmental disorders, such as hand flapping and echolalia (Jacobsen & Rapoport, 1998).

Studies of cognitive/neuropsychological functioning

In this section, we will review studies of various aspects of cognition in schizophrenic children. Cognition refers to the active perception, translation, rehearsal, storage, and retrieval of information, and higher-order processes in which a broader context influences the processing of specific information.

Cognition encompasses attention, perception, memory, language, and think-ing. Over the last decade, information processing models have been increasing-ly used to provide a unifying framework for the study of diverse aspects of cognition. These models emphasize the structures and processes by which individuals register, encode, select, maintain, transform, store, and retrieve information. Early information processing models emphasized the role of structural limitations on cognitive functions. In contrast, modern information processing models acknowledge the role of processing resources (capacity) in setting limits on the information processing that can be carried out in a fixed unit of time. Processing resources are broadly conceptualized as the limited fuels, processes, and skills that are available at a given moment to enable performance of cognitive tasks (Hirst & Kalmar, 1987). The findings of the following studies are consistent with the hypothesis that schizophrenic children have limitations in the availability or allocation of their resources, which impair their ability to perform well on a wide range of cognitive tasks.

Schizophrenic children, like schizophrenic adults, typically suffer from a mild, generalized cognitive impairment. This impairment is reflected in the somewhat lower scores they obtain on tests of general intellectual functioning. For example, the average Full Scale IQ of schizophrenic children in two recent studies was 81 (Spencer & Campbell, 1994) and 87 (Asarnow et al., 1994a), compared to an average score of 100 in the general population. It is thought that superimposed upon this mild generalized deficit is a more severe deficit in some *specific* aspect of cognition.

The presence of a relatively specific deficit (i.e., impaired performance in certain functions and *relatively* better performance in others) in schizophrenia is vividly illustrated by a comparison (Asarnow et al., 1987) of the performance of non-retarded autistic and schizophrenic children on the Wechsler Intelligence Scale for Children – Revised (WISC-R), a standardized measure of intellectual functioning (Wechsler, 1974). Children's performance on the WISC-R can be summarized by three independent factors that have been consistently found to account for most of the variance on this test. These factors are called "Verbal Comprehension", "Perceptual Organization", and "Distractibility" (Kaufman, 1979; Sattler, 1974). In the Asarnow et al. (1987) study, the average Full Scale IQs of the schizophrenic and autistic children were within the low average range and similar to each other. The groups differed dramatically, however, in the pattern of their factor scores.

Fig. 7.2 summarizes the performance of the two groups across individual subtest scores (expressed as standard scores) grouped according to their loading on the three factors. The autistic and schizophrenic children scored in the low

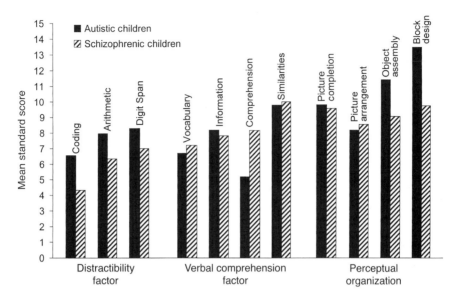

Fig. 7.2. Mean WISC-R subtest standard scores for non-retarded autistic and schizophrenic children. Reprinted with permission from the *Journal of Child Psychology and Psychiatry* (1987), **28**, 273–80. Copyright 1987, Association for Child Psychology and Psychiatry.

average range and did not differ significantly from each other on the Verbal Comprehension and Perceptual Organization factors. However, the schizophrenic children had significantly lower scores than the autistic children on the Distractibility factor. The mean score of the schizophrenic children on this factor was more than 1 standard deviation below the mean of the standardization sample, and more importantly, significantly lower than the scores they obtained on the Verbal Comprehension and Perceptual Organization factors. Although there is dispute over the precise meaning of the Distractibility factor, the subtests included in this factor (Arithmetic, Coding, and Digit Span) make extensive demands on controlled attentional processes because of their requirements for working memory, attention, and speed of responding (Sattler, 1974). The impairment on this factor appears to be relatively specific, as the schizophrenic children performed within the low average range on tasks tapping overlearned abilities (e.g., those tapped by the Verbal Comprehension factor).

Attention

Slow reaction time (RT) is one of the most consistently observed neurobehavioral characteristics of schizophrenic patients. Although a slow RT is diagnostically non-specific, the failure of schizophrenic patients to benefit from regularity (predictability) in the interval between the warning signal and the RT stimulus differentiates them from patients with other psychiatric disorders (Nuechterlein, 1977; Rist & Cohen, 1991). Many studies have shown a "cross-over" pattern in schizophrenic patients: at longer preparatory intervals (greater than 4 s) their RTs are slower under regular than under irregular conditions, whereas control subjects show the opposite pattern. This failure to benefit from regularity in the preparatory interval reflects an inability to maintain readiness to respond for more than a few seconds.

In a study of childhood onset schizophrenia at NIMH, Zahn et al. (1998) studied simple RT in schizophrenic and normal control children. Simple RT to tones with regular and irregular preparatory intervals of 2, 4, and 8 seconds was examined. Compared to controls, schizophrenic children had much slower RTs and a larger difference in overall RT between the regular and irregular series (RTs were significantly longer in the irregular than in the regular series). In addition, schizophrenic children had a larger increase in regular series RT than controls as the duration of the preparatory interval increased. "In general, the patients were well within the range of values for RT level and [preparatory interval] effects reported in previous studies on adults" (p. 101). Zahn et al. concluded that the performance of the children on the simple RT tasks was suggestive of a difficulty in sustaining attention.

In a second experiment, Zahn et al. (1998) measured RTs to lights and tones under three conditions defined by whether the warning and RT stimuli were in the same (ipsi-modal) or different (cross-modal) sensory modalities. The conditions were: (i) regular, in which all the stimuli were lights or all were tones; (ii) choice RT, in which the two types of stimuli were presented randomly, but were responded to with different hands; and (iii) cross-modal RT, in which the two types of stimuli were presented randomly, and each was responded to with the same, preferred hand. "The [cross-modal] condition differs from the regular condition in that there is stimulus uncertainty, whereas the choice condition additionally requires response selection" (p. 102). In studies of adults with schizophrenia, there is greater retardation in RT on cross-modal compared with ipsi-modal trials (Rist & Cohen, 1991; Sutton et al., 1961). Zahn et al. found that schizophrenic children showed a greater slowing than normal controls in the choice RT condition compared with the regular condition. The schizophrenic children did not show a greater deficit in the cross-modal condition overall, but did so only when the stimulus was a light. Zahn et al. interpret the differential effect of choice RT on schizophrenic children as supporting the hypothesis that "impairment in schizophrenia is greater as a function of the number of operations required for a response" (p. 104).

Children with schizophrenia were much slower than normal controls in

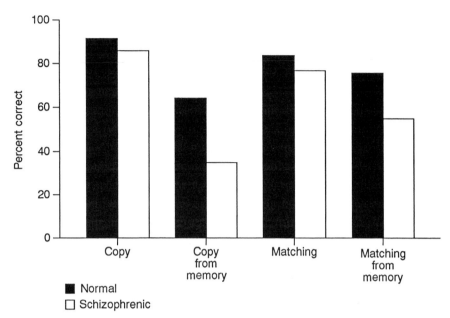

Fig. 7.3. Visual retention test and visual form discrimination test: mean scores for schizophrenic and normal control children when subjects copy or discriminate between designs in conditions with and without memory demands. Reprinted from *Schizophrenia Bulletin* (1994), **20**, 647–69.

both the simple and cross-modal RT paradigms. In general, Zahn et al.'s findings indicate that schizophrenic children show some of the same attentional dysfunctions as schizophrenic adults.

Perception

As noted above, schizophrenic children obtained low average scores on the WISC-R Perceptual Organization factor (Asarnow et al., 1987). The subtests included in this factor require subjects to arrange pictures similar to comic strip panels to make stories (Picture Arrangement), to identify missing parts in pictures of familiar objects (Picture Completion), to arrange the pieces of puzzles to create familiar objects (Object Assembly), and to arrange blocks to reproduce pictures of designs (Block Design). Schizophrenic children also performed within normal limits (Schneider & Asarnow, 1987) on the Benton Judgment of Line Orientation Task (Benton et al., 1975), which requires subjects to discriminate among lines differing in angular orientation.

In a recent study, we (Asarnow et al., 1994a) examined a circumscribed aspect of visual perception, form discrimination ability, using two other tasks developed by Benton. The first task, the Visual Retention Test (Benton, 1974) assesses form discrimination by requiring subjects to copy designs presented to them in a booklet. The second task, the Visual Form Discrimination Test (Benton et al., 1977), assesses form discrimination by means of a multiple choice format, which makes much fewer demands on graphomotor functions than does the Visual Retention Test. On the Visual Form Discrimination Test, subjects are required to select from four comparison designs the one that matches a sample design placed above. As can be seen in Fig. 7.3, schizophrenic and mental age-matched normal children did not differ in their ability to reproduce designs (Visual Retention Test) or to discriminate among simultaneously presented designs (Visual Form Discrimination Test).

Working memory

Memory demands were added to both Benton tasks in another condition of the study described by Asarnow et al. (1994a). On the Visual Retention Test, a 15-second delay was interposed between the presentation of the design and the point at which subjects were allowed to begin drawing the design. On the Visual Form Discrimination Test, the sample design was removed after a 10-second presentation, and subjects matched the comparison stimuli to their memory of the sample design. Thus, both tests required subjects to hold the sample stimulus in short-term memory before responding. As inspection of Fig. 7.3 reveals, schizophrenic children performed significantly worse than matched normal controls on both tests.

As noted previously, schizophrenic children also obtained scores on the WISC-R Digit Span (a measure of short-term verbal memory) that were significantly lower than scores obtained by subjects in the standardization sample of the WISC-R (Asarnow et al., 1987). More importantly, the scores of the schizophrenic children on Digit Span were significantly lower than their scores on the Verbal Comprehension factor of the WISC-R.

In a more recent study, we (Karatekin & Asarnow, 1998b) examined working memory in schizophrenic, ADHD, and age-matched normal children within the theoretical framework developed by Baddeley (e.g., 1996). According to Baddeley, working memory is a limited-capacity system that stores information for brief periods of time. It is thought to underlie a wide range of cognitive processes, from remembering a phone number for a few seconds to planning, learning, reasoning, and comprehension. Baddeley divides working memory into limited-capacity "sensory buffers" (which are responsible for maintaining verbal, spatial or visual information in memory for a few seconds at a time) and a "central executive" that provides strategic attentional control of the operation of the buffers and coordinates their activities. We measured verbal working memory on the Digit Span task. We assessed spatial working memory by presenting the children with a single dot on a page and asking them to remember the location of the dot 0 or 30 seconds later (Keefe et al., 1995). Both clinical groups showed verbal and spatial working memory deficits and did not differ on any measure. These results suggest that the capacity of the buffers holding verbal and spatial information is diminished in both disorders. However, as both types of working memory depend on the central executive, results can also be interpreted as indicating that both schizophrenic and ADHD children have limitations in the availability or allocation of central executive resources.

Language

As noted above, schizophrenic children scored within the low average range on the WISC-R Verbal Comprehension factor, which includes the Information, Similarities, Vocabulary, and Comprehension subtests (Asarnow et al., 1987). Schizophrenic children also scored (Asarnow et al., 1994a; Schneider & Asarnow, 1987) within the low average range on the Peabody Picture Vocabulary Test – Revised, a measure of receptive vocabulary (Dunn & Dunn, 1981).

However, schizophrenic children did show impairments on two other tasks that require the processing of auditory stimuli (Asarnow et al., 1994a). The first task, the Token Test from the Multilingual Aphasia Examination (Benton & Hamsher, 1989), screens for receptive aphasia by requiring subjects to follow oral instructions of increasing complexity (e.g., "touch the red square, then the yellow circle"). Schizophrenic children made significantly more errors than normal controls on this test. They had particular difficulty understanding complex grammatical transpositions or instructions that involved carrying out sequences of behavior involving multiple steps. Schizophrenic children also performed significantly worse than normal controls on the Seashore Rhythm Test (Seashore et al., 1960). This test measures the processing of non-linguistic, auditory stimuli by requiring subjects to reproduce (by tapping on a table) rhythms that are presented aurally.

The pattern of performance of the schizophrenic children on the Token and Seashore Rhythm Tests does not indicate central impairments in the primary processing of auditory stimuli. Rather, it appears that the errors made by schizophrenic children on these two tasks (one using linguistic and the other nonlinguistic stimuli) reflect impairments in attention and/or working memory, since the tasks require subjects to sustain attention and to remember sequences of verbal instructions (Token Test), or to reproduce sequences of nonverbal auditory stimuli (Seashore Rhythm Test).

Executive functions

One interesting executive function is guided visual search. Rey's Tangled Lines Test measures this function by requiring subjects to visually track a series of tangled lines that cross and overlap at multiple points (Rey, 1964). This test also makes demands on sustained attention and visual–motor coordination. We found that schizophrenic children showed a tendency to perform more slowly and to make more errors on Rey's Tangled Lines Test than normal children, matched on mental and chronological age (Schneider & Asarnow, 1987).

Numerous studies (e.g., Goldberg et al., 1987; Van der Does & Van den Bosch, 1992) have found that schizophrenic adults show deficits on the Wisconsin Card Sorting Test (WCST; Heaton, 1985). The WCST requires subjects to sort cards (which contain figures that differ in number, form, and color) according to sorting principles they have to discover on their own. This task makes extensive demands on verbal mediation and ability to engage in temporally extended problem solving. We administered the WCST to schizophrenic, autistic, and normal children (Schneider & Asarnow, 1987). Like schizophrenic adults, schizophrenic children made significantly more perseverative responses (sorts made according to a principle that is no longer correct or one that consistently leads to an incorrect response) than did normal subjects.

To isolate the cognitive impairments underlying the performance of the schizophrenic children on the WCST, subjects were explicitly taught the appropriate sorting principles halfway through this task (Schneider & Asarnow, 1987). Previous studies (e.g., Koh, 1978) had indicated that, when schizophrenic adults are taught the appropriate strategy, their performance can be normalized on certain memory tasks. However, the schizophrenic children in the Schneider and Asarnow study showed an *increased* number of nonperseverative errors (random responding) from the first to the second half of the WCST, whereas autistic and normal children showed no change (see Fig. 7.4). Thus, teaching schizophrenic children the relevant sorting principles led to a significant deterioration, *not a facilitation*, of their performance. Stuss et al. (1983) also found that a similar manipulation had a deleterious effect on the WCST performance of chronic schizophrenics with prefrontal leukotomies. In addition, K.M. Pueschel (1980, unpublished data) observed that providing verbal directions to schizophrenic adults impaired their performance on a hypothesis-testing task. These findings are reminiscent of Rodnick and Shakow's (1940) and Steffy's (1978) RT studies, which showed that providing relevant information to schizophrenic adults sometimes impaired their performance. The relevant information provided during the second half of the WCST in the Schneider and Asarnow study requires the momentary integration of informa-

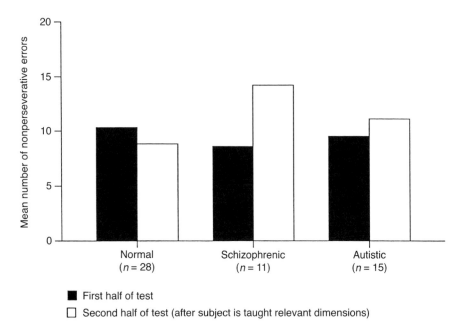

First half of test

Second half of test (after subject is taught relevant dimensions)

Fig. 7.4. Wisconsin Card Sorting Test: Mean number of non-perseverative errors made by schizophrenic, autistic and normal children before and after children were taught the relevant dimensions. Reprinted from *Schizophrenia Bulletin* (1994), **20**, 647–69.

tion from a variety of sources to direct an ongoing activity. Hence, providing task relevant information to the schizophrenic children, whose processing capacity may already be taxed, resulted in the seemingly paradoxical effect of further impairing their performance.

Visual information processing

The studies reviewed thus far suggest that simple perceptual functions and rote language skills are not impaired in schizophrenic children. In contrast, they perform poorly on tasks that place extensive demands on attention, working memory, and executive functions. Tasks like the WCST tap multiple cognitive processes. Which of these processes are responsible for the impaired performance shown by schizophrenic children on the broad range of cognitive/ neuropsychological tasks we have summarized? To isolate the cognitive processes impaired in these children, we conducted a series of studies of visual attention.

The first three experiments were aimed at determining which of the multiple cognitive processes tapped by the forced-choice Span of Apprehension task is impaired in children with schizophrenia (Asarnow & Sherman, 1984). The Span of Apprehension task was developed by Estes and Taylor (1964) to provide an index of the rate of visual information processing. This task detects dysfunction not only in actively psychotic schizophrenic patients but also in individuals vulnerable to schizophrenia, including schizophrenic adults in clinical remission and unaffected first-degree relatives of schizophrenic probands (for review see Asarnow et al., 1991).

In Experiment I, schizophrenic children, mental age-matched normal children, and younger normal children were administered the same Span of Apprehension task used in studies of adult schizophrenics and their relatives. Subjects were told that either a *T* or an *F* would be flashed briefly (for 50 milliseconds) on a backward projection screen along with other letters. They were instructed to report after each trial which of the two target letters had been presented. The target stimulus was embedded in arrays containing 0, 2, 4 or 9 *non-target* letters. Subjects received four scores, which represented the number of correct detections of the target stimuli for each array size. Schizophrenic and younger normal children obtained significantly lower scores than mental age-matched normal children on the 5- and 10-letter arrays of the Span task but not on the 1- or 3-letter arrays.

The results of Experiment I suggested that all three groups of subjects were engaged in serial search while performing the partial-report Span task. Serial search demands focal attention; it involves directing attention "serially to different locations, to integrate the features registered within the same spatio-temporal spotlight into a unitary percept" (Treisman & Gelade, 1980, p. 134). Because it requires mental effort, serial search makes extensive demands on processing resources. One of the defining characteristics of a serial mode of processing is that there is an incremental cost (in the form of increased RT or errors) when subjects are required to detect targets in arrays containing increasing numbers of distractors. This is exactly what happened on the Estes and Taylor Span of Apprehension task in Experiment I. As the number of distractors increased from 0 to 2 to 4 to 9, target detection rates decreased in all groups (see Fig. 7.5). The fact that the schizophrenic and the younger normal children showed a greater "cost" with increased number of distractors than did the mental age-matched normal children suggests that their serial search was either initiated more slowly or employed less efficiently than that of the older normal group.

A convergent result emerged from Experiment II. The subjects' search strategy was studied in this experiment by modifying the stimulus matrix so that each target stimulus appeared eight times in each quadrant of the screen. Both schizophrenic and mental age-matched normal children showed a significantly greater probability of correctly detecting the target when it was in the

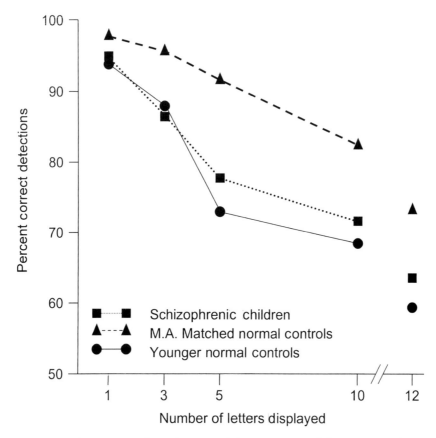

Fig. 7.5. Partial report span of apprehension task from Asarnow and Sherman (1984) from *Child Development*.

upper quadrants than when it was in the lower quadrants. This result suggests that both the schizophrenic and older normal children consistently began their serial search in the upper quadrants, and that their iconic image of the stimulus display faded before they could adequately process the lower quadrants.

In Experiment III, subjects were administered the full-report version of the Span of Apprehension task, which required them to report as many letters as they could from the display. Compared to the partial-report Span task, the full-report task makes greater demands on iconic memory (a large capacity visual memory store that holds information for 200–400 milliseconds) and immediate memory, but fewer demands on serial search and processing resources. Schizophrenic children were able to report as many letters as mental age-matched normal children on the full-report task, suggesting that impairments on the partial report version are not attributable to a deficiency in iconic memory.

In a follow-up study, we tested whether the impairment of schizophrenic children on the partial-report Span task is due to a delay in initiation of search or to a slow rate of serial search (Karatekin & Asarnow, 1998a). These hypotheses were tested within the framework of a Treisman's feature integration theory, which provides a model for the role of attention in visual search. We administered subjects two search tasks from Treisman and Souther (1985) that use the same stimuli but differ in their attentional requirements. According to feature integration theory, one task requires attention to be distributed over the whole display (parallel search), whereas the other requires attention to be focused (serial search). This distinction has been supported by behavioral, electrophysiological, and other neurobiological evidence (e.g., Luck and Hillyard 1990). To estimate rate of search, we recorded items searched per unit time. To estimate the duration of initiation of search, we took advantage of the fact that the basic oculomotor system is intact in schizophrenia and recorded time to make the first saccade on each trial. If schizophrenic children were slow to initiate their search, they should also be slow to start making a saccade. To test the specificity of findings, we compared schizophrenic children to age-matched children with Attention-Deficit/Hyperactivity Disorder (ADHD) and to chronological age-matched normal children. Results showed (i) delayed initiation of search in ADHD, but not in schizophrenic children; and (ii) a clear dissociation between intact parallel search rates and slowed serial search rates in both clinical groups. These results narrowed down the source of the search impairment in schizophrenia to a slow rate of serial search.

Next, we investigated deployment of visual attention under less constrained conditions in the same children by recording their eye movements to thematic pictures (Karatekin and Asarnow, 1998a). For each picture, the children were asked three questions varying in amount of structure. We determined if schizophrenic children would stare or scan too extensively and if their scan patterns would be differentially affected by the questions. The key measures were time spent viewing relevant and irrelevant regions, fixation duration, and distance between fixations. ADHD children had slightly shorter fixations than normal children on the question requiring the most detailed analysis (e.g., "how old is each person?"), suggesting that they had difficulty sustaining focused attention even over a few hundred milliseconds. Schizophrenic children looked at fewer relevant, but not more irrelevant, regions than normal children on all questions. They tended to stare more (i.e., fixate longer and traverse a shorter distance), but only on the least constrained question ("what is happening in this picture?"). The parameters of their eye movements were normalized on questions directing their attention to specific regions. Finally, the three groups did not differ in terms of which region they looked at first, indicating that they were all able to comprehend the gist of the pictures fairly rapidly.

These studies of visual information processing converge on the conclusion that the basic mechanisms controlling parameters of eye movements are intact in schizophrenic children. Initial stages of their search were also intact in the two studies of eye movements. They appeared to engage in the same processes as normal children when searching for externally provided targets. They were not unduly distracted by irrelevant details. In contrast, they appeared to suffer from limitations in cognitive resources necessary for higher levels of visual processing, which may have slowed their rate of serial search. They may have also narrowed their attention excessively when engaged in cognitively effortful or self-guided search. Finally, they had difficulty testing hypotheses about thematic scenes under unconstrained conditions, which suggests that they have an impairment in the top-down, self-guided control of visual attention.

Link of cognitive impairments to formal thought disorder (FTD) and discourse skills

FTD is a set of clinical signs (e.g., illogical thinking, loose associations and incoherence) that captures how a patient presents his/her thoughts to a listener and is one of the hallmarks of schizophrenia. Of the few studies that have examined FTD in schizophrenic children (e.g., Cantor et al., 1982; Kolvin et al., 1971), only two have used reliable and valid instruments that take into account the normal development of cognitive skills tapped by FTD (Arboleda & Holzman, 1985; Caplan et al., 1989). The importance of examining FTD from a developmental perspective is underscored by Caplan et al.'s (1989) finding that illogical thinking occurred more frequently in normal children under age 7 than in normal children older than age 7, and that a significant proportion of *normal* children under age 7 showed levels of illogical thinking comparable to those of schizophrenic children. In contrast, incoherence and poverty of content of speech, two other signs of FTD, were not found in younger normal children. Incoherence occurred infrequently in schizophrenic children as well; this FTD sign is also rare in adult schizophrenic patients (Andreasen & Olsen, 1982). The presence of poverty of content of speech is a consistent finding in schizophrenic adults (Andreasen & Grove, 1986), but not in schizophrenic children. The low base rate of poverty of content of speech in schizophrenic children could reflect developmental factors. Latency-age children use non-discursive and unelaborated speech. It is possible that children must be competent users of discursive speech for a reliable rating of poverty of content to be made (Caplan et al., 1989).

To present the listener with coherent information, a speaker needs to use linguistic devices such as cohesion and reference patterns to tie together his or her clauses (Halliday & Hasan, 1976). These linguistic devices enable the listener to follow who and what the speaker is referring to and how what the speaker says relates to what was said previously. Caplan et al. (1992) used Halliday and Hasan's analysis of cohesion to compare schizophrenic children to mental age-matched normal subjects. Findings showed that schizophrenic children, like schizophrenic adults, spoke less than normal controls and did not provide the listener with enough links to previous utterances (cohesive ties) or references to people, objects, or events mentioned in earlier utterances (referential cohesion). Schizophrenic children also broke the flow of the conversation by referring to people, objects or events in their immediate surrounding and by not focusing on the ongoing conversation (exophora). Like adult schizophrenics with thought disorder (Rochester & Martin, 1979), schizophrenic children with loose associations confused the listener by the unclear and ambiguous ways they referred to people, objects, and events (unclear/ambiguous reference).

Schizophrenic children had three discourse deficits that distinguished their speech from that of schizophrenic adults (Caplan et al., 1992). These children provided the listener with fewer connectives between contiguous clauses (conjunction) and with less repetition of words or word roots (lexical cohesion) than normal children. They also appeared to omit part of a previous clause on the presumption that the listener retained enough information from the clause (ellipsis). By using fewer conjunctions, less lexical cohesion and ellipsis than normal children, schizophrenic children made it difficult for the listener to piece together the parts of their speech.

Studies of the cognitive and discourse correlates of FTD provide a link between the cognitive impairments detected by certain cognitive/neuropsychological tasks and the clinical manifestations of schizophrenia. One such study (Caplan et al., 1990a,b) found that neither loose associations nor illogical thinking was correlated with WISC-R Full Scale IQ, indicating that these two signs of FTD are not simply reflecting a general intellectual deficit. Instead, loose associations were correlated with the WISC-R Distractibility and Verbal Comprehension factors. Illogical thinking, on the other hand, was not correlated with any of the WISC-R factors. Instead, illogical thinking, but not loose association, was related to impairments on the Span of Apprehension. Caplan et al. (1990a) hypothesized:

It is possible that the requirement to present the listener with logical reasoning taxes the schizophrenic child''s momentary processing capacity. In contrast, the child with loose associations unpredictably changes the topic of conversation without preparing the listener for the topic change. The cognitive demands of this situation could reflect distractibility more than reduced momentary processing capacity (p. 174).

Caplan and her colleagues also studied the conservation skills of schizophrenia-spectrum children because the ability to conserve heralds the achievement of abstract and logical thinking (Caplan et al., 1990b). Caplan et al. found that schizophrenic and schizotypal children were impaired in conserving continuous and discontinuous matter (e.g., knowing that, when a large glass of popcorn is distributed into smaller glasses, the quantity of the matter does not change) but not in conserving other measures (e.g., conserving two-dimensional space, number, substance). In addition, inability to conserve matter in tasks involving containers was related to illogical thinking, whereas inability to conserve matter in tasks that did not involve a container was related to both illogical thinking and loose associations. Caplan et al. hypothesized that tasks involving containers made greater demands on processing capacity by forcing the children to screen out extraneous information.

Taken together, Caplan's studies revealed that children with the greatest deficits in processing resources (as indexed by performance on the partial-report Span of Apprehension task) tended to show illogical thinking and conservation deficits, and to break the flow of conversation to refer to the immediate environment. *"What do these three measures have in common? Instead of screening out extraneous stimuli from the testing environment and focusing on the linguistic context of the conversation, children with schizophrenia who have exophoria break the flow of conversation to refer to stimuli in the testing situation or environment . . .. The requirement to present the listener with logical reasoning, to focus on the linguistic context of a conversation, and to detect the invariance of matter despite the change in the container all tap cognitive processes that make extensive demands on processing resources"* (Caplan, 1994, p. 680). The correlations among these three measures may reflect this common demand.

Studies of event-related potentials (ERPs)

Psychophysiological studies of the processes involved in the mobilization and allocation of processing resources are important complements to the behavioral studies reviewed in this chapter. Several decades of studies of mental chronometry using ERPs have yielded a lexicon of ERP components with fairly well-established neurocognitive correlates (Donchin et al., 1978; Hillyard &

Kutas, 1983). These components can be used to parse the sequence of neuro-cognitive events in such a way as to determine more precisely the nature of information processing deficits in schizophrenic children and adults. Asarnow et al. (1995) summarized a series of studies in which cognitive-behavioral tasks, such as the partial-report Span of Apprehension and the Continuous Perform-ance Test (CPT), were administered to schizophrenic children. The major dependent variables in these studies were the ERPs elicited by the tasks.

These ERP studies in schizophrenic children focused on four components: contingent negative variation (CNV), processing negativity (Np), a late positive component (P300), and hemispheric asymmetry in the amplitude of the P1/N1 component complex. The CNV provides a measure of orienting, preparation, and readiness to respond to an expected stimulus. The Np is a family of negative components that occur within the first 400 milliseconds after the onset of a stimulus. It indicates the degree to which attentional and perceptual resources have been allocated to stimulus processing. Because Np waves occur contemporaneously with other components (P1, N1 and P2), they can best be seen in difference potentials resulting from the subtraction of non-attend ERPs from attend ERPs (Hillyard & Hansen, 1986; Naatanen, 1982). The P300 is a frequently studied index of the recognition of stimulus significance in relation to task demands. In the case of tasks as complex as the Span, the P300 is seen between 400 and 500 milliseconds post stimulus. Finally, visual P1/N1 compo-nents are typically larger over the right than the left cerebral hemisphere in normal individuals. This lateralization during visual information processing tasks could reflect either differences between the hemispheres in the strategic utilization of processing capacity, or a lateralized neural deficit.

Table 7.1 summarizes, by component, the ERP results from four studies of schizophrenic children. All of the studies summarized in this table resulted in rather large and robust performance differences between groups in both the accuracy and reaction times of signal detection responses. Thus, the cognitive-behavioral paradigms were successful in eliciting information processing defi-cits in the patients. Of interest were the ERP differences associated with the deficits.

CNV differences between normal and schizophrenic subjects were not consistently found across the four studies. In contrast, Np was found to be smaller in schizophrenic than in normal children in every study summarized in Table 7.1 in which it was measured. This deficit was seen in schizophrenic children on both the Span of Apprehension (Strandburg et al., 1984, 1991) and the CPT (Strandburg et al., 1990, 1994b) tasks. A diminished Np amplitude was the earliest consistent ERP index of schizophrenic information processing

Table 7.1. Summary of evoked potential studies of schizophrenic children

Paper[a]	Task	CNV	Np	P300 amplitude	P1/N1 asymmetry
1984	Span	Norm > schiz	Norm > schiz[b]	Norm > schiz	Norm > schiz
1990	CPT[c]	Norm = schiz	—	Norm > schiz	Norm > schiz
1991	Span	Norm = schiz	Norm > schiz	Norm > schiz[d]	Norm > schiz
1994a	CPT	Norm = schiz	Norm > schiz	Norm > schiz	Norm > schiz

[a] Authors of all papers are Strandburg et al.

[b] Larger task-difficulty increase in N1 amplitude in normals than schizophrenics.

[c] Continuous Performance Test.

[d] Normals had larger P300 than schizophrenics for targets in the single-target CPT.

deficit to be observed in these studies. Both Michie et al. (1990) and Baribeau-Braun et al. (1983) have argued that Np amplitude reductions in schizophrenics reflect faulty allocation of processing resources.

Reduced amplitude P300 has been found in schizophrenic adults in many studies using a variety of experimental paradigms (for review see Pritchard, 1986). As can be seen in Table 7.1, a lower P300 amplitude was consistently observed in schizophrenic children on the Span of Apprehension and the CPT. Latency of the P300 component was also measured in two studies (results not shown in Table 7.1). Whereas one study found longer P300 latencies in schizophrenic than in normal children (Strandburg et al., 1994b), another study found no differences between normal and schizophrenic adults (Strandburg et al., 1994a). The majority of ERP studies have reported normal P300 latency in schizophrenic adults (Pritchard, 1986).

Absence of right lateralized P1/N1 amplitude in visual ERPs was a consistent finding in all four studies of schizophrenic children on the CPT and Span of Apprehension tasks. Abnormally lateralized electrophysiological responses, related either to a lateralized dysfunction in schizophrenics or to a pathology-related difference in information processing strategy, is a consistent aspect of childhood-onset schizophrenia.

Working hypothesis

Our survey of a broad range of neuropsychological functions and detailed studies of visual attention generally yielded converging results. The tasks that elicit impaired performance in schizophrenic children tap diverse computational functions across sensory modalities. A key characteristic of these tasks is that they make extensive demands on processing resources. Thus, the pattern of performance of schizophrenic children on these tasks is consistent with the hypothesis developed in earlier reviews of cognitive/neuropsychological studies of schizophrenic children (Asarnow et al., 1994a; Asarnow et al., 1986; Sherman & Asarnow, 1985) and adults (Nuechterlein & Dawson, 1984) that schizophrenic individuals have subtle limitations in processing capacity.

It is important to recognize the inter-relationships among processing resources, speed of responding, attention, working memory, and executive processes (Asarnow et al., 1994a; Karatekin & Asarnow, 1998b). All of these refer to constructs that cut across discrete computational functions, enable the efficient processing of information, and depend on each other for optimum efficiency. Research is now needed to tease apart the overlap in the definitions of these constructs and to characterize the contribution of each factor to the pattern of impairments observed in schizophrenia.

Neurobiology

Neuroanatomy

A pioneering investigation by Frazier and colleagues (1996) at the NIMH Child Psychiatry Branch provides intriguing hints at what may be the neurobiological substrate for the pattern of neuropsychological impairments observed in children with schizophrenia. Frazier et al. compared brain MRIs of 21 schizophrenic children (mean age = 14.6 years) and 33 age-, sex-, height, and weight-matched normal children. All of the schizophrenic children met DSM-III-R criteria for schizophrenia and had their onset of psychotic symptoms before age 12 and had responded poorly to treatment with typical neuroleptic medications. Quantitative measurements were obtained for the cerebrum, the anterior frontal region, lateral ventricles, thalamus, caudate, putamen, and globus pallidus. Frazier et al. (1996) found that the total cerebral volume of schizophrenic children was 9.2% smaller than that of normal controls. The midsagittal thalamic area was also smaller in schizophrenic children than in controls. The caudate, putamen, and globus pallidus were larger in schizophrenic children than in controls, and the lateral ventricles tended to be larger in schizophrenic children than in controls. Globus pallidus enlargement was correlated with neuroleptic exposure and age at onset of psychosis. This pattern of findings has been frequently observed in adults with schizophrenia. These data provide compelling evidence of neurobiological continuity between childhood- and adult-onset schizophrenia. Furthermore, a comparison with a sample of males with ADHD and matched controls examined with identical procedures (Castellanos et al., 1994, 1996) suggests that these findings do not merely reflect a nonspecific pattern for children with neurobehavioral impairments. Children with ADHD did not share the pattern of abnormalities observed in children with schizophrenia.

Sixteen of the schizophrenic children in the Frazier et al. (1996) study were rescanned 2 years later (Rapoport et al., 1997). There was a significant increase in ventricular volume (by an average of 19%) and a significant decrease in midsagittal thalamic area (by 6%) in schizophrenic children during this period, whereas normal children did not show a comparable deterioration. The schizophrenic children with the greatest progressive increase in ventricular volume had the lowest levels of premorbid adjustment (e.g., delays in motor and language delays, early transient autistic features) and the highest levels of clinical symptoms at follow-up (assessed on the Brief Psychiatric Rating Scale; Overall & Gorham, 1961).

Neurotransmitters

For decades, theories of the biochemical basis of schizophrenia and the mechanism of action of antipsychotic drugs have focused on the role of dopamine. "The original dopamine hypothesis of schizophrenia was characterized by increased dopamine function. This hypothesis was based primarily on the correlation between the ability of neuroleptics to displace dopamine antagonists in vitro and their clinical potency" (Kahn & Davis, 1995, p. 1193). Over the past decade, the dopamine hypothesis has been re-examined and revised. A primary impetus for the re-examination was the recognition that certain core symptoms of schizophrenia – negative symptoms and cognitive deficits – are far less responsive to treatment with dopamine agonists than are positive psychotic symptoms. In addition, when dopamine agonists such as amphetamine are administered to non-psychiatric control subjects, they produce positive schizophrenic symptoms (e.g., hallucinations) but not the FTD usually associated with schizophrenia (Kahn & Davis, 1995). This finding suggests that some of the core symptoms of schizophrenia might be unrelated to increased dopamine activity. Recently, a number of investigators have suggested that schizophrenia is characterized not by a simple abnormality of the dopamine system, but rather by abnormal interactions among multiple monoaminergic systems, particularly between the serotonin and dopamine systems (Kahn & Davis, 1995).

Other investigators have proposed a central role for an excitatory neurotransmitter, the amino acid glutamate, in schizophrenia. Bunney et al. (1995) reported that compounds that block the glutamate receptor, such as phencyclidine (PCP), produce both positive and negative schizophrenic symptoms in normal individuals. Kim et al. (1980) postulated a deficiency in glutamatergic function and an increase in dopamine function, and suggested that dopamine interacts with glutamate to inhibit glutamatergic action in schizophrenia.

Remarkably few studies have examined neurotransmitters in children and adolescents with schizophrenia. The first study to examine monoamine metabolites in cerebrospinal fluid (CSF) in childhood onset schizophrenia was carried out by investigators from the Child Psychiatry Branch at NIMH. Jacobsen and colleagues (1997) examined 18 patients (mean age = 14.2 years) with an onset of schizophrenia before age 12. The children were treated with haloperidol or clozapine. CSF homovanillic acid (HVA), 5-hydroxyindoleacteic acid (5HIAA), and 3-methoxy-4-hydroxyphenylglycol (MHPG), and serum prolactin were measured during drug-free and antipsychotic medication conditions. "Studies of monoamine metabolites in later-onset schizophrenia have revealed that treatment response is associated with biphasic changes in CSF HVA following initiation of treatment with typical neuroleptics" (Jacobsen et al., 1997, p. 69). The NIMH group tested the hypothesis of continuity between childhood- and later-onset schizophrenia by simultaneously analyzing CSF from a sample of patients with adult-onset schizophrenia to permit a direct comparison of metabolite levels between these groups. Findings showed that concentrations of HVA, 5-HIAA, and MHPG did not differ significantly between drug-free and treatment conditions in schizophrenic children. There was a trend toward a significant correlation between reduction in HVA concentration after clozapine treatment and improvement in positive psychotic symptoms on the Scale for the Assessment of Positive Symptoms (Andreasen, 1984). In contrast, there was no correlation between changes in metabolic concentrations and clinical ratings after treatment with haloperidol. Patients with childhood and adult onset schizophrenia did not differ significantly in the change from drug-free to clozapine treatment in concentrations of HVA/5-HIAA and MHPG, or in ratios of HVA to 5-HIAA or HVA to MHPG. Although patients experienced significant clinical improvement with both haloperidol and clozapine, CSF monoamine metabolite concentrations and HVA/5-HIAA and HVA/MHPG ratios did not change significantly over six weeks of either haloperidol or clozapine treatment. These findings highlight the complexity of the biochemical events mediating significant clinical changes and the difficulty of studying the neurochemistry of this disorder.

The NIMH group concluded that the absence of significant differences between childhood and adult onset schizophrenic patients in the effects of clozapine on CSF monoamine metabolites suggests neurobiologic continuity between the childhood and adult onset forms of the disorder. However, because they were unable to obtain CSF samples from normal children, the NIMH group could not determine if the levels of monoamine metabolites observed in the schizophrenic children were abnormal.

At UCLA, we have used magnetic resonance spectroscopy (MRS), a non-invasive neuroimaging technique, to measure the ratios of N-acetyl-aspartate (NAA) thought to measure the functional integrity of neurons, glutamate, and choline to creatine in schizophrenic children (Thomas et al., 1998). MRS spectra were measured in the frontal and occipital lobes of 12 children meeting DSM-III-R criteria for schizophrenia and 12 chronological age-matched healthy children. We hypothesized that differences in the metabolic ratios of schizophrenic and normal children would occur in the frontal but not the occipital lobes. Consistent with this prediction, the ratios of NAA, choline, and glutamate to creatine were reduced in the frontal lobes of schizophrenic children compared to controls. In contrast, there were no significant reductions in the metabolic ratios obtained from the occipital gray matter of schizophrenic children. Unfortunately, the overlap of glutamate and NAA peaks limited the precision of glutamate determination with standard techniques. In addition, we did not obtain estimates of the absolute concentration of metabolites. Nonetheless, the results of this study should stimulate further MRS investigations of protonated metabolites. The preliminary finding of decreased levels of cerebral glutamate in the frontal lobes of schizophrenic children is consistent with the glutamate hypothesis of schizophrenia.

In summary, the few studies that have examined neurotransmitters and brain metabolites in children with schizophrenia have tended to find the same abnormalities observed in adult-onset schizophrenia. Clearly, however, more research is needed in this area.

Neurodevelopmental model

Retrospective studies of the neurobehavioral antecedents of psychotic symptoms, cross-sectional studies of neurobehavioral functioning, FTD and communication impairments, and research on neurobiology in schizophrenic children provide some intriguing findings that can inform neurodevelopmental models of schizophrenia. Retrospective studies of neurobehavioral development in schizophrenic children indicate that they manifest certain neurobehavioral impairments well in advance of the first onset of psychotic symptoms. During infancy and early childhood, their language acquisition is slow and gross motor functioning is impaired. Somewhat later, they show impairments in fine motor coordination. These neurobehavioral impairments may be early manifestations of the brain lesions posited by neurodevelopmental models of schizophrenia. Expressive language and motor skills are subserved by structures in the frontal lobes. It is in these areas where many of the early brain lesions are also found (Weinberger, 1987).

If subtle neurobehavioral impairments reflect early damage to the frontal lobes, an interesting question arises: Why is there a delay in the production of psychotic symptoms? Is there some level of functional connectivity required between the frontal lobes and other parts of the brain, particularly the occipital and temporal lobes, to generate hallucinations? Presumably, that degree of functional connectivity is not required to support simple motor and language functions.

There is an interesting disparity between the results of our detailed cross-sectional neurobehavioral assessments and the results of retrospective studies of neurobehavioral development prior to the onset of psychotic symptoms. As noted above, a great majority of schizophrenic children were slow to acquire expressive language. For example, the children were delayed in speaking in two- and three-word phrases. Curiously, the results of the neuropsychological evaluations conducted when schizophrenic children were 9 years of age revealed that simple expressive and receptive language skills were among the *least* impaired functions in these children. It appears that the early impairments in language function were delays, not static neuropsychological deficits. On the other hand, when schizophrenic children had to process complex verbal and non-verbal information (e.g., by holding it in short-term memory while they executed a sequence of actions), their performance was impaired. Placing cognitive systems under time pressure (i.e., increasing the amount of information that must be processed in a fixed unit of time) increases demands on processing resources (Kahneman, 1973). This constellation of findings – a delay in the acquisition of certain skills and residual problems when the skills have to be performed under conditions that involve more complex processing – may offer important insights into the nature of neurobehavioral impairments in schizophrenia.

What mechanisms could produce this constellation of delayed acquisition of skills, which are not necessarily deployed efficiently even when acquired? Impairments still can be revealed, for example, by putting the system under time pressure. The developmental delays might be an analogue of a delay of atomatization of skills.

An informative parallel to the concept of developmental delays can be found in studies examining the acquisition of skilled motor performance and perceptual discrimination learning. It appears that schizophrenic children are most likely to be delayed in acquiring skills (e.g., speaking in two- and three-word utterances) that are at the cusp of development (that is, emerging skills that are just coming on line developmentally). It is not the case that the schizophrenic children are unable to speak in two- and three-word utterances. Instead, they are delayed in the acquisition of the skill, since they can speak in two- and three-word utterances some months later.

Developmental delays may be analogous to the delay in learning a skill. Why should schizophrenic children show delays in learning skills? An intriguing answer to this problem emerges from the earlier hypothesis that schizophrenic children have a reduced processing capacity. Controlled processes are used when an individual is first attempting to learn a skill. For example, on tasks like the Span of Apprehension, controlled processes modify long-term memory and are used to search the arrays and decide responses. With practice, these responses become automated; that is, they make fewer demands on processing resources. In this way, the limited controlled processing system lays down the "stepping stones" of automatic processing (Schneider et al., 1984). Reduced processing resources can lead to deficient development of automatic operations. In particular, they can lead to a delay in the time taken to make a task automated (i.e., resource free). Perhaps the developmental delays we have observed in schizophrenic children represent, on a broader time scale, the longer time it takes schizophrenic individuals to automate certain information processing tasks.

REFERENCES

Achenbach, T.M. & Edelbrock, C.S. (1983). *Manual for the Child Behavior Checklist and the Revised Behavior Profile*. Burlington, VT: Department of Psychiatry, University of Vermont.

American Psychiatric Association (1980). *Diagnostic and Statistical Manual of Mental Disorders* (DSM-III), 3rd edn. Washington, DC: APA.

American Psychiatric Association (1987). *Diagnostic and Statistical Manual of Mental Disorders* (DSM-III-R), 3rd edn, Revised. Washington, DC: APA.

Andreason, N.C. (1984). *Scale for the Assessment of Positive Symptoms (SAPS)*. Iowa City, IA: The University of Iowa.

Andreasen, N.C. & Olsen, S. (1982). Negative versus positive schizophrenics: definition and validation. *Archives of General Psychiatry*, **39**, 789–94.

Andreasen, N.C. & Grove, W.M. (1986). Thought, language, and communication in schizophrenia: diagnosis and prognosis. *Schizophrenia Bulletin*, **12**, 348–59.

Arboleda, C. & Holzman, P.S. (1985). Thought disorder in children at risk for psychosis. *Archives of General Psychiatry*, **39**, 789–94.

Asarnow, J.R. & Ben-Meir, S. (1988). Children with schizophrenia spectrum and depressive disorders: a comparative study of premorbid adjustment, onset pattern and severity of impairment. *Journal of Child Psychology and Psychiatry*, **29**, 477–88.

Asarnow, J.R., Tompson, M.C., & Goldstein, M. (1994). Childhood onset schizophrenia: a follow-up study. *Schizophrenia Bulletin*, **20**, 599–617.

Asarnow, R.F. & Sherman, T. (1984). Studies of visual information processing in schizophrenic children. *Child Development*, **55**, 249–61.

Asarnow, R.F. & Asarnow, J.R. (1994). Childhood onset schizophrenia: editors' introduction. *Schizophrenia Bulletin*, **20**, 561–97.

Asarnow, R.F., Sherman, T., & Strandburg, R.J. (1986). The search for the psychobiological substrate of childhood onset schizophrenia. *Journal of the American Academy of Child Psychiatry*, **26**, 601–14.

Asarnow, R.F., Tanguay, P.E., Bott, L., & Freeman, B.J. (1987). Patterns of intellectual functioning in non-retarded autistic and schizophrenic children. *Journal of Child Psychology and Psychiatry*, **28**, 273–80.

Asarnow, R.F., Granholm, E., & Sherman, T. (1991). Span of apprehension in schizophrenia. In *Handbook of Schizophrenia, Vol 5: Neuropsychology, Psychophysiology and Information Processing*, ed. S. Steinhauer, J. Gruzelier, & J. Zubin, pp. 335–70. New York: Elsevier Science Publishers.

Asarnow, R.F., Asamen, J., Granholm, E., Sherman, T., Watkins, J.M., & Williams, M. (1994). Cognitive/neuropsychological studies of children with a schizophrenic disorder. *Schizophrenia Bulletin*, **20**, 647–70.

Asarnow, R.F., Brown, W., & Strandburg, R. (1995). Children with a schizophrenic disorder: neurobehavioral studies. *European Archives of Psychiatry and Clinical Neurosciences*, **245**, 70–9.

Baddeley, A. (1996). The fractionation of working memory. *Proceedings of the National Academy of Sciences of the United States of America*, **93**, 13 468–72.

Baribeau-Braun, J., Picton, T.W., & Gosselin J. (1983). Schizophrenia: a neurophysiological evaluation of abnormal information processing. *Science*, **219**, 874–6.

Benton, A.L. (1974). *Revised Visual Retention Test*, 4th edn. New York: Psychological Corporation.

Benton, A.L. & Hamsher, K. de S. (1989). *Multilingual Aphasia Examination*, 2nd edn. Iowa City, IA: Benton Laboratory of Neuropsychology, Division of Behavioral Neurology, Department of Neurology, University Hospitals.

Benton, A.L., Hannay, H.J., & Varney, N.R. (1975). Visual perception of line direction in patients with unilateral brain disease. *Neurology*, **25**, 907–10.

Benton, A.L., Hamsher, K. de S., & Stone, B. (1977). Visual Retention Test: Visual Form Discrimination. Iowa City, IA: Division of Behavioral Neurology, Department of Neurology, University Hospitals.

Buchsbaum, M.S., Nuechterlein, K.H., Haier, R.J., Wu, J., Sicotte, N,, Hazlett, E., Asarnow, R., Potkin, S., & Guich, S. (1990). Glucose metabolic rate in normals and schizophrenics during the Continuous Performance Test assessed by Positron Emission Tomography. *British Journal of Psychiatry*, **156**, 216–27.

Bunney, B.G., Bunney, Jr. W.E., & Carlsson, A. (1995). Schizophrenia and glutamate. In *Psychopharmacology: The Fourth Generation of Progress*, ed. F.E. Bloom & D.J. Kupfer, pp. 1205–14. New York: Raven Press.

Cantor, S., Evans, J., Pearce, J., & Pezzot-Pearce, T. (1982). Childhood schizophrenia: present but not accounted for. *American Journal of Psychiatry*, **139**, 758–63.

Caplan, R. (1994). Communication deficits in childhood schizophrenia spectrum disorders. *Schizophrenia Bulletin*, **20**, 671–83.

Caplan, R., Foy, J.G., Sigman, M., & Perdue, S. (1990b). Conservation and formal thought disorder in schizophrenic and schizotypal children. *Development and Psychopathology*, **2**, 183–92.

Caplan, R., Guthrie, D., Fish, B., Tanguay, P.E., & David-Lando, G. (1989). The Kiddie Formal Thought Disorder Rating Scale: clinical assessment, reliability, and validity. *Journal of the American Academy of Child and Adolescent Psychiatry*, **28**, 408–16.

Caplan, R., Foy, J.G., Asarnow, R.F., & Sherman T. (1990a). Information processing deficits of schizophrenic children with formal thought disorder. *Psychiatry Research*, **31**, 169–77.

Caplan, R., Guthrie, D., & Foy, J.G. (1992). Communication deficits and formal thought disorder in schizophrenic children. *Journal of the American Academy of Child and Adolescent Psychiatry*, **31**, 151–9.

Castellanos, F.X., Giedd, J.N., Eckburg, P., Marsh, W.L., Vaituzis, C., Kaysen, D., Hamburger, S., & Rapoport, J.L. (1994). Quantitative morphology of the caudate nucleus in Attention-Deficit Hyperactivity Disorder. *American Journal of Psychiatry*, **151**, 1791–6.

Castellanos, F.X., Giedd, J.N., Marsh, W.L., Hamburger, S.D., Vaituzis. A.C., Dickstein, D.P., Sarfatti, S.E., Vauss, Y.C., Snell, J.W., Lange, N., Kaysen, D., Krain, A.L., Ritchie, G.F., Rajapakse, J.G., & Rapoport, J.L. (1996). Quantitative brain magnetic resonance imaging in Attention-Deficit Hyperactivity Disorder. *Archives of General Psychiatry*, **53**, 607–16.

Donchin, E., Ritter, W., & McCallum, W. (1978). Cognitive psychophysiology: the endogenous components of the ERP. In *Event-Related Brain Potentials in Man*, ed. E. Callaway, P. Tueting, & S. Koslow, pp. 349–442. New York: Academic Press.

Dunn, L.M. & Dunn, L.M. (1981). Peabody Picture Vocabulary Test-Revised. Circle Pines, Minnesota, American Guidance Service.

Estes, W.K. & Taylor, H.A. (1964). A detection method and probabilistic models for assessing information processing from brief visual displays. *Proceedings of the National Academy of Sciences of the USA*, **52**, 446–54.

Fish, B. & Ritvo, E.R. (1979). Psychoses of childhood. In *Basic Handbook of Child Psychiatry: Disturbances in Development*, Vol. 2, ed. J.D. Noshpitz, pp. 249–304. New York: Basic Books.

Frazier, J.A., Giedd, J.N., Hamburger, S.D., Albus, K.E., Kaysen, D., Vaituzis, A.C., Rajapakse, J.C., Lenane, M.C., McKenna, K., Jacobsen, L.K., Gordon, C.T., Breier, A., & Rapoport, J.L. (1996). Brain anatomic magnetic resonance imaging in childhood onset schizophrenia. *Archives of General Psychiatry*, **53**, 617–24.

Goldberg, T.E., Weinberger, D.R., Berman, K.F., Pliskin, N.H., & Podd, M.H. (1987). Further evidence for dementia of the prefrontal type in schizophrenia? A controlled study of teaching the Wisconsin Card Sorting Test. *Archives of General Psychiatry*, **44**, 1008–14.

Gottesman, I.E. & Shields, J. (1982). *Schizophrenia: The Epigenetic Puzzle*. Cambridge, UK: Cambridge University Press.

Halliday, M.A.K. & Hasan, R. (1976). *Cohesion in English*. London: Longman.

Heaton, R. (1985). *Wisconsin Card Sorting Test*. Odessa, FL: Psychological Assessment Resources.

Hillyard, S.A. & Kutas, M. (1983). Electrophysiology of cognitive processing. *Annual Review of Psychology*, **34**, 33–61.

Hillyard, S.A. & Hansen, J.C. (1986). Attention: electrophysiological approaches. In *Psychophysiology: Systems, Processes and Applications*, ed. M.G.H. Coles, E. Donchin, & S.W. Porges, pp. 227–43. New York: Guilford Press.

Hirst, W. & Kalmar, D. (1987). Characterizing attentional resources. *Journal of Experimental Psychology: General*, **116**, 68–81.

Jacobsen, L.K. & Rapoport, J.L. (1998). Childhood-onset schizophrenia: implications of clinical and neurobiological research. *Journal of Child Psychology and Psychiatry*, **39**, 101–13.

Jacobsen, L.K., Frazier, J.A., Malhotra, A.K., Karoum, F., McKenna, K., Gordon, C.T., Hamburger, S.D., Lenane, M.C., Pickar, D., Potter, W.Z., & Rapoport, J.L. (1997). Cerebrospinal fluid monoamine metabolites in childhood-onset schizophrenia. *American Journal of Psychiatry*, **154**(1), 69–74.

Kahn, R.S. & Davis, K.L. (1995). New developments in dopamine and schizophrenia. In *Psychopharmacology: The Fourth Generation of Progress*, ed. F.E. Bloom & D.J. Kupfer, pp. 1193–203. New York: Raven Press.

Kahneman, D. (1973). *Attention and Effort*. Englewood Cliffs, NJ: Prentice-Hall.

Karatekin, C. & Asarnow, R.F. (1998a). Components of visual search in childhood-onset schizophrenia and Attention-Deficit/Hyperactivity Disorder (ADHD). *Journal of Abnormal Child Psychology*, **26**(5), 367–80.

Karatekin, C. & Asarnow, R.F. (1998b). Working memory in chilhood-onset schizophrenia and Attention-Deficit/Hyperactivity Disorder (ADHD). *Psychiatry Research*, **80**, 165–76.

Karatekin, C. & Asarnow, R.F. (2000). Exploratory eye movements to pictures in childhood-onset schizophrenia and Attention-Deficit/Hyperactivity Disorder (ADHD). *Journal of Abnormal Child Psychology*, in press.

Kaufman, A.S. (1979). *Intelligent Testing with the WISC-R*. New York: Wiley.

Keefe, R.S.E., Roitman, S.E.L., Harvey, P.D., Blum, C.S., DuPre, R.L., Prieto, D.M., Davidson, M., & Davis, K.L. (1995). A pen-and-paper human analogue of a monkey prefrontal cortex activation task: spatial working memory in patients with schizophrenia. *Schizophrenia Research*, **17**, 25–33.

Kim, J.S., Kornhuber, H.H., Schmid-Burg, K., & Holzmuller, B. (1980). Low cerebrospinal fluid glutamate in schizophrenic patients and a new hypothesis of schizophrenia. *Neuroscience Letter*, **20**, 379–82.

Koh, S.D. (1978). Remembering of verbal materials by schizophrenic young adults. In *Language and Cognition in Schizophrenia*, ed. S. Schwartz, pp. 55–99. Hillsdale, NJ: Erlbaum.

Kolvin, I., Garside, R.F., & Kidd, J.S.H. (1971). Studies in the childhood psychoses, IV: parental personality and attitude and childhood psychoses. *British Journal of Psychiatry*, **118**, 403–6.

Kovelman, J.A. & Scheibel, A.B. (1986). Biological substrates of schizophrenia. *Acta Neurologica Scandinavica*, **73**, 1–32.

Luck S.J. & Hillyard, S.A. (1990). Electrophysiological evidence for parallel and serial processing during visual search. *Perception and Psychophysics*, **48**, 603–17.

Michie, P.T., Fox, A.M., Ward, P.B., Catts, S.V., & McConaghy, N. (1990). Event-related potential indices of selective attention and cortical lateralization in schizophrenia. *Psychophysiology*, **27**, 207–27.

Naatanen, P. (1982). Processing negativity: an evoked potential reflection of selective attention. *Psychological Bulletin*, **92**, 605–40.

Nasrallah, H.A. (1990). Magnetic resonance imaging of the brain: clinical and research applications in schizophrenia. In *Search for the Causes of Schizophrenia*, Vol. 11, pp. 257–74. Berlin: Springer-Verlag.

Nuechterlein, K.H. (1977). Reaction time and attention in schizophrenia: a critical evaluation of the data and theories. *Schizophrenia Bulletin*, **3**, 373–428.

Nuechterlein, K.H. & Dawson, M.E. (1984). Information processing and attentional functioning in the developmental course of schizophrenic disorders. *Schizophrenia Bulletin*, **10**, 160–203.

Overall, J.E. & Gorham, D.E. (1961). The Brief Psychiatric Rating Scale. *Psychological Reports*, **10**, 799–812.

Pritchard, W.S. (1986). Cognitive event-related potential correlates of schizophrenia. *Psychological Bulletin*, **100**, 43–66.

Rapoport, J.L., Giedd, J., Kumra, S., Jacobsen, L., Smith, A., Lee, P., Nelson, J., & Hamburger, S. (1997). Childhood-onset schizophrenia: progressive ventricular change during adolescence. *Archives of General Psychiatry*, **54**, 897–903.

Rey, A. (1964). *L'Examen Clinique en Psycologie* [*The Clinical Exam in Psychology*]. Paris: Presses Universitaires de France.

Rist, F. & Cohen, R. (1991). Sequential effects in the reaction times of schizophrenics: crossover and modality shift effects. In *Handbook of Schizophrenia*, Vol. 5: *Neuropsychology, Psychophysiology and Information Processing*, ed. S.R. Steinhauer, J.H. Gruzelier, & J. Zubin, pp. 241–71. New York: Elsevier Science Publishers.

Rochester, S.R. & Martin, J.R. (1979). *Crazy Talk: A Study of the Discourse of Schizophrenic Speakers*. New York: Plenum.

Rodnick, E.H. & Shakow, D. (1940). Set in the schizophrenic as measured by a composite reaction time index. *American Journal of Psychology*, **97**, 214–25.

Sattler, J.M. (1974). *Assessment of Children's Intelligence*. Philadelphia: W.B. Saunders.

Schneider, S.G. & Asarnow, R.F. (1987). A comparison between the cognitive/neuropsychological impairments of non-retarded autistic and schizophrenic children. *Journal of Abnormal Child Psychology*, **15**, 29–46.

Schneider, W., Dumais, S.T., & Shiffrin, R.A. (1984). Automatic and controlled processing and attention. In *Varieties of Attention*, ed. R. Parasuraman, J. Beatty, & J. Davies, pp. 1–27. San Diego: Academic Press.

Seashore, C.E., Lewis, D., & Sactveit, J.G. (1960). *Seashore Measures of Musical Talents*. New York: Psychological Corporation.

Sherman, T. & Asarnow, R.F. (1985). The cognitive disabilities of the schizophrenic child. In *Children with Emotional Disorders and Developmental Disabilities: Assessment and Treatment*, ed. M. Sigman, pp. 153–70. New York: Grune & Stratton.

Spencer, K.S. & Campbell, M. (1994). Children with schizophrenia: diagnosis, phenomenology, and pharmacotherapy. *Schizophrenia Bulletin*, **20**, 713–25.

Steffy, R.A. (1978). An early cue sometimes impairs process schizophrenic performance In *The Nature of Schizophrenia: Approaches to Research and Treatment*, ed. L.C. Wynne, R.L. Cromwell, & S. Matthysse, pp. 225–32. New York: Wiley.

Strandburg, R.J., Marsh, J.T., Brown, W.S., Asarnow, R.F., & Guthrie, D. (1984). Event-related potential concomitants of information processing dysfunction in schizophrenic children. *Electroencephalography and Clinical Neurophysiology*, **57**, 236–53.

Strandburg, R.J., Marsh, J.T., Brown, W.S., Asarnow, R.F., Guthrie, D., & Higa, J. (1990). Event-related potential correlates of impaired attention in schizophrenic children. *Biological Psychiatry*, **27**, 1103–15.

Strandburg, R.J., Marsh, J.T., Brown, W.S., Asarnow, R.F., Guthrie, D., & Higa, J. (1991). Reduced attention-related negative potentials in schizophrenic children. *Electroencephalography and Clinical Neurophysiology*, **79**, 291–307.

Strandburg, R.J., Marsh, J.T., Brown, W.S., Asarnow, R.F., Higa, J., & Guthrie, D. (1994b). Continuous processing-related ERPs in schizophrenic and normal children. *Biological Psychiatry*, **35**, 525–38.

Strandburg, R.J., Marsh, J.T., Brown, W.S., Asarnow, R.F., Guthrie, D., & Higa, J. (1994a). Reduced attention-related negative potentials in schizophrenic adults. *Psychophysiology*, **31**, 272–81.

Stuss, D.T., Benson, D.F., Kaplan, E.F., Weir, W.S., Naesser, M.A., Liberman, I., & Ferrill, D. (1983). The involvement of orbitofrontal cerebrum in cognitive tasks. *Neuropsychologia*, **21**, 235–48.

Sutton, S., Hakerem, G., Zubin, J., & Portnoy, M. (1961). The effect of shift of sensory modality on serial reaction time: a comparison of schizophrenics and normals. *American Journal of Psychology*, **74**, 224–32.

Thomas, M.A., Ke, Y., Levitt, J., Caplan, R., Curran, J., Asarnow, R., & McCracken, J. (1998). Frontal lobe proton MR spectroscopy of children with schizophrenia. *Journal of Magnetic Resonance Imaging*, **8**, 841–6.

Treisman, A.M. & Gelade, G. (1980). A feature-integration theory of attention. *Cognitive Psychology*, **12**, 97–136.

Treisman, A. & Souther, J. (1985). Search asymmetry: a diagnostic for preattentive processing of separable features. *Journal of Experimental Psychology: General*, **114**, 285–310.

Van der Does, A.J. & Van Den Bosch, R.J. (1992). What determines Wisconsin Card Sorting performance in schizophrenia? *Clinical Psychology Review*, **12**, 567–83.

Watkins, J.M., Asarnow, R.F., & Tanguay, P.E. (1988). Symptom development in childhood onset schizophrenia. *Journal of Child Psychology and Psychiatry*, **29**, 865–78.

Watt, N.F. & Lubensky, A.W. (1976). Childhood roots of schizophrenia. *Journal of Consulting and Clinical Psychology*, **44**, 363–75.

Wechsler, D. (1974). *Wechsler Intelligence Scale for Children – Revised Manual.* New York: Psychological Corporation.

Weinberger, D.R. (1987). Implications of normal brain development for the pathogenesis of schizophrenia. *Archives of General Psychiatry,* **44**, 660–9.

Zahn, T.P., Jacobsen, L., Gordon, C.T., McKenna, K., Frazier, J.A., & Rapoport, J.L. (1998). Attention deficits in childhood-onset schizophrenia: reaction time studies. *Journal of Abnormal Psychology,* **107**, 97–108.

8

Psychosocial factors: the social context of child and adolescent-onset schizophrenia

Joan R. Asarnow, Martha C. Tompson and
the late M:chael J. Goldstein

Introduction

Scientific advances over recent years have contributed to an emerging consensus that schizophrenia is a biologically based disorder. This biologically based view has been complemented, however, by accumulating research demonstrating that: (i) the disorder has a profound effect on the adolescent's psychosocial functioning, and (ii) the psychosocial environment in which an adolescent develops has a major impact on the expression of the disorder (for review, see Asarnow, 1994). Furthermore, the current emphasis on treating adolescents within the least restrictive setting has highlighted the stressors involved in rearing adolescents with schizophrenia and the need to attend to stress levels and coping efforts among parents, siblings, and other family members who are critical partners in the treatment process.

This chapter focuses on psychosocial factors in child and adolescent onset schizophrenia with the goal of highlighting promising psychosocial treatment strategies. We begin by examining current knowledge with respect to the psychosocial functioning of adolescents with schizophrenia. Secondly, we review current models for the psychosocial treatment of schizophrenia. Thirdly, we turn to the implications of current knowledge for the psychosocial treatment of adolescents with schizophrenia and conclude by offering suggestions regarding future directions for clinical research and treatment.

Schizophrenia in adolescence: psychosocial functioning and developmental progressions

Consider the following descriptions of the psychosocial impairments experienced by adolescents with schizophrenia:

Impaired academic and school functioning

All of a sudden I couldn't read or write or do maths anymore. Everything was so confusing because I couldn't understand anything that was going on around me (Anonymous, 1994, p. 587). My behavior was annoying, and my explanations were seen as fanciful lies to cover up my disruptive behavior (Lovejoy, 1982, p. 605).

Impaired peer adjustment

I really couldn't get along with anyone. That was when kids first began calling me "retard" (Anonymous, 1994, p. 587). My classmates quickly noticed that I was "different" and reacted to me differently . . .. My classmates ridiculed my efforts and I reacted to their rejection by isolating myself from them, knowing that I did not belong (Lovejoy, 1982, p. 605).

Impaired family adjustment and family stress

Unless my parents come down hard on me, I never get things done. One of them has to supervise me with all my homework . . . (Anonymous, 1994, p. 588).

Impaired social interaction

I never smiled or had any expression on my face. I had a blank look in all my school pictures (Anonymous, 1994, p. 588).

These descriptions of the experiences of children struggling with schizophrenia are consistent with accumulating research documenting the psychosocial impairments experienced by adolescents with schizophrenia. As illustrated in these descriptions, adolescents suffering from schizophrenia show early anomalies that frequently lead to rejection by peers, difficulties in school, and stress on family members. Recent research supports these clinical descriptions as summarized below.

Follow-up studies

Perhaps the most compelling data demonstrating the social impairments that characterize adolescents with schizophrenia are derived from the completed follow-up studies. To date, results are available from three follow-up studies of early-onset schizophrenia and one comprehensive case record study of children receiving psychiatric care both during childhood and as adults. Without exception, these studies highlight the severe psychosocial impairments observed among adolescents with schizophrenia. For example, Werry et al. (1991) found that, over the course of a 1–16 year follow-up interval (average follow-up interval of roughly 5 years), 90% of their sample showed either chronic schizophrenia or two or more schizophrenic episodes. Only 17% of the sample was in school full-time or had full-time employment. Moreover, the average level of general adaptive functioning (GAF) was 40, reflecting a relatively severe level of impairment (major impairment in several areas or some impairment in reality testing or communication).

Secondly, Eggers and Bunk (1997) recently presented impressive 42-year follow-up data for their sample of patients with childhood-onset schizophrenia. They found a somewhat higher rate of complete remission, 25%. However, 50% of the sample was judged to be in poor remission, to be chronically psychotic, or to have developed a severe residual syndrome.

Thirdly, in our 2 to 7-year follow-up study of childhood-onset schizophrenia (Asarnow, Tompson & Goldstein, 1994a), we found substantial recovery in 22% of our sample. However, 44% of our sample showed minimal improvement or a deteriorating course based on ratings of global adjustment. Our somewhat more optimistic picture of outcome may have been associated with the fact that this was a recently treated sample; 94% of children were treated with antipsychotic medications and all of the children received some form of psychosocial intervention. Additionally, the sample included a small group of children who on follow-up appeared to have schizoaffective disorders. If these cases were dropped from the sample, 50% of the sample would be rated as showing minimal to no improvement, a figure that is roughly identical to that reported by Eggers and Bunk (1997).

Fourthly, results of Zeitlin's (1986) case record study indicate considerable continuity between psychosis in childhood and adulthood, with nine of ten patients diagnosed with psychoses during childhood also presenting with psychoses as adults (90%). Eight of these ten patients received diagnoses of schizophrenia as children, while the other two were diagnosed with manic depressive disorder as children. All but two of the children who presented with non-acute onset of schizophrenia, continued to present with schizophrenia as adults. Alternatively, four of the six children with acute onset of schizophrenia received non-schizophrenic adult diagnoses.

Premorbid adjustment and predictors of outcome

Studies that have examined premorbid adjustment also highlight the social dysfunctions associated with childhood onset schizophrenia. For example, all of the follow-up studies reviewed above have emphasized the fact that the more characteristic insidious onset observed in child vs. adolescent onset schizophrenia is associated with greater impairment. Additionally, Asarnow et al. (1994) found relatively low levels of premorbid adjustment among adolescents with schizophrenia, as compared to adolescents with major depression, particularly in the areas of peer relationships, scholastic performance, school adaptation, and interests. These data are consistent with Eggers and Bunk's (1997) observation that childhood onset psychoses were often predated by earlier psychiatric symptoms and signs of behavioral disturbance, as well as Werry et al.'s (1991) report of higher rates of premorbid personality abnormalities among psychotic adolescents who received follow-up diagnoses of schizophrenia, as compared to psychotic adolescents who received follow-up diagnoses of bipolar disorder.

Importantly, Werry et al. (1991) found that premorbid adjustment was the best predictor of outcome in their schizophrenic sample, again underscoring the prognostic significance of social competence measures. Similarly, Eggers and Bunk (1997) reported that a more insidious as opposed to acute course, a variable which is likely associated with premorbid dysfunction, was associated with a more negative prognosis. Earlier age of onset, particularly before 12 years of age, was also associated with more severe social dysfunction in the Eggers and Bunk (1997) sample.

Family stress

Clinical observations underscore the stress experienced by many families attempting to rear children with schizophrenia. These observations in conjunction with research indicating that stress within the family environment is associated with more negative outcomes among adults with schizophrenia (Kavanagh, 1992), underscore the importance of clarifying the impact of family risk and protective factors on the course of schizophrenia among adolescents. To date, however, this area has received minimal research attention.

The scant data that do exist on the family environments of schizophrenic adolescents do present a picture of stress and distress. It is unclear, however, whether the levels of stress seen in families of schizophrenic adolescents differ from those seen in families of adolescents with other disorders. Additionally, evidence that family variables predict outcome among adolescents with schizophrenia has not yet emerged. In a series of studies conducted in our laboratory, we have begun to document the family environmental correlates of childhood onset schizophrenia and schizotypal personality disorder (SPD), a syndrome considered to fall within the schizophrenia spectrum. SPD is characterized by oddities of thought and perception that represent milder variants of those seen in full blown schizophrenic disorders. Our studies have shown that children with schizophrenia or SPD tend to show elevated rates of thought disorder during direct family interactions, suggesting that characteristic schizophrenic symptoms tend to intrude into family interactions (Tompson et al., 1997). Parents of schizophrenic and SPD children also tend to show elevated levels of thought disorder during the same interaction task, relative to parents of normal controls (Tompson et al., 1997). Parents of schizophrenic and SPD children were also found to show elevated levels of communication deviance, an index of difficulties associated with a failure to establish and maintain a shared focus of attention (Asarnow et al., 1988b). While it is unclear whether these measures of communication difficulties and thought disorder reflect parental reactions to a disturbed child, shared genetic vulnerabilities to schizophrenia, or some other environmental factor; these data do underscore the fact that family transactions involving schizophrenic adolescents are more likely to be characterized by communication difficulties and disordered thinking than are family transactions involving non-disturbed adolescents.

Numerous studies have shown higher relapse rates among schizophrenia patients returning to homes where there are high levels of contact with relatives rated as high in expressed emotion (EE) as compared to patients residing with low EE relatives (Kavanagh, 1992). Contrary to findings with adults, however, our data indicate relatively low levels of parental EE based on ratings of criticism and emotional overinvolvement on the Five Minute Speech Sample Expressed Emotion (FMSS-EE) measure (Asarnow et al., 1994b). Whereas 23% of families of our schizophrenic and SPD adolescent were rated as high EE, the most comparable adult study found a rate of 44% high EE among families of adults with schizophrenia (Miklowitz et al., 1989). Indeed, the rate of overall EE among parents of schizophrenic and SPD adolescent in our sample was comparable to that seen in parents of normal controls. However, the type of EE differed as a function of child diagnostic status. Whereas high EE parents of schizophrenic and SPD adolescent were rated high based on criticism, high EE parents of normal controls tended to be classified based on high scores on the emotional overinvolvement measure, underscoring the differences in the family processes that characterize families rearing normal (non-disturbed) adolescent as opposed to families rearing adolescent with schizophrenia or SPD.

Interactional data on our sample further indicate a tendency for parents of schizophrenic and SPD adolescents to express more harsh criticism towards their children in a family problem-solving task, as compared to parents of depressed adolescents and parents of normal controls (Hamilton et al., 1997). However, in this context it is important to note that parents of depressed adolescents displayed high rates of criticism on the FMSS EE measure (Asarnow et al., 1994a), and their children displayed high rates of negative behavior during the problem-solving task (Hamilton et al., 1997). Consequently, it may be that the more negative behavior of the depressed adolescent during the family interaction may have served to suppress critical behavior as parents attempted to manage the negative behavior of their depressed children.

Additionally, negative parent affective style during the family problem-solving task (a composite measure based on the presence of harsh criticism, guilt induction, or six or more intrusive statements) was found to be associated with lower levels of social competence and academic performance in our overall sample of children with schizophrenia or SPD, children with depressive disorders, and normal controls (Hamilton et al., 1997). This suggests that parents whose children show competence deficits are most likely to respond with criticism or other negative behaviors during family interactions underscoring the strong links between child characteristics and parent reactions.

Another dimension examined in our laboratory is family burden, or the impact of the child's dysfunction on family members (Asarnow & Horton, 1990). Results indicated that parents of children with schizophrenia and SPD reported high levels of burden and disruption, as did parents of children with depressive disorders. There were no differences in reported burden as a function of child diagnosis. The greatest impact of the child's impairment was felt on the family life dimension (87% of mothers and 88% of fathers). A large proportion of mothers also described moderate to extreme impact on their social lives (55%) and in their personal relationships (41%). These dimensions appear to be somewhat more protected in fathers. Work functioning was the least disrupted by the child's dysfunction, although 39% of mothers and 34% of fathers reported moderate to severe impact on work functioning. Significant predictors of reported burden/disruption for mothers were the absence of supportive intimate relationships and non-acute (insidious) onset of disorder. When asked about the strategies that they used to cope with their children's illnesses, parents most frequently described active cognitive coping strategies such as "I'd just tell myself to take one day at a time" or "I'd remind myself that lots of people have it much worse". When asked how they would advise other parents with similar problems, however, given the advantage of hindsight, most parents advised seeking community resources and treatment for helping their children.

Treatment strategies for schizophrenia in adolescents

Despite the dearth of controlled treatment trials for adolescents suffering from schizophrenia, accumulating clinical and research data highlight some major issues with respect to the treatment of schizophrenia in adolescent. First, the

Three-phase

Model of treatment

current emphasis on treating adolescents within the least restrictive setting and reducing hospitalizations and residential care have resulted in many more adolescents with schizophrenia being treated within their families and communities. In this context, the three-phase model of treatment (e.g., Goldstein & Miklowitz, 1995) is useful: (i) during the *acute* phase the emphasis is on bringing acute psychotic symptoms under control through a combination of medication and inpatient care, (ii) during the *stabilization* phase outpatient pharmacologic and psychosocial treatment is employed with the goal of stabilizing the adolescent's clinical state, and (iii) during the *maintenance* phase the emphasis is on helping the adolescent to maintain a stable state through continuing multimodal treatment. Because the acute phase of treatment emphasizes pharmacological treatment, readers are referred to excellent reviews of the pharmacologic treatment of acute psychotic states in adolescents with schizophrenia (e.g., Kumra et al., 1996; Remschmidt et al., 1994; Spencer & Campbell, 1994). The present review will focus on psychosocial treatment during the stabilization and maintenance phases of treatment.

Three primary psychosocial intervention approaches investigated for adults with schizophrenia include (i) individual psychotherapy, (ii) family-focused interventions, and (iii) skills building strategies. These approaches may prove particularly applicable to the treatment of adolescents with schizophrenia and are discussed below.

Individual psychotherapy

The role of individual psychotherapy in treating adolescents with schizophrenia remains to be determined. Extant data does not support the efficacy of intensive psychodynamic therapy for adults with schizophrenia, and indeed, some studies have documented a potentially detrimental effect of "uncovering" strategies for individuals with schizophrenia (Mueser & Berenbaum, 1990). However, supportive reality-oriented therapy interventions have shown some promise (Rockland, 1993; Scott & Dixon, 1995). In a comprehensive and well-controlled study addressing these issues, Stanton and colleagues (1984) compared an intensive, insight-oriented treatment, in which therapy sessions took place three times weekly, to one time a week supportive and reality oriented treatment. While the two treatment groups did not differ on symptom measures over the two year follow-up period, those patients in the reality focused, supportive therapy spent less time in the hospital and demonstrated better role functioning, as assessed by time spent in full-time work, occupational level, number of job changes and assumption of household responsibilities (Gunderson et al., 1984). Because this study did not include a no-therapy control group, we can conclude that reality-oriented approaches were superior to psychodynamic approaches, but additional data are needed to clarify whether supportive psychotherapy yields significantly more gains than no treatment or alternative treatment approaches. It is also important to note that none of these studies focused on adolescents with schizophrenia, and results may not generalize to younger populations.

More recently, attempts have been made to operationalize individual treatment interventions for schizophrenia. For example, Hogarty and colleagues (1995) have designed Personal Therapy, a specific psychotherapy approach for individuals with schizophrenia. The therapy is supportive, educational and skills building. It is conducted in three, graduated phases, which vary in length and intensity depending on the needs of the patient. Phase I occurs during the stabilization period and emphasizes supportive therapy strategies. During this phase, the therapist "joins" with the patient, builds a therapeutic alliance, enters into a treatment contract which outlines treatment goals, and begins the process of psychoeducation. Phase II begins when patients have stabilized positive symptoms and living situations, have achieved a low maintenance neuroleptic dose and a rudimentary understanding of schizophrenia, and have sufficient attention and coping skills. This second stage of therapy focuses on patients "development of self-awareness regarding affective, cognitive, and behavioral states and increasing personal competence at self-regulation and management" (Hogarty et al. 1995, p. 385). Patients learn self-monitoring of prodromal signs and strategies for coping with affective dysregulation. While this phase focuses on self-awareness, it also addresses problems in social perception, assisting patients in learning to evaluate social situations. Phase III begins when patients continue to be stable, have some insight into the role of stress in schizophrenia, can identify a cue of their own stress level, can participate in role plays and homework, and demonstrate evidence of accurate social perception. This final stage continues to emphasize education with further focus on individual prodromal symptoms. Additional attention is also turned to increasing coping skills in social interaction and on building criticism management and conflict resolution skills. Personal Therapy is conceptualized as a long-term, individualized process in which therapists continually recognize the possibility of decompensation and attend to cognitive limits of the patient. While final results of this study have not yet been reported, initial findings (Hogarty et al., 1995) indicate that 90% of those participating in a trial of Personal Therapy completed phase I and advanced to Phase II. About 50% advanced from Phase II to Phase III.

Table 8.1. Components of first generation family treatments

(i) Engagement of the family in a no-fault atmosphere early in the treatment process

(ii) Education about schizophrenia that included information about:

    a. vulnerability stress models

    b. etiologic theories

    c. variations in course and prognosis

    d. rationales for different treatments

(iii) Recommended strategies for coping with the disorder

(iv) Communication training aimed at improving:

    a. general communication clarity

    b. ways of providing positive and negative feedback within the family

(v) Problem-solving training aimed at enhancing:

    a. daily management of problems and hassles

    b. management of stressful life events

    c. general problem-solving skills

(vi) Crisis intervention during periods of:

    a. severe stress for 1 or more family members

    b. early warning signs of possible recurrence

Source: Adapted from Goldstein & Miklowitz, (1995).

Family interventions

Family interventions have been one of the most highly investigated psychosocial treatment strategies for individuals with schizophrenia. Beginning in the late 1970s, a series of studies were conducted which showed that family "psychoeducational" treatment when combined with maintenance pharmacotherapy was effective in reducing relapse among adults with schizophrenia in the short term, 9 months to 1 year after discharge from hospital (Goldstein & Miklowitz, 1995). These family treatments were designed to address the specific problems that patients and families confront during the posthospitalization period. Techniques emphasized in this first generation of psychoeducational family treatments were based on empirical data showing links between intrafamilial processes and the risk of recurrence, rather than derived from specific theories or traditional family therapy techniques. Components shared by most of these treatments are listed in Table 8.1. It is important to note, however, that while almost all first generation family treatments shared the components listed in Table 8.1, these treatments did vary along several dimensions including length of treatment, whether treatment was provided at home or in a clinic setting, and the major focus of the intervention (e.g., crisis intervention, behavioral skills training, psychoeducation).

Fig. 8.1 summarizes the results of six studies comparing first generation "psychoeducational" family treatments to either individual treatment, medication only, or customary care protocols (Falloon, et al., 1982; Goldstein et al., 1978; Hogarty et al., 1986, 1991; Leff et al., 1982, 1989; Randolph et al., 1994; Tarrier et al., 1988). Inspection of this figure reveals dramatic effects in favor of family treatment. Across all six studies, family treated cases consistently exhibited lower relapse rates than those not receiving family treatment.

Results from three recent studies provide additional information on the effects of family treatment. First, early results have been reported from the NIMH Treatment Strategies Study (TSS; Schooler et al., 1997), a large multisite study that examined the effects of (i) three medication strategies termed standard dose, low dose, and intermittent dose (i.e., drugs were reintroduced at early signs of a recurrence), and (ii) two psychosocial strategies: (a) a "supportive family management" condition which included both a psychoeducational workshop for relatives and a monthly supportive group which ran for a 2-year period, and (b) "applied family management" which included "supportive family management" plus the addition of a 1-year intensive in-home family intervention program modeled after Falloon et al.'s behavioral family management program. In addition to the intensive in-home intervention, relatives in the applied family management condition also had access to the resources provided through the supportive family management condition, and relatives in the applied family management and supportive conditions attended the supportive relatives groups at comparable rates. Results generally indicate no advantage for the more intensive applied family management condition, over the less intensive supportive family management condition. Further, the addition of the more intensive family condition did not lead to improved outcomes in the low dose or intermittent medication condition, suggesting that adding an intensive family treatment does not permit the successful application of "riskier" pharmacological strategies. However, psychoeducational workshop attendance was a significant predictor of continuation into the maintenance phase of treatment, suggesting that family involvement is useful. Because of the absence of a non-family involved or treated condition, and the fact that the supportive family management condition provided relatives with the opportunity for consistent support over a 2-year period, this study does not permit us to identify the active ingredients in an effective family treatment program. However, the results of other studies (Cozolino et al., 1988; Tarrier et al., 1988) showing that the effects of brief education and involvement programs for relatives tend to have limited effectiveness over a sustained period, underscore the need to further clarify the

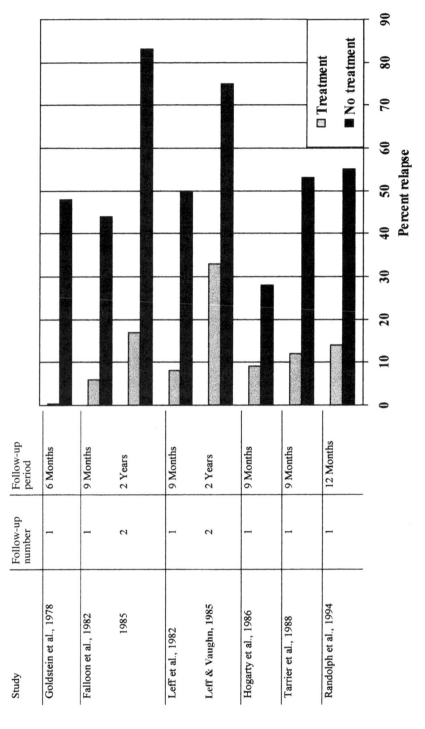

Fig. 8.1. Six family treatment studies with adult schizophrenic patients: relapse rates.

critical components required to generate optimal family intervention programs.

The second recent study, completed on the adolescent unit at the Amsterdam Medical Center (Linszen, 1993), compared a family intervention program modeled after Falloon et al. (1985) with a "standard care" condition. The "standard care" condition employed in this study was a combination of drug therapy and a rich form of individual supportive treatment, which employed a psychoeducational model in which patients were educated about their disorder, taught to recognize stressors, learned coping mechanisms for the recognition of prodromal signs and symptoms of disorder, and learned about the hazards of substance abuse and medication self-management. Thus, this study examined whether adding a family component yielded improvements relative to an intense individually focused treatment session. It is further important to note that both treatments were conducted within a comprehensive care system in which patients stayed an average of 13.5 weeks in the hospital, followed by a 3-month day hospital treatment period, and 9 months of outpatient care after leaving day treatment. Very low relapse rates were observed, 16% over a 12-month period, with no between group differences.

McFarlane et al. (1995) examined the relative advantages of psychoeducation conducted in multiple-family versus single family groups. In a first pilot study, McFarlane et al. (1995) found lower relapse rates among patients from the multiple-family groups (12.5% at 12 months, 25% at 24 months), as compared to patients from the single-family groups (23.5% at 12 months, 47.1% at 24 months). Furthermore, relapse rates were lower in both of these conditions than those for patients who received a multiple-family approach not based on a psychoeducational model (42.9% at 12 months, 42.9% at 24 months). Early results from a multicenter trial comparing multiple-family and single-family psychoeducational groups appear consistent with the early findings, although not as dramatic.

Collectively, the data reviewed above provide strong support for the utility of involving families in the treatment of adolescent with schizophrenia, although there may be examples where very rich forms of individually based treatments emphasizing psychoeducation and coping skills (Linszen, 1993) yield comparable effects. With children and adolescents, family involvement is likely to be particularly critical as most adolescents reside with their families and are more dependent on family members than are older adults. Based on extant data, however, it is too soon to determine if any one format for family treatment is most effective (Tompson et al. (in press)). Indeed, optimal family treatment formats may vary depending on patient characteristics, including age, phase of a particular episode, or lifetime history of the schizophrenic disorder.

Skills building models

Skills training approaches employ behavioral techniques to teach individuals with schizophrenia requisite skills for establishing interpersonal relationships and living in the community (Liberman & Kopelowicz, 1995). Specific skills that have been the focus of attention include social skills (e.g., conversational) and self-management skills (e.g., hygiene, medication management). Skills building approaches, which can be implemented in groups or using an individual format, have focused goals and specified behavioral techniques, and emphasize in vivo practice to facilitate generalization (Liberman, 1994). A noteworthy example of a skills building model is one developed at the UCLA Clinical Research Center for Schizophrenia and Psychiatric Rehabilitation (Liberman et al., 1986). This approach uses a group format and includes between five and ten patients and one or two therapists. Groups focus on learning specific skills, including medication management, leisure and recreation, self-care and personal hygiene, food preparation, and money management. These groups include modeling, role playing, and rehearsal of skills. More complex social skills are broken down into teachable pieces, practiced extensively, and finally practiced in more complex sequences.

While patients are clearly able to learn social skills during such training, data on the impact of such interventions on symptoms are mixed (for review, see Bellack & Mueser, 1993). In a meta-analysis of studies using social skills training with schizophrenia patients, Benton and Schroeder (1990) reviewed all studies published between 1972 and 1988. Results indicated strong effects of social skills training on increasing assertiveness, decreasing social anxiety and increasing rates of hospital discharge. However, significantly weaker effects were found on ratings of general functioning, self-reported symptoms and relapse rates. It should be noted that most studies included in this analysis were conducted in an inpatient setting, and study selection criteria were tilted toward those individuals with both chronic and severe psychopathology, limiting the generalizability of these findings. Examining skills training in 14-day hospital patients, Bradshaw (1993) exposed half the patients to several coping skills modules – managing physiological arousal, time management, cognitive restructuring and social skills training. At the end of training, the seven patients who received the training showed significantly more improvement across treatment, as measured by change in Global Adjustment Score, than patients treated using a problem-solving model.

Four controlled trials have examined the efficacy of social skills training (SST). The first of these (Bellack et al., 1984) compared two groups of patients in a 12-week day hospital program – those who received supplemental SST for three hours per week and those who did not. While the two groups did not differ symptomatically at post-test, at 6-month follow-up, SST patients reported fewer symptoms. However, 12-month rehospitalization rates did not differ – approximately 50% in both groups. The second study compared group SST to a "holistic health" condition in long-term State hospital patients (Liberman et al., 1986). While patients in SST demonstrated better social adjustment, there was no difference in relapse rates at 2-year follow-up. In a group of VA patients on low-dose neuroleptic treatment, Eckman et al. (1992) compared group SST to a supportive group therapy. SST yielded a slight advantage over supportive therapy in symptom reduction during the first six months, but this may be due to the higher symptoms reported by this group at the outset of treatment. In a well-designed and executed study, Hogarty and colleagues (Hogarty et al., 1986, 1991) evaluated four treatment groups: (i) family psychoeducational treatment, (ii) SST, (iii) family psychoeducational treatment and SST, and (iv) medication only. Relapse rates at the 1-year follow-up were lower in SST (20%) and family psychoeducational treatment (19%) than relapse rates in the medication only group (38%). The effects appeared to be additive, as patients who received both psychosocial treatments had no relapses in the first year. Two-year follow-up data, however, revealed some loss of treatment effectiveness, as relapse rates in the SST group increased compared to the medication only condition (50% vs. 62%, respectively). The family treated groups showed similar relapse rates at the 2-year follow-up (family alone = 29%; family + SST = 25%).

The psychosocial treatment of adolescents with schizophrenia

The literature reviewed above documents both the psychosocial impairment associated with schizophrenia in adolescence and the promise of psychosocial treatment strategies that have been evaluated among adults with schizophrenia. There is an urgent need for additional research to clarify optimal treatment strategies for adolescents with schizophrenia. However, based on the preceding review, several approaches would appear to hold particular promise for adolescents and merit evaluation.

Family interventions

First, the strong evidence supporting the efficacy of psychoeducational family treatments underscores the potential of this approach for adolescents who, by virtue of their developmental stage, are even more dependent on their families than adults. While these family treatments will clearly require adaptation to the developmental level of the adolescent, it may be useful to review five critical issues addressed in psychoeducational family treatments for psychotic patients and strategies for addressing these issues (Goldstein, 1995).

First, patients and families must integrate the psychotic experience. In addressing this issue, therapists review the signs and symptoms of the disorder, encourage each member to share his/her experience of the phenomenology of psychotic experiences, clarify how differences in family members' perceptions of these experiences come about, review the nature of life events that could have served as triggers for the most recent episode, and present the vulnerability-stress model as a system for understanding how psychosis comes about. Secondly, families and patients need to accept vulnerability to future episodes. This process is facilitated by presenting data about probability of recurrence and encouraging expressions of feelings about the possibility of recurrence. Often this involves the use of analogies to other chronic medical disorders, identifying both risk (e.g., drug use, poor coping skills) and protective factors (e.g., medication compliance, social support), and emphasizing ways in which risk and protective factors may be controlled. Thirdly, both patients and family members must accept the patients' dependence on psychotropic medications for symptom control. This issue is addressed in the family psychoeduational approach by presenting information on neurotransmitter models of psychosis, explaining how drugs reduce vulnerability by modifying problematic neurotransmitter states, encouraging discussion of negative side effects and ways of managing them, and encouraging discussion of non-compliance when it occurs so that it can be addressed in the therapy. Fourthly, therapists must help family members and patients to understand the significance of life events as stressors for psychotic relapse. Strategies for addressing this issue include reviewing the stressful life events occurring before each prior episode, having patients and families rank their impact and significance, attempting to identify categories into which stressors might fit (e.g., losses, interpersonal difficulties), helping family members predict which life events are likely to occur, and engaging in anticipatory planning to address these stressors. Finally, families must learn to distinguish ongoing personality traits and styles from signs and symptoms of schizophrenia. Therapists can review the patients prior accomplishments from both the premorbid and intermorbid periods, help them to discriminate normal variations in mood and behavior from prodromal signs, identifying continuities in personality style over the lifespan of the patient, and distinguish between residual psychotic states and individual personality traits. Such issues must be approached with special care among adolescents, where the precursors of psychosis may be difficult to disentangle from the development of other personal qualities. Further, links to theories of etiology and course will have to be adapted to the cognitive level and attention span of the adolescent.

Interventions aimed at promoting social skill and competence

The social skills deficits observed among adolescents with schizophrenia in conjunction with the impairment observed both in premorbid adjustment and in social competence during episodes underscores the need for interventions targeting social skill and competence. Skills building modules such as those developed by Liberman et al. (1986); Liberman (1994); Liberman & Kopelowicz, 1995); Bellack et al. (1984); Bellack and Mueser (1993), as well as Hogarty's "personal therapy" (Hogarty et al., 1995) provide promising examples of this approach. These interventions, which emphasize skill building and developing competencies, should logically lead to decreases in the stresses and strains of daily living. Given research demonstrating that the occurrence of stressful life events is associated with an elevated risk of florid psychotic episodes (e.g. Ventura et al., 1989), one could hypothesize that skills training might both enhance social rehabilitation and decrease the risk of relapse and/or progressive psychosis by reducing the level of environmental stress. Although systematic evaluations of the efficacy of skill building approaches with young populations are urgently needed, many specialized school, hospital, and day treatment programs do target daily living skills such as social skills, stress management, and adaptive behavior (see, for example, Remschmidt et al., 1994). Additional research is clearly needed to evaluate the efficacy of skills training interventions for adolescents with schizophrenia.

Importance of early intervention

Like data with adults, emerging data on child and adolescent samples underscores the social morbidity associated with schizophrenia. There are also some data to support the notion that childhood-onset is associated with a more malignant form of the illness (e.g., Werry et al., 1991). Research with adults further provides some evidence to suggest that early pharmacologic and psychosocial treatments that control psychotic symptoms and keep patients socially active may reduce deterioration and improve outcome (see McGlashan & Johannessen, 1996). For example, recent studies have highlighted the fact that many adults experience relatively lengthy periods of untreated illness around the time of their first episodes. In one study (Johnstone et al., 1996), the mean duration of untreated illness among first episode patients was 151 weeks, and the mean duration of untreated psychosis was 52 weeks. These figures are consistent with Eggers and Bunk's (1997) description of delays between the age of first psychiatric symptoms, age of first psychotic symptoms, and age at first hospitalization. Importantly, however, research with adults indicates that the longer the untreated illness the worse the outcome (for review, see McGlashan & Johannessen, 1996). The mechanisms underlying the apparent decline in treatment responsiveness over time, however, remain to be clarified. From a neurodevelopmental perspective, factors such as neural deterioration and decreased brain plasticity have been postulated (McGlashan & Johannessen, 1996). Alternatively, from a psychosocial perspective, given that untreated illness is associated with deterioration in social functioning and deficits in learning and mastery of social tasks, child and adolescent onset schizophrenia is likely to be associated with a failure to acquire key social skills and to master critical developmental tasks. Thus, a period of untreated illness is likely to lead to developmental disruptions which have a profound impact on the psychosocial adaptation of the adolescent.

These data support the need for early intervention strategies. There are some recent demonstrations of promising early interventions strategies. Most notably, the landmark Buckingham Project conducted by Falloon and colleagues (Falloon et al., 1996) offers a promising approach to prevention and early intervention. By integrating a comprehensive mental health service with an effective primary care program, Falloon et al. developed a screening and consultation program aimed at early detection of individuals showing prodromal symptoms of schizophrenia. An educational program was developed to assist family practitioners in detecting prodromal symptoms and a ten-item screening interview and eight-item prodromal checklist were used to aid family practitioners in screening patients. Mental health service staff were readily accessible for immediate consultation and further evaluation of the patient. A more extensive evaluation was conducted which included systematic interviews such as the Present State Examination (PSE). This evaluation was designed to provide (i) a more comprehensive evaluation of patient symptoms as well as information needed for differential psychiatric diagnosis, (ii) interviews with family members and friends aimed at providing additional information about the patient and assessing the strengths and resources for home-based clinical management, and (iii) assessments of the strengths and vulnerabilities of caregivers and the degree to which they appeared willing and capable of coping with the stress of caring for the identified "patient."

Once a patient was identified, an integrated crisis management plan was individually tailored to the needs of each patient within a clinical management protocol that included three major components. First, within 24 hours of identification an informal psychoeducational seminar was presented to the patient and key caregivers. This seminar provided a rationale for the early intervention program and emphasized positive outcomes, the value of support from family and friends, and the benefits of 24-hour in-home care. Secondly, home-based stress management training was conducted with the goals of identifying stressors and enhancing patient and caregiver coping and problem resolution strategies. Although the level of support was tailored to the stated needs of the patients and caregivers, the behavioral family therapy model (Falloon et al., 1982) was generally employed to further develop communication and problem-solving. Thirdly, where indicated by the presence of clearly identified symptoms likely to respond to medication, the family practitioner was advised to prescribe a minimum effective dose. When used, drug therapy was time limited and generally less than 1 week. Once the patient's prodromal symptoms had remitted, the intensity of treatment was reduced. However, regular weekly in-home meetings were continued as a means of monitoring and bolstering the abilities of the patient and caregivers to cope with existing stresses and problems. The final phase of treatment emphasized recognition of prodromal symptoms and wallet-sized cards were designed that listed one to three signs of a likely prodromal episode as well as procedures for contacting family practitioners and mental health therapists. Periodic mental health monitoring was continued over a 24-month period, with booster sessions as needed. Patients were returned to routine monitoring by the family practitioner when they had been free of psychiatric symptoms and disability for 24 months.

The Falloon et al. (1996) study was essentially an open trial, and there are no data on outcome among individuals who were identified and not treated using the prevention protocol. However, the annual incidence of first episodes of schizophrenia in Buckingham County during the 4 years of the project was markedly lower, 0.75 per 100 000, than the annual incidence rate of 7.4 per 100 000 during 1974 and 1975. Although these results need to be interpreted with caution due to the design and case finding limitations of the study (see Falloon et al., 1996; McGlashan, 1996; McGlashan & Johannessen, 1996), the Buckingham Project provides an exciting example of one approach to early intervention and prevention of the devastating cycle of dysfunction and deterioration experienced by all too many victims of schizophrenia. This approach could be extended to younger populations and adapted for the needs of adolescent showing prodromal signs of schizophrenia.

Conclusions

In conclusion, the research reviewed above demonstrates that adolescents suffering from schizophenia show early social impairments that often lead to rejection by peers, difficulties in school, and stress on family members. Major advances have been made in knowledge regarding the efficacy of alternative psychosocial strategies for the treatment of schizophrenia among adults. In this chapter, we have discussed several promising approaches to the psychosocial treatment of adult schizophrenia that merit evaluation for adolescents. These include (i) family interventions emphasizing psychoeducation and coping skills, (ii) individual and group interventions designed to build skills and competencies, and (iii) early intervention strategies. Common features shared by these interventions include a focus on the present, an emphasis on promoting the patient's gradual reintegration into the family and community, and the reorganization of family and community resources to facilitate the management of the illness. Given the absence of controlled trials of psychosocial interventions for adolescents with schizophrenia, a major question that needs to be addressed is whether psychosocial treatment strategies that have proved efficacious for adults with schizophrenia will also prove effective for adolescents struggling with this disorder.

Recent years have also witnessed advances in knowledge regarding optimal pharmacotherapy for adolescents with schizophrenia. Current data support the importance of pharmacotherapy in the treatment of adolescent with schizophrenia (Kumra et al., 1996; Remschmidt et al., 1994; Spencer & Campbell, 1994; Spencer et al., 1992). However, there are still relatively few controlled trials of medication for schizophrenia in adolescents, complete remission of schizophrenic symptoms and associated disabilities is rare, and extant data suggest that adolescents may be sensitive to the adverse effects of neuroleptics (e.g., extrapyramidal side effects, weight gain, galactorrhea) as well as clozapine (e.g., neutropenia, seizures). This underscores the importance of integrated multicomponent treatment approaches that include both pharmacologic and psychosocial components. Future research is urgently needed to clarify optimal strategies for combining psychosocial and pharmacologic treatment strategies for adolescents.

Finally, current trends in the organization of services for adolescents with mental disorders has emphasized community and in-home care, as efforts have been made to treat adolescents within the least restrictive setting. Various models have been promoted for organizing treatment services including (i) family preservation which emphasizes time-limited in-home and community interventions aimed at mobilizing resources for treating the adolescent within his/her family and community (e.g., Henggeler, Melton & Smith, 1992), (ii) comprehensive coordinated systems of care that emphasize interagency collaboration and service integration in the treatment of disturbed adolescents (Stroul & Friedman, 1996), and (iii) wrap-around services where child and family teams are developed to identify those treatment services (medication, psychosocial treatment, school placement) and community resources (child care, respite care, community support) that are most likely to maximize recovery and rehabilitation within the community (VanDenBerg & Grealish, 1996). These models share an emphasis on the need to find creative ways to organize services to meet the complex needs of severely disturbed adolescents. Adolescents with schizophrenia rank among our most severely disturbed and impaired adolescents. They will clearly represent frequent utilizers of mental health services and will require a complex array of services (e.g., medication, therapy, school, skills training). In the past, adolescents with schizophrenia and SPD have tended to be frequent utilizers of inpatient and residential care (Asarnow et al., 1988b) and residential care is associated with a high rate of replacement in residential settings (Asarnow et al., 1996). The current shift to community-based care and decreased availability of residential beds will clearly require changes in the way we care for adolescents with schizophrenia. Future research is needed to clarify the advantages and disadvantages of these different approaches to service delivery, as well as to identify optimal strategies for organizing services for adolescents with schizophrenia.

Acknowledgment

This chapter is dedicated to Michael J. Goldstein. He was a beloved colleague, mentor, and friend. His work inspired efforts to understand how families could aid in the prevention and treatment of schizophrenia and other major mental disorders.

REFERENCES

Anonymous (1994). First person account: Schizophrenia with childhood onset. *Schizophrenia Bulletin*, **20**, 587–90.

Asarnow, J.R. (1994). Annotation: childhood-onset schizophrenia. *Journal of Child Psychology and Psychiatry*, **35**, 1345–71.

Asarnow, J.R. & Horton, A.A. (1990). Coping and stress in families of child psychiatric inpatients:

parents of children with depressive and schizophrenia spectrum disorders. *Child Psychiatry and Human Development*, **21**, 145–57.

Asarnow, J.R., Goldstein, M.J., & Ben-Meir, S. (1988a). Parental communication deviance in childhood onset schizophrenia spectrum and depressive disorders. *Journal of Child Psychology and Psychiatry*, **29**, 825–38.

Asarnow, J.R., Goldstein, M.J., Carlson, G.A., Perdue, S., Bates, S., & Keller, J. (1988b). Child-onset depressive disorders: a follow-up study of rates of rehospitalization and out of home placement among child psychiatric inpatients. *Journal of Affective Disorders*, **15**, 245–53.

Asarnow, J.R., Tompson, M., & Goldstein, M.J. (1994a). Childhood-onset schizophrenia: a follow-up study. *Schizophrenia Bulletin*, **20**, 599–618.

Asarnow, J.R., Tompson, M., Hamilton, E.B., Goldstein, M.J. & Guthrie, D. (1994b). Family-expressed emotion, childhood-onset depression, and childhood-onset schizophrenia spectrum disorders: is expressed emotion a nonspecific correlate of child psychopathology or a specific risk factor for depression? *Journal of Abnormal Child Psychology*, **22**, 129–46.

Asarnow, J.R., Aoki, W., & Elson, S. (1996). Children in residential treatment: a follow-up study. *Journal of Clinical Child Psychology*, **25**, 209–14.

Bellack, A.S. & Mueser, K.T. (1993). Psychosocial treatment for schizophrenia. *Schizophrenia Bulletin*, **19**, 317–36.

Bellack, A.S., Turner, S.M., Hersen, M., & Luber, R.F. (1984). An examination of the efficacy of social skills training for chronic schizophrenic patients. *Hospital and Community Psychiatry*, **35**, 1023–8.

Benton, M.K. & Schroeder, H.E. (1990). Social skills training with schizophrenics: a meta-analytical evaluation. *Journal of Consulting and Clinical Psychology*, **58**(6), 741–7.

Bradshaw, W.H. (1993). Coping-skills training versus a problem-solving approach with schizophrenic patients. *Hospital-and-Community-Psychiatry*, **44**(11), 1102–4.

Cozolino, L.J., Goldstein, M.J., Nuechterlein, K.H., West, K.L., & Snyder, K.S. (1988). The impact of education about schizophrenia on relatives varying in expressed emotion. *Schizophrenia Bulletin*, **14**, 675–87.

Eckman, T.A., Wirshing, W.C., Marder, S.R., Liberman, R.P., Johnston-Cronk, K., Zimmermann, K., & Mintz, J. (1992). Technique for training schizophrenic patients in illness self-management: a controlled trial. *American Journal of Psychiatry*, **149**, 1549–55.

Eggers, C. & Bunk, D. (1997). The long-term course of childhood-onset schizophrenia: a 42-year follow-up. *Schizophrenia Bulletin*, **23**, 105–17.

Falloon, I.R.H., Boyd, J.L., & McGill, C.W. (1982). Family management in the prevention of exacerbation of schizophrenia: a controlled study. New England Journal of Medicine, **306**, 1437–40.

Falloon, I.R.H., Boyd, J.L., McGill, C.W., Williamson, M., Razani, J., Moss, H.B., Gilderman, A.M., & Simpson, G.M. (1985). Family management in the prevention of morbidity of schizophrenia: clinical outcome of a two-year longitudinal study. *Archives of General Psychiatry*, **42**, 887–986.

Falloon, I.R.H., Kydd, R.R., Coverdale, J.H., & Laidlaw, T.M. (1996). Early detection and intervention for initial episodes of schizophrenia. *Schizophrenia Bulletin*, **22**, 271–82.

Goldstein, M.J. (1995). Psychoeducation and relapse prevention. *International Clinical Psychopharmacology*, **9**(Suppl. 5), 59–69.

Goldstein, M.J. & Miklowitz, D.J. (1995). The effectiveness of psychoeducational family therapy in the treatment of schizophrenic disorders. *Journal of Marital and Family Therapy*, **21**(4), 361–76.

Goldstein, M.J., Rodnick, E.H., Evans, J.R., May, P.R.A., & Steinberg, M. (1978). Drug and family therapy in the aftercare of acute schizophrenia. *Archives of General Psychiatry*, **35**, 1169–77.

Gunderson, J.g., Frank, A.F., Katz, H.M., Vannicelli, M.L., Frosch, J.P., & Knapp, P.H. (1984). Effects of psychotherapy in schizophrenia: II. Comparative outcome of two forms of treatment. *Schizophrenia Bulletin*, **10**, 564–96.

Hamilton, E.B., Asarnow, J.R. & Tompson, M.C. (1997). Social, academic, and behavioral competence of depressed children: relationship to diagnostic status and family interaction style. *Journal of Youth and Adolescence*, **26**, 77–87.

Henggeler, S.W., Melton, G.B., & Smith, L.A. (1992). Family preservation using multisystemic therapy: an effective alternative to incarcerating serious juvenile offenders. *Journal of Consulting and Clinical Psychology*, **60**, 953–61.

Hogarty, G.E., Anderson, C.M., Reiss, D.J., Kornblith, S.J., Greenwald, D.P., Javna, C.D., Madonia, M.J., & the EPICS Schizophrenia Research Group (1986). Family psychoeducation, social skills training and maintenance chemotherapy in the aftercare treatment of schizophrenia: I. One-year effects of a controlled study on relapse and expressed emotion. *Archives of General Psychiatry*, **43**, 633–42.

Hogarty, G.E., Anderson, C.M., Reiss, D.J. Kornblith, S.J., Greenwald, D.P., Ulrich, R.F., & Carter, M. (1991). Family psychoeducation, social skills training, and maintenance chemotherapy in the aftercare of schizophrenia II. Two-year effects of a controlled study on relapse and adjustment. *Archives of General Psychiatry*, **4**, 340–7.

Hogarty, G.E., Kornblith, S.J., Greenwald, D., DiBarry, A.L., Cooley, S., Flesher, S., Reiss, D., Carter, M., & Ulrich, R. (1995). Personal therapy: a disorder-relevant psychotherapy for schizophrenia. *Schizophrenia Bulletin*, **21**(3), 379–93.

Johnstone, E.C., Connelly, J., Frith, C.D., Lambert, M.T. Owens, D.G. (1996). The nature of "transient" and "partial" psychoses: findings from the Northwick Park "Functional" Psychosis Study. *Psychological Medicine*, **26**(2), 361–9.

Kavanagh, D.J. (1992). Recent developments in expressed emotion and schizophrenia. *British Journal of Psychiatry*, **160**, 601–20.

Kumra, S., Frazier, J., Jacobsen, L., McKenna, K., Gordon, C.T., Lenane, M., Hamburger, S., Smith, A., Albus, K. Alaghband-Rad, J., & Rapoport, J.L. (1996). Childhood-onset schizophrenia: a double blind clozapine-haloperidol comparison. *Archives of General Psychiatry*, **53**, 1090–7.

Leff, J. & Vaughn, C. (1985). *Expressed Emotion in Families: Its Significance for Mental Illness*. New York: Guilford Press.

Leff, J., Kuipers, L., Berkowitz, R., Eberlein-Fries, R., & Sturgeon, D. (1982). A controlled trial of social intervention in the families of schizophrenic patients. *British Journal of Psychiatry*, **141**, 77–80.

Leff, J., Berkowitz, R., Shavit, N., Strachan, A., Glass, I., & Vaughn, C. (1989). A trial of family therapy v. a relatives group for schizophrenia. British Journal of Psychiatry, **154**, 58–66.

Liberman, R.P. (1994). Psychosocial treatments for schizophrenia. Psychiatry, **57**, 104–14.

Liberman, R.P. & Kopelowicz, A. (1995). Basic elements in biobehavioral treatment and rehabilitation of schizophrenia. International Clinical Psychopharmacology, **9**(Suppl. 5), 51–8.

Liberman, R.P., Mueser, K.T., Wallace, C.J., Jacobs, H.E., Eckman, T., & Massel, H.K. (1986). Training skills in psychiatrically disabled: learning coping and competence. Schizophrenia Bulletin, **12**, 631–47.

Linszen, D.(1993). Recent onset schizophrenic disorders: outcome, prognosis and treatment. Unpublished doctoral dissertation, University of Amsterdam, Netherlands.

Lovejoy, M. (1982). Expectations and the recovery process. Schizophrenia Bulletin, **8**, 605–9.

McFarlane, W.R., Lukens, E., Link, B., Dushay, R., Deakins, S.A., Newmark, M., Dunne, E.J., Horen, B., & Toran, J. (1995). Multiple family groups and psychoeducation in the treatment of schizophrenia. Archives of General Psychiatry, **52**, 679–87.

McGlashan, T.K. (1996). Early detection and intervention in schizophrenia: research. Schizophrenia Bulletin, **22**(2), 327–45.

McGlashan, T.H. & Johannessen, J.O. (1996). Eartly detection and intervention with schizophrenia: Rationale. Schizophrenia Bulletin, **22**, 201–22.

Miklowitz, D.J., Goldstein, M.J., Doane, J.A., Nuechterlein, K.H., Strachan, A.M., Snyder, K.S., & Magana, A.M. (1989). Is expressed emotion an index of a transactional process? I. Relative's affective style. Family Process, **28**, 153–67.

Mueser, K.T. & Berenbaum, H. (1990). Psychodynamic treatment of schizophrenia: is there a future? Psychological Medicine, **20**, 253–62.

Randolph, E.T., Eth, S., Glynn, S.M., Paz, G.G., Leong, G.B., Shaner, A.L., Strachan, A., Van Vort, W., Escobar, J.I., & Liberman, R.P. (1994). Behavioral family management in schizophrenia: outcome of a clinic-based intervention. British Journal of Psychiatry, **164**, 501–6.

Remschmidt, H.E., Schulz, E., Martin, M., Warnke, A., & Trott, G.E. (1994). Childhood-onset schizophrenia: history of the concept and recent studies. Schizophrenia Bulletin, **20**, 727–46.

Rockland, L.H. (1993). A review of supportive psychotherapy, 1986–92. Hospital and Community Psychiatry, **44**(11), 1053–60.

Schooler, N., Keith, S., Severe, J., Matthews, S., Bellack, A., Glick, I., Hargreaves, W., Kane, J., Ninan, P., Frances, A., Jacobs, M., Lieberman, J., Mance, R., Simpson, & G., Woerner, M.(1997). Relapse and rehospitalization during maintenance treatment of schizophrenia. Archives of General Psychiatry, **54**, 453–63.

Scott, J.E. & Dixon, L.B. (1995). Psychological interventions for schizophrenia. Schizophrenia Bulletin, **21**, 621–30.

Spencer, E.K. & Campbell, M. (1994). Children with schizophrenia: diagnosis, phenomenology, and pharmacotherapy. Schizophrenia Bulletin, **20**, 713–26.

Spencer, E.K., Kafantaris, V., Padron-Gayol, M.V., Rosenberg, C.R., & Campbell, M. (1992). Haloperidol in schizophrenic children: Early findings from a study in progress. Psychopharmacology Bulletin, **28**(2), 183–6.

Stanton, A.J., Gunderson, J.G., Knapp, P.H., Frank, A.F., Vannicelli, M.L., Schnitzer, R., &

Rosenthal, R. (1984). Effects of psychotherapy in schizophrenia: I. Design and implementation of a controlled study. *Schizophrenia Bulletin*, **10**, 520–51.

Stroul, B.A. & Friedman, R.M. (1996). The system of care concept and philosophy. In *Children's Mental Health: Creating Systems of Care in a Changing Society*, ed. B.A. Stroul & R.M. Friedman. Baltimore, MD: Paul H. Brookes.

Tarrier, N., Barrowclough, C., Vaughn, C., Bamrah, J.S., Porceddu, K., Watts, S., & Freeman, H. (1988). The community management of schizophrenia: a controlled trial of a behavioral intervention with families to reduce relapse. *British Journal of Psychiatry*, **153**, 532–42.

Tompson, M.C., Asarnow, J.R., Hamilton, E.B., Newell, L.E., & Goldstein, M.J. (1997). Children with schizophrenia-spectrum disorders: thought disorder and communication problems in a family interactional context. *Journal of Child Psychology and Psychiatry*, **38**, 421–9.

VanDenBerg, J.E. & Grealish, E.M. (1996). Individualized services and supports through the wraparound process: philosophy and procedures. *Journal of Child and Family Studies*, **5**, 7–21.

Ventura, J., Nuechterlein, K.H., Lukoff, D., & Hardesty, J. (1989). A prospective study of stressful life events and schizophrenic relapse. *Journal of Abnormal Psychology*, **98**, 407–11.

Werry, J.S., McClellan, J.M., & Chard, L. (1991). Childhood and adolescent schizophrenic, bipolar, and schizoaffective disorders: a clinical and outcome study. *Journal of the American Academy of Child and Adolescent Psychiatry*, **30**, 457–65.

Zeitlin, H. (1986). *The Natural History of Psychiatric Disorder in Children*. Institute of Psychiatry Maudsley Monographs, 29. Oxford: Oxford University Press.

9

Treatment and rehabilitation

Helmut Remschmidt, Matthias Martin, Klaus Hennighausen, and Eberhard Schulz

Neuroleptic (antipsychotic) agents and their properties

Typical or classical neuroleptics are agents with an antipsychotic effect that have been introduced into clinical practice since the antipsychotic effect of chlorpromazine was detected (Delay et al., 1952). In consequence of this discovery, several other neuroleptics (high potency typical neuroleptics) were developed that had stronger antipsychotic properties, mainly on productive (positive) symptoms, but had no advantage according to the improvement of negative schizophrenic symptoms. At the same time they caused more severe extrapyramidal side effects (EPS) such as acute dystonia, parkinsonism, akathisia, and tardive dyskinesia. These observations led to the hypothesis that the antipsychotic efficacy is closely related to the development of EPS. The introduction of these classical, high potentcy, neuroleptics was a revolution in the treatment of schizophrenia and related disorders. It was soon revealed that, in spite of a good effect in the majority of schizophrenic cases, between 30 and 40% of the patients did not respond to the neuroleptic medication mainly caused by the persistence of negative schizophrenic symptoms. These so-called non-responders or pharmaco-resistant patients are still an enormous problem in clinical psychiatry. The reported rate of non-responders in adult psychiatry is similar to that found in child and adolescent psychiatry, where about 40% of the children and adolescents with schizophrenia do not respond to classical neuroleptic medication (Remschmidt, 1993a,b). A new era of pharmacological treatment has been opened up with the introduction of atypical antipsychotics such as clozapine. Up to 60% of non-responders to typical neuroleptics improved under clozapine. In the reduction of productive symptoms, atypical neuroleptics are comparable to classical neuroleptics (Kahn et al., 1993). Additionally, they are more effective according to the improvement of negative symptoms, and their antipsychotic properties are not linked to EPS (i.e., causing fewer EPS while having the same or even better efficacy).

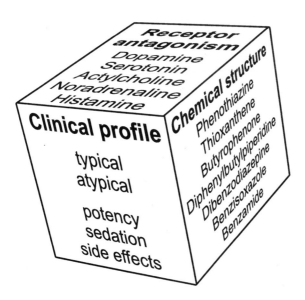

Fig. 9.1. Dimensions for the classification of neuroleptic agents.

Classification of neuroleptics

Neuroleptic (antipsychotic) agents can be classified according to three main principles: chemical structure, receptor binding profile and clinical profile. The clinical profile covers several areas of action such as neuroleptic potency, sedation, side effects, but also some aspects of interaction with the central nervous system receptors. This has led to the classification of neuroleptics into two groups: typical and atypical neuroleptics. Typical or classical neuroleptics have been found to be effective mainly in the positive symptoms of schizophrenia and cause extrapyramidal side effects (EPS). Both effects have been attributed to their high dopamine receptor antagonism (esp. D_2). In contrast, atypical neuroleptics have a different receptor affinity pattern, targeting not only dopamine receptors but also serotoninergic, alpha-adrenergic, muscarinic and histaminergic receptors (see Fig. 9.2). The alternative classifications are demonstrated in Fig. 9.1, which will be the basis for the following description of the neuroleptic treatment in child and adolescent schizophrenia.

Chemical structure

Chemical structure should not be the major feature for the classification of neuroleptics, because for many substances, there is no clear relationship between the chemical structure and the clinical action profile. The history of the development of neuroleptics is interesting, but demonstrates very clearly

Table 9.1. Major neuroleptic compounds classified according to their chemical substance classes

Chemical class	Compound	Brand name
Phenothiazines		
– Aliphatic	Chlorpromazine	*Megaphen*®[D], *Thorazine*®[CAN, US], *Largactil*®[UK, F]
	Levomepromazine = Methotrimeprazine	*Neurocil*®[D], *Nozinan*®[UK, CAN, US, F, Be, It, Ch, NL], *Levoprome*®[US]
	Promethazine	*Atosil*®[D], *Phenergan*®[US, UK, Be, Ch, NL]
– Piperidines	Thioridazine	*Melleril*®[D, UK, US, F, Be, NL, Ch, It], *Mellaril*®[CAN, US]
– Piperazines	Perphenazine	*Decentan*®[D, It], *Trilafon*®[CAN, US, Be, NL, Ch], *Fentazin*®[UK], *Etrafon*®[CAN, US], *Trilafan*®[F]
	Fluphenazine (-Decanoate)	*Lyogen*®[D], *Dapotum*®[D], *Prolixin*®[CAN, US], *Permitil*®[CAN, US], *Modecate*®[UK, CAN]
	Perazine	*Taxilan*®[D]
Thioxanthenes	Flupent(h)ixol (-Decanoate)	*Fluanxol*®[D, CAN, US, F, Ch], *Depixol*®[UK]
	Chlorprothixene	*Truxal*®[D], *Taractan*®[D, US, F]
Butyrophenones	Haloperidol (-Decanoate)	*Haldol*[D, UK, US, CAN, F, Ch, NL, Be, It, Is, Port], *Haldol-Decanoat(e)*®[D, UK, US, F, It, Ch]
	Benperidol	*Glianimon*®[D], *Anquil*®[UK], *Frenactil*[F, Be]
	Pipamperone	*Dipiperon*®[D, F, Ch, NL, Be]
Diphenylbutylpiperidines	Pimozide	*Orap*[D, UK, US, CAN, F], *Opiran*®[F]
	Fluspirilene	*Imap*®[D], *Redeptin*®[UK]
Dibenzodiazepines	Clozapine	*Leponex*®[D, F, Be], *Clozaril*[UK, US, CAN]
(Thieno-)Benzodiazepines	Olanzapine	*Zyprexa*®[D, UK, US, CAN]
Dibenzothiepines	Zotepine	*Nipolept*®[D], *Lodpin*[Jap]
Dibenzothiazepines	Quetiapine fumarate	*Seroquel*®[UK, US, CAN]
Benzisoxazoles	Risperidone	*Risperdal*®[D, UK, US, CAN, F]
Benzamides	Sulpiride	*Dogmatil*®[D, F, Be, NL, E, Jap], *Dolmatil*®[UK], *Sulpitil*®[UK]
	Tiapride	*Tiapridex*®[D], *Equilium*®[F], *Tiapridal*®[F, Be]

The following abbreviations are used to indicate in which country the compound is available under the given brand name: Be=Belgium, CAN=Canada, Ch=Switzerland, D=Germany, E=Spain, F=France, It=Italy, Is=Iceland, Jap=Japan, NL=The Netherlands, Port=Portugal, UK=United Kingdom, US=United States of America.

that many of these compounds were discovered by chance and not by systematic chemical experiment. Nevertheless, the development of modern atypical neuroleptics shows that systematic alterations of heterotricyclic compounds may be successful, as demonstrated by the development of clozapine and olanzapine. Classification according to chemical structure usually distinguishes several groups, shown in Table 9.1. Of course, both the receptor binding pattern and the clinical profile depend on the chemical structure of the compound, but properties other than the chemical structure class have a higher relevance for classification. For the purposes of treatment, we found that the classification of typical and atypical neuroleptics is the most useful one and this is therefore used in this chapter with a subdivision into a subgroup with high neuroleptic potency and another subgroup showing moderate or low neuroleptic potency.

Receptor binding and clinical profile

The receptor binding profile is essential for the pharmacological action and for the clinical efficacy of all neuroleptic agents. Fig. 9.2 gives an overview of the receptor binding profile of the most important neuroleptic (antipsychotic) compounds, subdivided into the three groups: typical high-potency neuroleptics, typical moderate and low-potency neuroleptics, and atypical neuroleptics covering five relatively newly developed compounds.

Typical and atypical neuroleptics

As far as the mechanism of action is concerned, all neuroleptics were thought to function according to the dopamine hypothesis of schizophrenia (Van Rossum, 1966), which postulated a hyperactivity of central dopaminergic neurotransmission that could be blocked by the dopamine receptor antagonism of neuroleptic agents. According to this theory, based on the observation that all neuroleptic agents were functioning in this way, the existence of EPS was thought to be a necessary condition for the antipsychotic effects of neuroleptics. This hypothesis provided an animal model for developing new substances and testing their antipsychotic properties (e.g., the apomorphine test, induction of catalepsy). Moreover, the dose–response relationships in animals provided information about the likely clinical dose range for patients. Consequently, the search for new neuroleptic agents followed the line of extrapyramidal side effects. This was indeed successful but accordingly restricted the development of new neuroleptic agents to only one type – dopamine receptor antagonists.

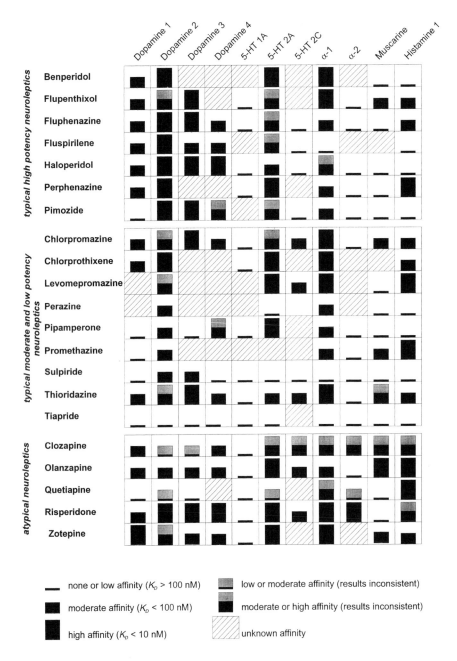

Fig. 9.2. Radioreceptor binding profiles (adapted from Arima et al., 1986; Bymaster et al., 1996; Degner & Rüther, 1998; Ebert, 1997 Kretschmar & Stille, 1995; Leysen et al., 1988; Schotte et al., 1995; Seeman, 1993; Sokoloff et al., 1992; Van Tol et al., 1991). In-between affinities (e.g., moderate to high affinity) indicate that some studies found a moderate affinity and others a high affinity.

Typical high potency neuroleptics
This group covers several chemically different compounds and is characterized by a high affinity to D_2 receptors, a moderate affinity to D_1 receptors, some of the compounds also showing high or moderate affinity to D_3 and D_4 receptors. As far as the receptors of the serotoninergic system are concerned, this group is characterized by a moderate to high affinity to 5-HT_{2A} receptors, a low affinity to other 5-HT receptors and a moderate to high affinity to $alpha_1$ receptors, which is associated with autonomic side effects such as hypotension and tachycardia. Some compounds, such as perphenazine, fluphenazine, and flupenthixol, are characterized by a moderate to high affinity to the $histamine_1$ receptor, which is associated with the effects of sedation and weight gain.

Typical moderate and low potency neuroleptics
The main difference of this group of neuroleptics in comparison to the typical high-potency neuroleptics is their lower affinity to D_1 and D_2 receptors. Additionally, a somewhat higher affinity to $alpha_1$ receptors, and for some compounds a moderate or high affinity to histamine receptors can also be found. In comparison with the typical high-potency neuroleptics, these compounds are characterized clinically by a lower rate of extrapyramidal reactions, more pronounced sedation and increased anticholinergic side effects. However, there are remarkable differences between the different compounds in their receptor binding (Fig. 9.2) as well as in their clinical profile (Table 9.2).

Atypical neuroleptics
These have a receptor profile different from both groups of typical neuroleptics. The relation of dopaminergic to serotoninergic affinity (and others) as well as the relation of D_2 to D_4 receptor affinity has been proposed as being responsible for their different clinical action, characterized by a very low rate of extrapyramidal side effects, and moderate to low sedation effects. Clozapine was originally not thought to have an antipsychotic efficacy because of the absence of extrapyramidal side effects. Its now well-established antipsychotic efficacy was termed as atypical with respect to the above-mentioned dopamine hypothesis of schizophrenia. The different receptor profile involving the dopaminergic, serotoninergic, glutaminergic, and alpha-adrenergic systems led to new considerations and hypotheses on the etiology of schizophrenia (Kornhuber & Weller, 1994). For compounds that were considered to act according to this different mechanism, the term "atypical neuroleptics" was introduced.

Table 9.2. Effects of neuroleptics

	Sedation	Anticholinergic reaction	Extrapyramidal reaction	Positive symptoms	Negative symptoms	Neuroleptic potency	Usual oral dose (usual depot dose i.m.)
Typical high potency neuroleptics							
Benperidol	+	+	++(+)	++	++	100	1–6 mg/day
Flupenthixol	+	+	++(+)	++	++	50	2–10 mg/day
(-decanoate)							(20–100 mg/2–4 weeks)
Fluphenazine	+(+)	+	+++	+++	++	30	5–20 mg/day
(-decanoate)							(12.5–100 mg/2–4 weeks)
Fluspirilene	+	+	+++	+++	++	300	(2–10 mg/week)[a]
Haloperidol	+	+	+++	+++	++	60	2–20 mg/day
(-decanoate)							(50–300 mg/2–4 weeks)
Perphenazine	++	+(+)	++(+)	+++	++	8	12–64 mg/day
(-enanthate)							(50–200 mg/2 weeks)
Pimozide	+	+	+++	+++	++	50	4–20 mg/day
Typical moderate and low potency neuroleptics							
Chlorpromazine	+++	+++	++	+++	++	1	150–600 mg/day
Chlorprothixene	+++	+++	+(+)	+(+)	++	0.8	150–600 mg/day
Levomepromazine	+++	+++	+(+)	++	++	0.8	75–600 mg/day
Perazine	++	++(+)	+	++	++	0.5	75–600 mg/day
Pipamperone	++	+	+			0.2	120–360 mg/day
Promethazine	+++	+++	+				50–400 mg/day
Sulpiride	+	+(+)	+(+)	++	+++	0.5	100–800 mg/day

Thioridazine	+++	+++	+(+)	++	0.7	200–700 mg/day
Tiapride	+	+	+	+		300–600 mg/day
Atypical neuroleptics						
Clozapine	+++	+++	+	+++	(0.5–2)	25–600 mg/day
Olanzapine	++	++	+	+++	(8–20)	5–20 mg/day
Quetiapine	+(+)	+	+(+)	+++		150–750 mg/day
Risperidone	+	+	+	+++	(5)	1–12 mg/day
Zotepine	++	++	+(+)	+++	(2)	75–300 mg/day

+ none or low.

++ moderate.

+++ high.

[a] available only as depot neuroleptic.

(Adapted from Arvanitis & Miller (1997); Baldessarini (1996); Beasley et al. (1997); Benkert & Hippius (1996); Berner & Schönbeck (1987); Bezchlibnyk-Butler & Jeffries (1991); Casey (1997); Claus et al. (1992); Degner & Rüther (1998); Demisch & Staib (1994); Frangos et al. (1978); Kaplan & Sadock (1994); Kretzschmar & Stille (1995); Petit et al. (1996); Remschmidt (1992); Schönhofer & Schwabe (1992); Tamminga et al. (1997).

These atypical neuroleptics include a group of chemically different compounds, characterized by the following properties:

– a different receptor binding profile as compared with classical neuroleptics (relatively lower binding to dopamine receptors in comparison to 5-HT$_{2A}$ and alpha$_1$ receptors), which is claimed to be responsible for a different action;
– low extrapyramidal side effects as a consequence of this receptor profile;
– efficacy also with regard to negative symptoms in contrast to classical neuroleptics;
– absence of hyperprolactinemia.

However, the homogeneity of the group is to be considered as preliminary. As can be seen in Figs. 9.2 and 9.3 and in Table 9.2, there are some marked differences between the compounds according to their receptor binding profiles, therapeutic effects, and side effects.

Indications and contraindications

Indications

The use of typical neuroleptics has been proposed for a wide range of diagnoses and conditions. We therefore restrict this paragraph to those indications that are closely related to the antipsychotic properties. In this context there exist the following indications:

– acute treatment of schizophrenic disorders;
– maintenance treatment and relapse prevention of schizophrenic disorders;
– acute treatment and maintenance treatment of schizo-affective disorders;
– treatment of organic and symptomatic mental disorders with psychotic features;
– treatment of mental and behavioral disorders due to psychoactive and other substance use.

Further indications for neuroleptics include acute treatment of manic episodes and bipolar affective disorders, maintenance treatment of bipolar affective disorders when lithium and anticonvulsants (carbamazepine and valproate) have failed, pervasive developmental disorders, Gilles de la Tourette's syndrome, tic disorders, mental retardation, self-injurious behavior, motion sickness and preparation for anesthesia.

Contraindications

Contraindications for the use of neuroleptics include acute intoxications with sedative agents (antidepressants, analgesics, hypnotics, tranquilizers), and alcohol. Patients with leukopenia should not be medicated with tricyclic neuroleptics (mainly clozapine). If drugs with high anticholinergic properties are used, pylorus stenosis, glaucoma and prostatic hypertrophy must be excluded. Parkinson's syndrome, seizures, allergic reactions, diseases of the hematological system, hypotension or cardiovascular diseases, liver and kidney diseases, prolactin-dependent tumors, asthma or bronchospasm and pheochromocytoma are further restrictions.

Special considerations for atypical neuroleptics

The main indications for atypical neuroleptics are the acute and maintenance treatment of schizophrenic disorders with an emphasis on the treatment of refractory and chronic schizophrenic disorders. However, due to the lower risk of extrapyramidal side effects such as tardive dyskinesias, there is a tendency to a wider range of indications for some of the atypical neuroleptics. Favorable effects in drug-induced psychoses have been demonstrated for olanzapine. Clozapine is effective in the treatment and relapse prevention of manic episodes and bipolar disorders. However, these states and disorders have not yet been established as therapeutic indications. This is likely to occur, however, in the near future.

Receptor binding and clinical profiles

Typical neuroleptics

As demonstrated in Fig. 9.2, typical neuroleptics are subclassified into high neuroleptic potency groups with accordingly high D_2 receptor affinity and a moderate to low neuroleptic potency group that has also a relative high affinity to the D_2 receptors. The high affinity to D_2 receptors is responsible for a high rate of extrapyramidal side effects such as acute dystonia, parkinsonism, akathisia, and tardive dyskinesia. Table 9.3 demonstrates the pharmacological and behavioral effects with regard to receptor binding. As this table demonstrates, receptor blockade of the D_2 receptors in the mesolimbic–mesocortical system leads to a reduction of positive symptoms in schizophrenia, whereas blockade of the D_2 receptors in the nigro-striatal system causes the extrapyramidal motoric side effects (EPS). A further characteristic of all typical or classical neuroleptics is hyperprolactinemia, which is caused by D_2 receptor blockade in the tubero-infundibular system. The antiemetic effect, in contrast, is caused by receptor blockade of the D_2 receptors in the postrema area. It can be concluded that the D_2 receptor blockade in different areas of the brain has different pharmacological and behavioral effects.

Table 9.3. Profile-linked effects

Receptor blockade	Effects
D_1	Reduction of aggression and self-injury
D_2 (mesolimbic–mesocortical system)	Reduction of productive symptoms in schizophrenia
D_2 (nigro-striatal system)	EPS
D_2 (tubero-infundibular system)	Gynaecomastia, galactorrhea
D_2 (hypothalamic system)	Hypothermia
D_2 (Postrema area)	Antiemetic
D_4	Reduction of productive and negative symptoms in schizophrenia, no EPS
5-HT_{1A}	Increase in heart rate and respiratory rate, decrease in blood pressure
5-HT_{2A}	Reduction of negative symptoms in schizophrenia, Reduction of EPS, weight gain
5-HT_{2C}	Antiparkinsonian effects
$\alpha 1$	Autonomic side effects (e.g., hypotension, tachycardia); sedation
$\alpha 2$	Vasodilatation, fall in blood pressure, increased noradrenaline release
Muscarinic	Reduction of EPS, pharmacologically induced delirium
H_1	Somnolence, sedation, weight gain

Adapted from Breese et al. (1990); DiFrancesco (1994); Fox et al. (1998); Göthert et al. (1996); Janssen & Awouters (1995); Rang & Dale (1991).

Table 9.2 demonstrates the overall actions of the three groups of neuroleptics in three domains: sedation, anticholinergic actions and extrapyramidal reactions. Typical high-potency neuroleptics show the most pronounced extrapyramidal reactions, with low anticholinergic and sedative effects. Typical moderate and low-potency neuroleptics are characterized by a high degree of sedation and anticholinergic side effects. As can also be seen in Fig. 9.3, there are remarkable differences between the different compounds, but there is also a more or less general characteristic which applies to all of the compounds grouped together.

Atypical neuroleptics

As Fig. 9.2 demonstrates, the receptor binding profile of the five atypical neuroleptics is mainly characterized by a higher $5\text{-HT}_2/D_2$ binding ratio in comparison with classical neuroleptics. This profile is responsible for their

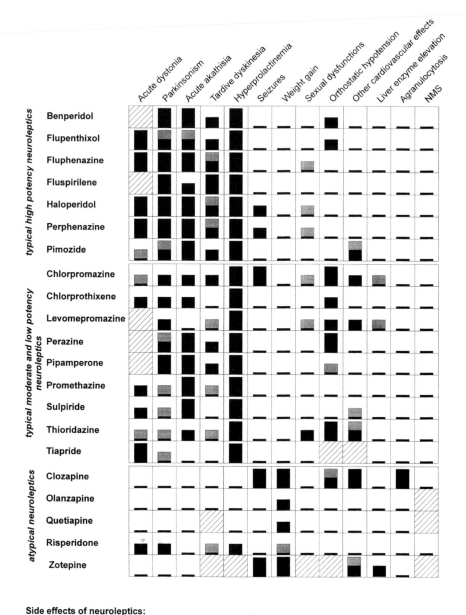

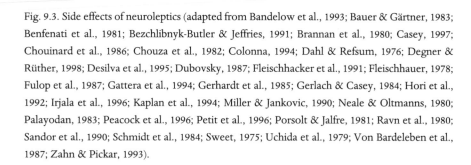

Fig. 9.3. Side effects of neuroleptics (adapted from Bandelow et al., 1993; Bauer & Gärtner, 1983; Benfenati et al., 1981; Bezchlibnyk-Butler & Jeffries, 1991; Brannan et al., 1980; Casey, 1997; Chouinard et al., 1986; Chouza et al., 1982; Colonna, 1994; Dahl & Refsum, 1976; Degner & Rüther, 1998; Desilva et al., 1995; Dubovsky, 1987; Fleischhacker et al., 1991; Fleischhauer, 1978; Fulop et al., 1987; Gattera et al., 1994; Gerhardt et al., 1985; Gerlach & Casey, 1984; Hori et al., 1992; Irjala et al., 1996; Kaplan et al., 1994; Miller & Jankovic, 1990; Neale & Oltmanns, 1980; Palayodan, 1983; Peacock et al., 1996; Petit et al., 1996; Porsolt & Jalfre, 1981; Ravn et al., 1980; Sandor et al., 1990; Schmidt et al., 1984; Sweet, 1975; Uchida et al., 1979; Von Bardeleben et al., 1987; Zahn & Pickar, 1993).

different clinical actions in comparison to typical high-potency and typical moderate and low-potency neuroleptics. The clinical profile is demonstrated in Table 9.2 and can be charaterized by a very low frequency of extrapyramidal reactions applying more or less to all of the five compounds listed in this figure, and their effect on negative schizophrenic symptoms. On the other hand, atypical neuroleptics have a higher rate of anticholinergic side effects than do typical high potency neuroleptics. Sedative effects are not homogenous in this group. For instance, clozapine, which has nearly no extrapyramidal side effects, is a highly sedative compound and also shows remarkable anticholinergic reactions. Olanzapine shows these side effects to a lesser extent but risperidone does not at all.

Pharmacological treatment

Acute psychotic states

There is general agreement among child and adolescent psychiatrists that the treatment of schizophrenic psychoses has to use a multimodal approach including medication, psychotherapeutic and family-oriented interventions and, in chronic cases, also rehabilitation. However, during the acute phase of the disorder, inpatient treatment and an adequate neuroleptic medication are required as the most important components. In spite of reports that some patients with acute and first episode schizophrenia can be treated as outpatients or daypatients (Jaffa, 1995; Tolbert, 1996) inpatient treatment is still the standard procedure.

During this first inpatient phase of treatment, drug treatment is the central component, and there is evidence that the antipsychotic drugs used in adults are also effective in childhood and adolescent onset schizophrenia. But, there may also be differences with regard to dosage and metabolism, which have not yet been investigated. So, the principles of pharmacotherapy of acute psychotic states in children and adolescents are based mainly on clinical experience.

Until recently, only typical high-potency neuroleptics, which have been found to be effective against positive symptoms such as delusions and hallucinations and which had also a normalizing effect with regard to agitation, aggression, tension, and formal thought disorders were used for acute psychotic states. The most frequently used compound is still haloperidol from the butyrophenone group. Other substances quite often used are fluphenazine, perphenazine, flupenthixol and (only in Germany) perazine. Antipsychotic medication should always be initiated in a low dose. Dosages should be increased until improvement of symptoms or the maximum recommended dosage is reached. When a sufficient symptom improvement is achieved, a readjustment of the dosage is recommended, because for maintenance treatment lower dosages are often effective. In cases where the disorder is already chronic and a readmission takes place, an existing treatment with typical moderate and low-potency neuroleptics such as perazine or thioridazine can be continued in a medium or higher dosage. If the acute psychotic state is complicated by aggression, tension and psychomotor agitation, a typical high-potency neuroleptic (e.g., haloperidol) can be combined with typical moderate and low-potency neuroleptics, such as levomepromazine or chlorprothixene, or alternatively for a limited time with a benzodiazepine. To avoid sedation or cognitive blunting, the necessity for this comedication should be reviewed regularly. The antipsychotic effects and the dosages of some frequently used neuroleptics are shown in Table 9.2.

Another important strategy in the pharmacological treatment of acute psychotic states is the differentiation of positive and negative symptoms. It has been demonstrated that both kinds of symptoms can precede the onset of the schizophrenic disorder (Remschmid et al., 1995). Where the positive symptom treatment response is adequate, but there has been no or little effect on negative symptoms, a switch from typical to atypical neuroleptics should be considered. Table 9.2 demonstrates the pharmacological profile of different neuroleptics with regard to their efficacy on positive symptoms, negative symptoms, sedation, anticholinergic effects and extrapyramidal side effects. As the table demonstrates, most typical neuroleptics are effective against positive symptoms, but not negative symptoms. This is the domain of the atypical neuroleptics, which also have the advantage of a lower risk of severe extrapyramidal side effects. Because of this advantage, atypical neuroleptics are increasingly being used as first-choice neuroleptics.

Fig. 9.4 shows a decision tree for the neuroleptic treatment of child and adolescent schizophrenia. Treatment is initiated with either typical or atypical antipsychotic medication. Depending on the individual reaction (efficacy and side effects), the decisions for switching or maintaining the present medication are made. Only after two different compounds are not effective or not tolerated may treatment with clozapine be initiated.

Prevention of relapses

Schizophrenic disorders in children and adolescents as well as in adults are characterized by a high risk of relapses. These are sometimes triggered by emotional stress, adverse life events, but also by positive emotional experiences. Such an occasion is, for instance, falling in love which very often triggers a psychotic relapse in adolescents.

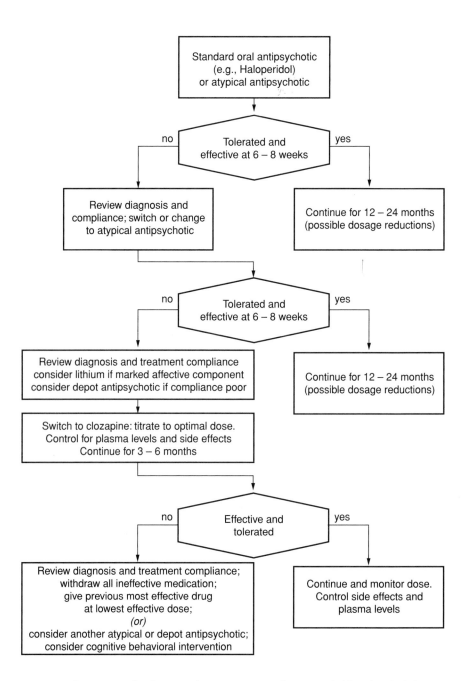

Fig. 9.4. A decision tree for the neutroleptic treatment selection in childhood and adolescence (adapted and modified from Clark and Lewis, 1998).

With regard to these factors, it is very important to anticipate a relapse prevention by either maintaining low dose oral medication or by switching to a depot neuroleptic. Especially when compliance is a problem, a depot medication is recommended. The depot neuroleptics that have been useful for these purposes have a quite similar receptor and efficacy profile and are mainly effective against positive symptoms, but are also helpful against autistic behaviour, withdrawal and psychomotor uneasiness. Frequently used depot neuroleptics are haloperidol-decanoate, fluphenazine-decanoate and fluspirilene. They are given as an intramuscular injection, the duration of efficacy is between one and four weeks. Depot neuroleptics are given in relatively low dosages. They should be used for a timespan of 1 or 2 years after the first episode in order to prevent a relapse which very often impedes reintegration and worsens the long-term prognosis. During childhood and adolescence, relapse prevention is even more important than in adulthood as the majority of the patients have not yet finished school or started a professional career. Therefore, the possibility of continuing school or professional training is extremely important.

Side effects

The selection of a neuroleptic agent for the treatment of schizophrenic disorders cannot only take into consideration the antipsychotic effects. The avoidance of unwanted side effects is of equal importance. As Fig. 9.3 demonstrates, the most pronounced side effects of typical neuroleptics are the extrapyramidal symptoms (EPS). This applies in particular to all compounds subsumed under the heading of typical high-potency neuroleptics and, to some extent, also to compounds classified as typical moderate and low-potency neuroleptics. All typical neuroleptics are characterized by hyperprolactinemia, due to D_2 receptor blockade in the tubero-infundibular system. Other notable side effects are:

- epileptic seizures, in particular with haloperidol, perphenazine, chlorpromazine, zotepine and clozapine;
- orthostatic hypotension, a very common side effect, particularly in low to moderate potency neuroleptics;
- other cardiovascular effects.

Extrapyramidal side effects
Neuroleptic potency and extrapyramidal side effects
The reported rates of EPS in adults vary between 25% and 75% after the use of typical high potency neuroleptics. For adolescents, rates between 30 and 40%

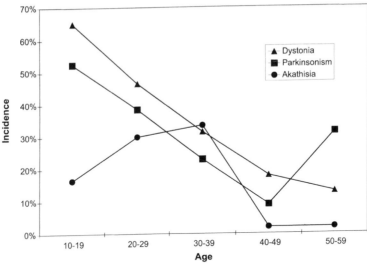

Fig. 9.5. Incidence rates of extrapyramidal symptoms in dependance of age (adapted from Nissen et al., 1998, reprinted with permission).

have been reported. Variations in reported prevalence may be due to a lack of consistency in the definition of cases, neuroleptic prescribing practices, study design, and the demographics of the population being studied.

The most important extrapyramidal side effects in children and adolescents are acute dystonia (incidence about 65%, higher in males than in females), parkinsonism (50%), akathisia (15%), and tardive dyskinesia (5%). The incidence of EPS depends on age and gender. This is demonstrated in Fig. 9.5. Extrapyramidal side effects are, in many cases, an extreme handicap for the successful treatment of schizophrenia. In many patients, they are associated with a high level of anxiety and contribute significantly to non-compliance. The risk of developing tardive dyskinesia (TD) is estimated with 4% per year of antipsychotic medication. The prevalence of TD is higher in older patients and in females.

This observation is especially important for child and adolescent psychiatrists who treat younger patients. Other risk factors for EPS are: male sex, use of high-potency neuroleptics and previous dystonic reactions in a patient. The probability of developing EPS depends to a large extent on the potency of neuroleptics.

Typical neuroleptics
Typical neuroleptics have been classified from a clinical point of view into high-potency, medium-potency, and low-potency neuroleptics. This

classification was based on the dopamine-hypothesis of schizophrenia which claimed that this disorder was associated with a hyperdopaminergic activity, related in particular to the D_2 receptor.

Accordingly, a number of D_2 antagonists were developed, the prototype being haloperidol. The neuroleptic potency was defined in relation to the neuroleptic threshold causing extrapyramidal symptoms.

Typical high-potency neuroleptics

This group of neuroleptic agents has a high antipsychotic effect but also has a high risk for extrapyramidal symptoms, whereas the behavior effect is not so pronounced, and there is also a diminished risk of cardiovascular side effects. They can be used in lower doses and can be combined effectively with benzodiazepines if behavioral control is needed. The low risk of cardiovascular side effects, however, led to their use in inappropriately high doses. Recent research has shown that high neuroleptic doses do not lead to a more rapid or better recovery from psychoses, which can be better achieved through the addition of benzodiazepines such as lorazepam to a lower neuroleptic dose. This has shown to achieve the same degree of behavioral control (Remington, 1997).

Typical low and medium-potency neuroleptics

The compounds classified under this heading have, compared with high-potency neuroleptics, a lower antipsychotic effect, a diminished risk of extrapyramidal side effects, pronounced behavioral effects (sedation in the case of agitation and depression), but a high risk of cardiovascular side effects, particularly in the form of postural hypotension and tachycardia. Further disadvantages are the lack of depot formulations and ocular changes while using high dosages, e.g., pigmentary retinopathy with thioridazine in dosages above 800 mg/day.

Table 9.2 shows the major effects of these two groups of neuroleptic agents.

Atypical neuroleptics

The so-called novel neuroleptics are defined as compounds that have no or a low risk of inducing extrapyramidal side effects. They are effective in a substantial proportion of patients who are refractory to typical neuroleptics and are also effective with regard to negative symptoms (Remschmidt et al., 1994b, 1999). These effects are due to a different profile of action which is not mainly based on a dopamine receptor antagonism. Their effect seems to be also based predominantly on other receptor-binding profiles, including the serotoninergic and the adrenergic system. The most commonly used of the novel neuroleptics is clozapine. Risperidone, like clozapine, has more serotoninergic (5-HT$_2$) than D$_2$ antagonism. In comparison with the typical neuroleptics, risperidone has a very low risk of EPS, but a greater risk than clozapine. This is explained by its greater D$_2$ antagonism in comparison with clozapine. Other novel compounds include olanzapine, quetiapine, and zotepine. The side effect profile of these compounds is quite different from that of the typical neuroleptics and may be explained, at least in part, by effects related to their serotoninergic antagonism.

Fig. 9.3 shows the most common side effects of the most important novel neuroleptics derived from studies in adult schizophrenic patients. There are no comparable large studies in young age carried out with clozapine, risperidone or the other atypical neuroleptics. Symptoms are described in Table 9.4.

Acute dystonia

Over 90% of episodes of acute dystonia occur during the first 4 days of treatment (Remington, 1997). They may also occur within the first hours of treatment and can be potentially life-threatening, for instance, in the case of acute laryngeal–pharyngeal dystonia. Risk factors for the manifestation of acute dystonia are young male patients, the use of typical high-potency neuroleptics, a previous dystonic reaction and neuroleptic naive patients. As the risk is increased in younger patients, the initial prophylactic use of antiparkinsonian therapy is recommended, which can be gradually reduced and finally discontinued at the end of the first week, after the period of greatest risk (day 1 to 4) for acute EPS is over (Remington, 1997).

Parkinsonism

The clinical picture of parkinsonism comprises rigidity, akinesia and tremor. As with other extrapyramidal side effects, parkinsonism occurs to some extent in all patients treated with high-potency typical neuroleptics.

Akathisia

Akathisia is manifested by a combination of subjective and objective restlessness and occurs typically within the first 4 weeks of treatment or dose change, but may occur already in the first hours. It is often associated with anxiety or interpreted as a worsening of the psychotic disorder. It can also be associated with increased violence and self-harm.

The objective features comprise a hyperaroused state with restlessness or frank agitation. The phenomenon can best be observed when the patient is standing. In this position he or she frequently shifts his weight from one foot to

Table 9.4. Novel neuroleptics: most common side effects (%)

Drug	N	Dosage	Reference
Clozapine	126	600 mg/day	Kane et al. (1988)
Somnolence (24)		(mean peak dose)	
Tachycardia (17)			
Constipation (16)			
Dizziness (14)			
Olanzapine	64	7.5–12.5 mg/day	Tollefson et al. (1994)
Somnolence (30)		(dose range)	
Dizziness (9)			
Constipation (8)			
Weight gain (8)			
Risperidone	64	6 mg/day	Marder & Meibach (1994)
Headache (16)			
Rhinitis (16)			
Insomnia (13)			
Agitation (11)			
EPS (11)			
Quetiapine	286	400 mg/day	Hirsch (1994)
Somnolence (14)		(mean dose)	
Insomnia (10)			
Dry mouth (8)			
Agitation (7)			

From Remington (1997).

the other or shows a kind of "stationary pacing" of which he or she seems unaware. While sitting, akathisia can often be manifested by frequent shifts in position, or by shaking of the legs.

The subjective features can be very variable. Subjectively, akathisia is always a unpleasant and distressing experience. The patient can interpret the physical experience of akathisia in a psychotic way, thus describing electricity flowing through his body, which can be misinterpreted as a delusional experience. If the physician is unaware of this phenomenon, the symptoms may lead him to increase the dose of antipsychotic medication which, in turn, will increase akathisia (Kutcher, 1998). Thus, it is extremely important to be aware of this complication in every patient who is treated with antipsychotic agents. Direct observation of the patient is important for the diagnosis, but also direct questioning is necessary. The subjective evaluation can start with an open question as to how the patient is feeling and becoming more detailed, for example, "How are you feeling inside yourself?" or "Do your stomach or legs feel jumpy or shaky?".

Tardive dyskinesia (TD)

Tardive dyskinesia occurs after at least a 3-month period of neuroleptic medication. Its incidence is approximately 5% annually during the first 5 years of treatment. In contrast to former opinions, TD is not necessarily irreversible, although an effective treatment is not available. Tardive dyskinesia occurs more frequently in older patients than in younger ones, and occurs more frequently after a longer period of treatment than after a shorter one. Other risk factors are dosage of neuroleptic medication, cerebral trauma, and smoking. To our current knowledge, clozapine is the only neuroleptic agent that is not associated with the risk of TD.

Other side effects

An overview is given in Fig. 9.3 (side effect of neuroleptics) and in Table 9.4 (features and treatment of side effects). Since many of these side effects are not related purely to the substance class but more to individual substances, a detailed description can be found in the Section "Major compounds and their actions". Looking at the side effect profile (Fig. 9.3), the differences between the atypical neuroleptics in comparison to typical high-potency and typical moderate- and low-potency neuroleptics become evident. Clozapine, for instance, is characterized by the absence of, or very low, extrapyramidal side effects, but bears a high risk of epileptic seizures, leads to considerable weight gain in many patients and causes also, to some extent, orthostatic hypotension and other cardiovascular effects. The highest danger may be its effect on the hematological system, leading to agranulocytosis as the most severe complication. This complication can, however, be managed by a careful blood count monitoring which will be described later.

Olanzapine and quetiapine seem to have the lowest rate of side effects, but may not be as effective as clozapine with regard to positive and negative symptoms. Risperidone may cause extrapyramidal side effects such as parkinsonism and tardive dyskinesia, and is also characterized by the occurrence of hyperprolactinemia and, to some extent, weight gain. It does not cause hypotension or other cardiovascular side effects.

Treatment of side effects

There are no effective medications that are free from unwanted side effects. This applies also to all neuroleptic agents. Therefore, both the desired

Table 9.5. Features and treatment of side effects of neuroleptics

Reaction	Features	Treatment
Acute dystonia	Spasm of muscles of tongue, face, neck, back; may mimic seizures; not hysteria	Antiparkinsonian agents
Parkinsonism	Bradykinesia, rigidity, variable tremor, mask face, shuffling gait	Antipakinsonian agents
Akathisia	Motor and internal restlessness; not anxiety or agitation	Reduce dose or change drug: antiparkinsonian agents, benzodiazepines or propranolol may help
Tardive dyskinesia	Oral-facial dyskinesia; widespread choreoathetosis or dystonia	Prevention crucial; treatment unsatisfactory
Neuroleptic malignant syndrome (NMS)	Catatonia, stupor, fever, unstable blood pressure, myoglobinemia; can be fatal	Stop neuroleptic immediately: dantrolene or bromocriptine may help; antiparkinsonian agents are not effective
Anticholinergic effects	Dry mouth, constipation, glaucoma, pyloric spasms, bladder dysfunction	If necessary change to butyrophenones; in case of bladder dysfunction: carbachol
Elevation of liver enzymes, cholestatic icterus		In case of icterus discontinuation of neuroleptics
Agranulocytosis	Low/reduced white blood cell count	No neuroleptics, if necessary change to butyrophenones
Hyperprolactinemia	Gynecomastia, galactorrhea	Reduction of neuroleptics
Sexual dysfunction	Dysfunction of erection, libido or orgasm	Reduction of neuroleptics
Sedation		If unwanted: reduce or change drug
Seizures		Reduce or change drug, if needed antiepileptic drugs
Dermatological alterations	Skin allergy, photo-sensibilization	In case of skin allergy discontinuation of neuroleptics; dermatological therapy
Opthalmological alterations	Pigmentary retinopathies and corneal opacities	Change to butyrophenone
Alterations of glucose metabolism and eating behavior	Reduced tolerance of glucose, weight gain	If necessary reduce drug
Hypotension		Dihydroergotamine; reduce or change drug
Other cardiovascular effects	ECG alterations, arrhythmia	If necessary change to butyrophenones or discontinuation of agents

Adapted from Baldessarini (1996); Möller et al. (1989); Young et al. (1998).

pharmacological effects including efficacy and the profile of unwanted side effects have to be taken into account in the selection of an appropriate neuroleptic agent.

Table 9.5 reviews the most important side effects, their main features and the principles of treatment. Extrapyramidal side effects are considered first, followed by reactions involving other areas which are described in the next section of this chapter.

Treatment of extrapyramidal side effects

Neuroleptic-induced extrapyramidal side effects are a special problem in the treatment of children and adolescents with schizophrenia for several reasons. Young patients are often extremely irritated and anxious, because they cannot understand the symptoms. Parents are understandably extremely concerned and are often inclined to stop the medication. These factors contribute significantly to non-compliance.

The patient and parents should be given full information about the treatment procedure, including effects and the potential side effects of medication, before starting the treatment. This should also be documented in the patient's chart.

Acute dystonia

As the risk is increased in younger patients, the initial prophylactic use of antiparkinsonian therapy is recommended, which can be gradually reduced and finally discontinued at the end of the first week, covering the period of greatest risk (day 1 to 4) for acute EPS (Remington, 1997).

Parkinsonism

Parkinsonism is best treated by lowering the dosage of the antipsychotic agent or by adding an antiparkinsonian compound (biperiden (2–12 mg per day), benztropine (0.5–4 mg per day)). Antiparkinsonian therapy should not be continued indefinitely, as there is an increased risk of tardive dyskinesia. Antiparkinsonian therapy should therefore be discontinued, or at least given at a lower dose after 2–3 months.

Akathisia

As far as treatment of akathisia is concerned, traditional antiparkinsonian medications have, at most, a minor effect, but are often totally ineffective. In contrast, beta-blockers and benzodiazepines have been demonstrated to be effective. The choice between a benzodiazepine or a beta-blocker may be guided by the patient's medical history (Remington, 1997). For example, asthma is a contraindication to beta-blockers, and benzodiazepines should be avoided in cases at risk of substance abuse. Of the benzodiazepines, clonazepam has been tried successfully, starting with dosages of 0.5 mg given twice daily with a maximum daily dose of about 2 mg. Usually, after a few days, improvement or an interruption of akathisia can be achieved.

If a beta-blocker is to be used, propranolol can be administered, starting with 10 mg daily and increasing to a maximum of 30 mg/day. Propranolol should not be used in patients with diabetes or asthma. Heart rate and blood pressure should be monitored carefully. In addition to these pharmacological treatment strategies, psychosocial interventions are of great importance (Kutcher, 1998). These include a careful education about the potential onset of akathisia, detailed information about the medication for the children and their parents and, in case of inpatient treatment, careful observations of the patient and information about akathisia and treatment strategies for the staff.

Tardive dyskinesia

The treatment alternatives for tardive dyskinesia (TD) are all very unsatisfactory, therefore the prevention of TD plays an important role (e.g., selection of agent, adjustment of dosage, requirement for continuation of treatment). For patients with mild to moderate TD, therapeutic efforts primarily aim at minimizing neuroleptic exposure or using atypical neuroleptics. Patients with moderate to severe forms are more challenging. They often require medication to suppress their symptoms, however no treatment strategy has emerged that is unequivocally successful. Increasing the doses of typical neuroleptics may result in short-term improvement; however, there is no information on the long-term efficacy and risks of this strategy. The short-term suppressive effects of clozapine seem, at best, weak, but patients may improve with long-term treatment. Medications with relatively few side effects that may have suppressive efficacy in some patients include calcium channel blockers, clonidine, propranolol, tiapride, benzodiazepines, and vitamin E (Egan et al. 1997).

Fig. 9.6 presents a decision tree for the treatment of neuroleptic-induced extrapyramidal side effects and summarizes the above.

Treatment of other side effects

A detailed summary is given in Table 9.5. If serious side effects like neuroleptic malignant syndrome or agranulocytosis occur, specialists in intensive care or hematology should be consulted.

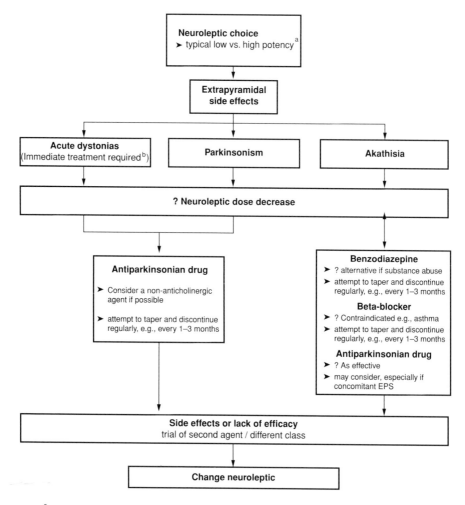

Fig. 9.6. Flow chart for the treatment of extrapyramidal symptoms (adapted from Remington, 1997).

Major compounds and their actions

The major compounds and the most common brand names are listed in Table 9.1. Haloperidol is the most widespread and common substance. Others are more or less prevalent in different countries. Chlorpromazine is included due to historical reasons and because it is widely used as a reference substance, e.g., for the calculation of equivalence dosages of neuroleptic potency. Nowadays it is no longer recommended for the treatment of schizophrenic disorders. The same applies for tiapride which is used in the treatment of movement disorders and in some countries in the treatment of Gilles de la Tourette's syndrome. Recommended dosage is shown in Table 9.2.

Typical neuroleptics

In general, high potency typical neuroleptics have good efficacy with positive symptoms but carry a high risk of inducing EPS. Moderate to low potency neuroleptics have good sedation properties with a higher risk of anticholinergic effects. For details see Table 9.2 and Fig. 9.3.

High potency neuroleptics

Butyrophenones (haloperidol, benperidol): Benperidol is the most potent neuroleptic agent. Both neuroleptics are used as antipsychotics and in the reduction of agitation. The most important side effects are EPS. Of all high potent neuroleptics, haloperidol is by far the most researched one in children and adolescents.

Diphenylbutylpiperidines (pimozide, fluspirilene): The most important indication for both substances is maintenance treatment of chronic schizophrenic psychosis. Fluspirilene is only available as depot medication. The most prominent side effects are EPS and, to some extent, cardiovascular effects.

Phenothiazines (perphenazine, fluphenazine): Indications are acute and chronic schizophrenic psychoses. Both substances seem to have a slightly higher rate of sexual dysfunction than other typical high potency neuroleptics. EPS is the most common and important side effect.

Thioxanthenes (flupenthixol): This is used especially in schizophrenic disorders with positive symptoms. In schizo-affective disorders it is an option when lithium and carbamazepine have failed. It may have higher antidepressive properties than other typical neuroleptics, and furthermore has been shown to reduce suicidal and self-injurious behavior.

Moderate and low potency neuroleptics

Benzamides (sulpiride (tiapride)): Indications include delusive psychosis, chronic schizophrenic disorders especially with lack of motivation. Further indications are as second line for depressive syndromes when antidepressants have failed. Additionally sulpiride has good antivertiginous and antiemetic effects, and induces little or no sedation.

Butyrophenones (pipamperone): Indications include agitation and sleep disorders. This substance has almost no anticholinergic activity, and has been widely evaluated clinically in children and adolescents.

Phenothiazines (levomepromazine, perazine, promethazine, thioridazine): Levomepromazine is used for the acute treatment of psychosis. It is highly sedative and has good analgesic properties and is therefore often used in combination with a high potency typical neuroleptic in the presence of aggressiveness, tension and psychomotor agitation. Promethazine has no antipsychotic properties and is used in sleep disorders and for sedation. Perazine and thioridazine are mainly used for maintenance therapy in chronic schizophrenic psychosis. Thioridazine has good antidepressive properties and a low rate of EPS. Perazine is, to our knowledge, only well established in Germany, where it is used in the treatment of schizophrenic psychoses and delusional disorders.

Thioxanthenes (chlorprothixene): Chlorprothixene is a well-established therapy for schizophrenic psychoses. In acute psychosis, it is usually combined with high-potency butyrophenones.

Atypical neuroleptics

In general, there is a lack of controlled studies on the use of atypical neuroleptics in children and adolescents. Only one controlled trial has been conducted with clozapine. Concerning the efficacy of risperidone and olanzapine, only open trials and case reports are available (for review, see Toren et al., 1998). There are even less data on quetiapine and zotepine. For details see Table 9.2 and Fig. 9.3.

Clozapine

Clozapine is a dibenzodiazepine derivative that shows, in spite of its structural similarity to imipramine, pharmacological effects that are more closely related to those of chlorpromazine than of imipramine. Clozapine differs in the following ways from classical antipsychotics (Coward, 1992): greater arousal inhibition activity, no inhibition of apomorphine- or amphetamine-induced stereotypic behavior, no induction of catalepsy, no dopaminergic or GABAergic supersensitivity on chronic administration, no depolarization, blocking of nigrostriatal dopamine neurons with chronic exposure, relatively high 5-HT$_2$ blocking ratio, less D$_2$, but greater D$_1$ and D$_4$ receptor blockade.

There are three main indications for clozapine in treatment of childhood and adolescent onset schizophrenia (Remschmidt et al., 1994a,b, 1999):

(i)   acute schizophrenic psychosis characterized by delusions, hallucinations, thought disorder, aggressive and acting-out behavior;

(ii)   chronic and therapy-refractory schizophrenic psychosis; and

(iii) symptom-suppression and prophylaxis of relapse in acute and chronic schizophrenic psychosis during long-term treatment.

In some countries the treatment guidelines for clozapine require that the patients have failed to respond to, or have not tolerated, standard neuroleptic medications. For example, in Germany and in the USA, two other standard neuroleptic agents have to be tested before clozapine treatment may be introduced. Because of the risk of agranulocytosis, the absence of any hematological anomaly (number of white blood cells more than 3500/mm^3, normal differential blood count) is required. Before initiating treatment, patients must have a baseline white blood cell and differential count. During treatment, white blood cell count has to be monitored (frequency and duration depends on the country, e.g., USA: weekly during the entire treatment and 4 weeks after discontinuation, UK: weekly during first 18 weeks and at least at 2-week intervals for the first year, then at least every 4 weeks and for 4 weeks after discontinuation, Germany: weekly for the first 18 weeks and subsequently every 4 weeks). Additionally, total and differential blood counts have to be administered if any symptoms or hints of an agranulocytosis occur (e.g., febrile infections, see Table 9.4).

Absolute contraindications
These include allergic hypersensitivity reactions against clozapine, known dysfunction of the hematological system (in particular undertreatment with clozapine or other neuroleptics or agents), acute intoxication or psychosis induced by agents with adverse CNS effects (especially alcohol, antidepressants or other neuroleptics, tranquilizers, hypnotics and opiates), severe cardiovascular, gastrointestinal or renal disease, intestinal atonia, and therapy-refractory epileptic seizures. Comedication with other substances that are known to induce leukopenia (e.g., carbamazepine, thioridazine).

Relative contraindications and special risk factors for clozapine treatment
These include pregnancy, brain dysfunction, glaucoma, prostate adenoma, comedications with substances that carry a risk of bone marrow suppression,

allergic reactions to other medications and combinations with depot-neuroleptics, especially of the tricyclic type.

Efficacy in short-term treatment
From studies in adult schizophrenics, it is evident that clozapine treatment has at least the same or a superior antipsychotic effect as compared to conventional neuroleptics. In some studies, clozapine was superior with regard to symptom reduction in severe and acute schizophrenic patients. Other studies demonstrated a superiority of clozapine as compared to chlorpromazine with regard to a reduction of negative symptoms such as emotional withdrawal and flattened affect, measured by BPRS (Brief Psychiatric Rating Scale) scores (Ekblom & Haggstrom, 1974). As the guidelines do not allow to use clozapine as a first-choice drug, most patients have been treated before with at least two other typical or atypical neuroleptics.

Only one controlled trial has assessed the efficacy of clozapine in child and adolescent psychiatry. Twenty-one (mean age 14.4 ± 2.9 years) adolescents with treatment refractive early onset schizophrenia received either clozapine (mean ($\pm$SD) final daily dose 176 ± 149 mg) or haloperidol (mean final daily dose 16 ± 8 mg) in a 6-week double-blind parallel comparison. Clozapine was found to be superior to haloperidol on all measures of psychosis, and showed a striking superiority for both positive and negative symptoms (Kumra et al., 1996).

Efficacy in maintenance treatment
Studies in adult schizophrenia concerning maintenance treatment have been especially interesting because the majority of the patients were non-responders to conventional neuroleptics. These studies demonstrate the superior efficacy of clozapine as maintenance treatment in therapy-refractory psychosis, treated by classical neuroleptics. Beyond that, it could be demonstrated that clozapine was effective in reducing recurrence rates and duration of hospitalization. The superior efficacy of clozapine has been demonstrated in adolescents suffering from chronic schizophrenia (Schulz et al., 1996, 1997).

Treatment recommendations and practical guidelines
Treatment recommendations are, in general, the same as in adult psychiatry and have to respect the guidelines of the producing company (Bleeham, 1993). We have modified these guidelines slightly for the younger age group of patients with early onset schizophrenia. These guidelines emphasize that the clozapine dosage must always be adjusted individually for each patient. The

lowest effective dose should be used, which should be assessed by careful titration. Administration is usually oral, parenteral administration is only available for intramuscular injection using the same dosages and is rarely used. In most cases, intramuscular injections can be replaced by oral administration after a few days.

Some general recommendations for clozapine treatment in childhood and adolescent onset schizophrenia have been formulated by a consensus conference of 13 German child and adolescent psychiatrists who have special expertise in clozapine treatment (Deutsche Gesellschaft für Kinder- und Jugendpsychiatrie, 1994). The main principles of this consensus conference were:

(i)   clozapine treatment is recommended in acute early-onset schizophrenia under clinical conditions;

(ii) at least one traditional neuroleptic agent administered for 4 to 6 weeks in an adequate dosage should have failed to improve the positive and/or negative symptomatology;

(iii) clozapine is also indicated with the occurrence of intolerable side effects of classical neuroleptics;

(iv) clozapine is also effective in chronic schizophrenia; and

(v)   no recommendation can, as yet, be given for relapse prevention because of inadequate data.

Olanzapine
Olanzapine was developed as a consequence of research seeking an antipsychotic agent with a similar receptor-binding profile as clozapine, but without its adverse side effects, especially agranulocytosis. Olanzapine interacts with a broad spectrum of receptors, including the dopamine, serotonin, muscarinic, adrenergic and histamine receptors. The receptor-binding profile is demonstrated in Fig. 9.2. This receptor profile is responsible for the advantages of this compound, but also for its side effects. In comparison with typical neuroleptics, the affinity of olanzapine for the family of dopamine receptors is relatively low, and for the serotonin receptors relatively high. Similar to clozapine, this may be explain why olanzapine is more effective with regard to negative and mood symptoms in schizophrenic patients. The adverse effects of olanzapine can also be explained by its receptor-binding profile. The anticholinergic effects result from its interaction with muscarinic receptors, whereas sedation can be attributed to the effects at histamine and adrenergic receptors. One of the most pronounced adverse effects is weight gain, which results from its antagonism to serotonin receptors. Finally, the reduced risk of

extrapyramidal side effects (EPS) has to do with the weak D_2 blockade, combined with the antimuscarinic action. This is important, because it suggests that, as a result of these properties, there might be a low risk for tardive dyskinesia. Compared with clozapine, the compound is characterized by a weaker action at the alpha-adrenergic receptors which accounts for the decreased risk of orthostatic hypotension.

Imaging studies in adult patients show that the threshold for extrapyramidal symptoms is approximately 80% occupancy of D_2 receptors. In the usual clinical dose range, haloperidol, for instance, occupies between 70 and 90% of the D_2 receptors, clozapine between 20 to 60%, and olanzapine around 60%. Olanzapine additionally occupies 80% of the 5-HT_2 receptors at a 10 mg daily dose. If the dose is increased above the recommended daily maximum of 20 mg, the binding profile becomes very similar to that of standard neuroleptics, with the consequent risk of EPS and loss of its advantages (Gardner, 1997).

In a recent study, Kumra et al. (1998) treated eight patients with early onset schizophrenia with olanzapine. The mean age of the group was 15.3 years, the mean duration of illness 4.6 years. The group was exceedingly ill, demonstrated by the rating score on the Brief Psychiatric Rating Scale of 53.2 ± 15.3 at baseline. The patients were described as being treatment-refractory after having used, on average, 2.3 different neuroleptic medications at intake. Four subjects had previously been responsive to clozapine; however, this medication had to be discontinued because of adverse side effects. The treatment period lasted for up to 8 weeks. The dosage was titrated on a weight-adjusted basis up to a maximum of 20 mg daily. The results of this trial demonstrated a significant improvement in symptomatology indicated by a 17% improvement of the BPRS, a 27% improvement on the Scale for the Assessment of Negative Symptoms, and a 1% improvement on the Scale for the Assessment of Positive Symptoms. In terms of the Clinical Global Impression Scale, three patients were rated as much improved and two as minimally improved. In the others, there was either no change or they became even worse. In a follow-up investigation (follow-up interval 3 to 14 months), half of the subjects continued olanzapine medication, the other half discontinued treatment because of an inadequate response. The adverse side effect was quite marked: Six out of eight patients suffered increased appetite, nausea, vomiting, headache, somnolence, sustained tachycardia and increased agitation. In five patients, constipation and concentration problems were observed, and seven out of eight patients suffered from insomnia and showed elevations of liver transaminase levels.

In conclusion, the effect of olanzapine in this group of patients was not very impressive, and the adverse side effects were quite substantial. In particular, a weight gain after a 6-week period of treatment of 3.4 ± 4.1 kg is quite striking, and would be a particular problem for adolescents.

Risperidone
Risperidone is a benzisoxazole derivative. Presumably the antipsychotic activity is mediated through a combination of a D_2 and 5-HT_{2A} receptor antagonism. Risperidone also binds with high affinity to alpha$_1$ and alpha$_2$ adrenergic receptors and to H_1 histaminergic receptors. Several investigations in adult patients have demonstrated a significant improvement of positive and negative symptoms comparable to the efficacy of haloperidol (for review, see Degner & Rüther, 1998). In a meta-analysis, it has been proposed that risperidone might have a higher efficacy than haloperidol in the improvement of negative symptoms (Carman et al., 1995). Flynn et al. (1998) conducted an open trial on treatment resistant schizophrenics (mean treatment duration: 12.1 weeks) 57 patients were treated with clozapine at a mean dose of 420 mg; and 29 received risperidone, at a mean dose of 7.75 mg. Their results indicated a better improvement of positive and negative symptoms in those treated with clozapine compared to risperidone. However, risperidone appeared to be more effective than the typical neuroleptics on both positive and negative symptoms, and on global psychopathology. In a controlled trial of 86 treatment refractive schizophrenic patients, risperidone has been shown to be as effective on positive and negative symptoms as clozapine (Bondolfi et al., 1998).

Until now there has been no controlled study on the use of risperidone in children and adolescents. Only one open trial has assessed its efficacy. Risperidone produced clinically and statistically significant improvement in ten schizophrenics on the Positive and Negative Symptom Scale for schizophrenia, the Brief Psychiatric Rating Scale, and the Clinical Global Impression at a mean daily dosage of 6.6 mg (range 4 to 10 mg). The reported side effects in this study included: mild somnolence during dose finding (eight of ten subjects), acute dystonic reaction (2/10), parkinsonism (3/10), mild oro-facial dyskinesia (1/10), blurred vision (1/10), impaired concentration (1/10), and weight gain (8/10, mean weight gain 4.85 kg). Throughout the study, electrolytes, blood cell count, liver enzymes, and ECG remained within normal limits (Armenteros et al., 1997). Several case studies also suggest a good efficacy of risperidone in child and adolescent schizophrenia (for review, see Toren et al., 1998). The overall side effect profile (see Fig. 9.3) and receptor binding profile (Fig. 9.2) suggest that risperidone may be more related to the typical neuroleptics. Thus, due to the dose-dependent of EPS, it has been questioned whether risperidone can really be called an atypical neuroleptic (Cardoni, 1995). It has been demonstrated that dosages of 10 mg/day or more cause EPS, which can be avoided by the administration of dosages below 6 mg/day (Marder & Maibach, 1994).

Two case histories

We describe here briefly two boys with early onset schizophrenia. Their treatment caused many problems, and they have now been followed up for 10 years.

The first case, R.K., was admitted as an inpatient at the age of 11 years 2 months with a mixture of symptoms including bizarre behavior, hallucinations, delusions, suicidal thoughts, anhedonia and depression. Several neuroleptics were tried, as shown in Table 9.6. Some typical neuroleptics such as perphenazine and haloperidol led to fairly good symptom reduction; however, several readmissions to the hospital were necessary because of severe relapses, mainly with positive symptoms.

In week 126, clozapine was introduced into the treatment regime (the boy was at that time 13 years 7 months). This led to a good symptomatic relief. In week 141, the patient was discharged to a rehabilitation centre where he is still living (1999). He is now 18 years 8 months old, has finished a school for special education and is now working 8 hours/day in a sheltered workshop in the rehabilitation center. Medication with clozapine continues at a dose of 400 mg/day. At the age of 18 years 5 months he had a grand mal seizure for the first time in his life. Since then, he has additionally received valproate (900 mg/day).

Psychopathology is now markedly different. The initial diagnosis of *paranoid schizophrenia* (F20.0) has now shifted to *residual schizophrenia* (F20.5). Table 9.6 demonstrates how difficult it was to find the right medication. Unfortunately, the atypical neuroleptic clozapine did not result in cure, and he continues to suffer from residual psychotic symptoms. It should be mentioned that there were many other components to his treatment, including family counseling, individual support as well as a comprehensive rehabilitation program. These are not described in detail, because the major focus of this case history is medication issues.

The second case history describes a boy (S.G.) with early onset schizophrenia. He was admitted at the age of 12 years 1 month with symptoms including social withdrawal, depression, mutism, eating problems, bizarre behavior, anergia, anhedonia, and affective flattening. The initial antidepressive medication (imipramine) was based on the assumption that he suffered from a depressive disorder, because on admission social withdrawal, eating problems

Table 9.6. Case history 1: R. K. *1980, male

Week 1		Admission as inpatient (Freiburg): Bizarre behavior, hallucinations, delusions, suicidal thoughts, social withdrawal, anergia, anhedonia, depression
Week 3	Perphenazine 16 mg/d	Reduction of "positive" and "negative" symptoms
Week 10	Discontinuation due to a temperature rise (infection)	Symptom worsening
Week 12	Perphenazine 20 mg/d	Again good symptom reduction
Week 30	Perphenazine 20 mg/d	Admission as inpatient (Marburg): hallucinations, delusions, compulsions, social withdrawal, anergia, anhedonia
Week 33	Haloperidol 24 mg/d	Symptom reduction
Week 46	Haloperidol 24 mg/d Chlorprothixene 50 mg/d	Discharged to a special rehabilitation centre (Leppermühle)
Week 123	Haloperidol 24 mg/d Chlorprothixene 50 mg/d	Readmission, Marburg: Prominent "positive" symptoms: hallucinations, delusions, compulsions, bizarre behavior, social withdrawal, anergia, anhedonia
Week 126	Clozapine 300 mg/d	Symptom reduction
Week 141	Clozapine 300 mg/d	Discharged to a special rehabilitation centre (Leppermühle)
Week 195 (follow-up)	Clozapine 300 mg/d Clozapine serum level: 100 ng/ml, clozapine-N-oxide: 36 ng/ml, N-desmethyl-clozapine: 134 ng/ml	Living as an inpatient in a rehabilitation centre, attending a special school for mentally ill children. *Psychopathology*: affective flattening, alogia, anergia, anhedonia, attentional impairment, no "positive" symptoms

Summary

Family history: Mother obesity, hypothyroidism; father no information available.

Diagnosis: Childhood psychosis according to ICD-10: F20.0.

Symptoms: Hallucinations, delusions, delusional ideas, suicidal thoughts, anhedonia, anergia affective flattening, social withdrawal, depression.

First schizophrenic symptoms (according IRAOS) with:	10 years 7 months.
First admission as inpatient with	11 years 2 months.
Admission to rehabilitation centre with	12 years.
First neuroleptic medication with	11 years 2 months.
First clozapine trial with	13 years 7 months.

and depression were the predominant symptoms. Under this medication the depressive symptoms, however, remained unchanged. Due to worsening of his bizarre behavior, anergia and affective flattening, a diagnosis of childhood schizophrenia was made. Sulpiride was tried with no benefit and then perazine which produced a moderate improvement. This medication had to be discontinued because of liver problems. In week 31, haloperidol was introduced with no improvement, followed again by sulpiride and again haloperidol. Finally, an atypical neuroleptic, clozapine, was administered but none of these medications showed any improvement. After a wash-out phase of 3 weeks, fluphenazine was prescribed with a remarkably good improvement, and the patient was discharged to a rehabilitation center in week 94. The details of the different trials of treatment are demonstrated in Table 9.7. The case was particularly interesting in that the schizophrenic symptomatology required for the diagnosis of paranoid schizophrenia developed only after 12 weeks of inpatient treatment, and that a partial remission was only achieved after the introduction of the sixth neuroleptic substance (fluphenazine).

Follow-up
The course of this patient's disorder was favorable. He did very well at the rehabilitation center, completed his higher education successfully and in 1999 was about to start University, studying theology. Medication was continued until the age of 20 and has now been discontinued for 6 months. Minor psychopathological symptoms with an irritable and cranky mood, and a mildly disorganized speech with circumstantiality are still present.

Conclusions

The following guidelines are suggested with regard to the use of antipsychotic medications (slightly modified from Remington, 1997 and from Remschmidt et al., 1996):

(i)   Typical and atypical neuroleptics are, to some extent, comparable with regard to their clinical efficiency; they differ, however, remarkably with regard to their side effect profile.

(ii) Conventional neuroleptics should be administered in adequate dosages, using the lowest dosage that is effective. To give an example with regard to the prototype of typical antipsychotics, the daily dosage of haloperidol should be in the range between 2 and 5 mg haloperidol equivalents per day, depending on age and weight.

(iii) It is imperative that children and adolescents who are treated with neuroleptics and their parents are informed about the disorder and the effects and side

Table 9.7. Case history 2: S. G. *1977, male

Week 1		Admission as inpatient: Social withdrawal, depression, mutism, eating problems, bizarre behaviour, anergia, anhedonia, affective flattening
Week 4	Imipramine 3 × 25 mg/d	No symptomatic improvement
Week 9	Discontinuation due to ECG-alterations	
Week 9	Sulpiride 3 × 50 mg/d	No symptomatic improvement
Week 12	Perazine 3 × 100 mg/d	Moderate improvement
Week 28	Discontinuation due to acute liver enzyme elevation (GOT: 85 U/1; GPT: 673 U/l; γ-GT: 29 U/1)	Symptom worsening (positive formal thought disorder, pressure of speech, delusional ideas, neologisms, thought blocking)
Week 31	Haloperidol 3 × 2 mg/d	No symptomatic improvement
Week 33	Sulpiride 3 × 100 mg/d	No symptomatic improvement
Week 40	Haloperidol 3 × 6 mg/d	No symptomatic improvement
Week 48	Clozapine 3 × 100 mg/d	No symptomatic improvement
Week 66	No medication	Symptom worsening
Week 69	Fluphenazine 3 × 4 mg/d	Good symptomatic improvement
Week 94	Fluphenazine 2 × 2 mg/d Fluphenazine-Decanoate 37.5 mg i.m. (2.5 weeks interval)	Discharged to a special rehabilitation centre
Week 192 (follow-up)	Fluphenazine-Decanoate 25 mg i.m. (3 weeks interval)	Living as an inpatient in a rehabilitation centre, attending a normal school. *Psychopathology*: affective flattening, anergia, anhedonia. No positive symptoms, except a slight formal thought disorder.

Family history: Uncle (maternal) schizophrenic psychosis; grandmother (maternal) depression.

Summary:

Diagnosis: Childhood psychosis according to ICD-10: F20.0.

Symptoms: Positive formal thought disorder, bizarre behavior, delusional ideas, pressure of speech, neologisms, anergia, anhedonia, affective flattening, social withdrawal, mutism, depression.

First schizophrenic symptoms (according to IRAOS) at	11 years 6 months.
First admission as inpatient at	12 years 1 month.
Admission to a rehabilitation center at	13 years 1 month.
First neuroleptic medication at	12 years 3 months.
First clozapine trial at	13 years.

Partial remission after the sixth neuroleptic substance (Fluphenazine).

effects of the medication. All this has to be documented in the patient's chart. Further, a careful monitoring of effects and side effects has to be carried out during long-term treatment.

(iv)   It has been useful to distinguish with regard to the treatment goal the antipsychotic effect from the effect on behavior. High-potency neuroleptics, for example, are mainly effective against the psychotic symptoms, whereas low potency neuroleptics have a more pronounced effect on behavior (e.g., sedation).

(v)   All neuroleptic medication has to start at low dosages and should be increased slowly in order to reach steady-state levels. The treatment should also not be interrupted suddenly.

(vi)   It is important to differentiate between non-response and non-compliance in the group of patients who do not respond to treatment.

(vii) First episode patients seem to be more sensitive to side effects and may require lower doses than chronic patients. At the same time, they usually respond better to treatment; however, most of them will experience another episode.

(viii) It is recommended that first episode patients should remain on neuroleptic therapy for a period of 1 to 2 years, the long-term dosage being low as a measure to prevent relapses.

(ix)   In case of acute dystonia, parkinsonism or akathisia, the therapy of choice is antiparkinsonian agents. If akathisia occurs, the drug should be given at a reduced dose or changed. Benzodiazepines or propranolol can also be helpful for akathisia.

Electroconvulsive treatment (ECT)

Since the initial administration of electroconvulsive treatment to adolescents (Heuyer et al., 1947/8), this treatment has been a matter of great controversy. Without doubt, this method is effective in mood disorders in adults and adolescents and is a life-saving treatment method in febrile catatonia. ECT, however, is rarely used as a treatment method for children and adolescents in spite of the established efficacy for the treatment of depression and bipolar disorders, and the endorsement in the use in children by the American Psychiatric Association (1990). Because of the relative lack of experience in the field with ECT in children and adolescents, American Psychiatric Association recommendations call for second opinions from psychiatrists not otherwise involved in the case, who are experienced in treating children/adolescents (one such individual for patients ages 13 to 17 and two for patients age 12 or under).

Table 9.8. Selected ECT publications since 1990

Study	Study design	n	Age range in years	Diagnoses	Outcome criteria	Response rate
Schneekloth et al. (1993)	Retrospective chart review	20	13–18	4 = Depression 4 = Bipolar 12 = Schizophrenia schizophreniform schizoaffective	Clinical impression	65%
Kutcher & Robertson (1995)	Retrospective controlled cohort	16	16–22	8 = Bipolar-manic 8 = Bipolar-depressed	Standardized rating scales	Significantly better than refusers
Ghaziuddin et al. (1996)	Retrospective	11	13–18	9 = Major depression 1 = Bipolar-depressed 1 = Organic mood disorder	Depression rating scores, global functioning score	64%
Moise & Petrides (1996)	Retrospective chart review	13	16–18	3 = Major depression 2 = Bipolar disorder 8 = Mixed diagnostic group	Clinical impression	76%
Cohen et al. (1997)	Retrospective chart review	21	14–19	10 = Major depression with psychotic symptoms 4 = Bipolar-mania 7 = Schizophrenia	Clinical impression	100% for depressed 75% for bipolar partial in schizophrenia
Walter & Ray (1997)	Retrospective chart review	42	14–18	14 = Major depression 14 = Psychotic depression 12 = Schizophrenia	Clinical impression	51% improvement across diagnoses
Strober et al. (1998)	Prospective	10	13–17	3 = Bipolar-depressed 7 = Major depression	Depression rating scores	60%

From Ghadziuddin (1998).

Results of recent studies

Recent reviews and original studies on the use of ECT in children and adolescents have suggested that this method is only rarely used in children and adolescents. Walter and Rey (1997), in their study on the frequency of ECT treatment between 1990 and 1996 in New South Wales, found only 0.93% of all ECT patients were under the age of 18. A survey of attitudes towards ECT in the UK revealed that less than 7% of child psychiatrists would even consider the use of ECT for their patients (Parmar, 1993).

In Table 9.8, selected ECT publications since 1990 are listed. This demonstrates that the response rates in different diagnoses vary from 51 to 100%, the latter with regard to severely depressed patients.

The major indication for ECT is not schizophrenia, but uni- and bipolar mood disorders. These patients show the highest response rates. The response rate in schizophrenia is much lower, with a symptom response of between 35 and 50%, whereas in schizoaffective disorders, a remission of around 75% was achieved (Walter & Rey, 1997; Rey & Walter, 1997). However, these results reflect findings from a very small group of schizophrenic and schizo-affective patients.

Similar results were obtained by Schneekloth et al. (1993), who reported significant improvements in patients with schizophreniform disorder (80%) and schizo-affective disorder (50%), but a response rate of only 35% in patients with schizophrenia. This is also in line with the study by Cohen et al. (1997), who reported a remarkable improvement in only three out of seven patients.

In studies with adult patients ECT has been shown to be far more effective in acute schizophrenia than in chronic and treatment refractory schizophrenia. The treatment effects are, in general, comparable to those of neuroleptic medication.

Adverse effects

As far as adverse effects are concerned, headache, nausea and vomiting and memory disturbances are most prominent.

Table 9.9 demonstrates the frequency of adverse side effects described in four recent studies. A major concern is epileptic seizures. They can be differentiated into tardive seizures (occurring after complete recovery from ECT) and prolonged seizures with a duration greater than 120 to 180 seconds. The first type of seizures is a rare complication, but has been described in a few cases (Ghaziuddin et al., 1996; Schneekloth et al., 1993). Prolonged seizures occured in 3 out of 13 patients in the study by Moise & Petrides (1996) and in 9.6% of 135 treatments of all patients in the study by Ghaziuddin et al. (1996). Seven of

Table 9.9. Side effects of ECT in children

Symptom	Cohel et al. (1997) % per patient	Walter & Rey (1997) % per patient	Ghadziuddin et al. (1996) patient	Kutcher & Robertson (1995) % of total treatments
Headache	42	65	80	53
Agitation	—	—	—	9
Nausea/vomiting	37	14	64	2
Confusion	—	18	0	18
Tardive seizure	0	0	9 (1 of 11 patients)	0
Disinhibition	26	—	0	0
Memory loss (subjective)	52	22	—	9
Memory loss (objective)	47	—	Significantly impaired digit and passage recall	—
Mania/hypomania	—	4	0	9

From Ghaziuddin (1998).

these 11 patients experienced at least one prolonged seizure. Because of the risk of seizures after ECT treatment, a thorough neurological investigation including EEG is required before the application of ECT.

Conclusions

On the background of current experience and reports in the literature, the following conclusions can be drawn (Ghaziuddin, 1998; Kutcher & Robertson, 1995; Walter & Rey, 1997):

(i)   ECT therapy is not a treatment of choice in schizophrenia. Its main indication is mood disorder in patients who are either unresponsive to, or unable to tolerate, conventional pharmacotherapy. Other psychiatric disorders with prominent mood symptoms such as schizoaffective disorders and probably therapy-resistant schizophreniform disorders may also show some improvement with ECT.

(ii) A careful physical and psychiatric evaluation including an EEG should be undertaken as an anaesthesiologist should be consulted.

(iii) The decision to undertake ECT should be supported by two psychiatrists uninvolved with the case management and experienced in the treatment of children and adolescents.

(iv) ECT treatment should be administered only in centers with a team of experienced experts, and should be carried out only in an inpatient setting, in view of the danger of tardive and prolonged seizures.

(v) Pre- and post cognitive assessments should be conducted including assessment 6 months following the last treatment. Measurement of preliminary response to ECT should occur around treatment six, at which time the possibility of changing from unilateral to bilateral electrodes may be considered (Ghaziuddin, 1998).

(vi) Information about the whole procedure, its possible side effects and alternative treatment methods must be provided to the patient (in an age-appropriate way) and to the parents. Both parents and patient should give their informed consent.

Psychotherapeutic measures (see also Chapter 8)

Cognitive psychotherapy and other behavioral approaches

Systematic behavioral interventions based on basic learning principles started in the 1970s, and were introduced into clinical settings under the name of the so-called "token economy program." They were administered individually as well as in groups and were mainly focused on the training of everyday activities such as self-sufficiency (e.g., clothing, hygiene, punctuality at school or at work) and the undertaking of certain duties (e.g., kitchen service, cleaning). Several of these token economy techniques were also used individually in order to control smoking, excessive eating, or even to influence those occupied by hallucinations and delusions.

Later on, the focus of behavioral therapy shifted towards more complex programs as, e.g., social skills training (Wallace et al., 1980; Brady, 1984a,b), which is based on an analysis of each patient's interpersonal strengths and weaknesses and forms a more individualized therapeutic approach. Social skills training for schizophrenic patients includes several techniques such as modeling prosocial behaviors, problem-centered group discussions, model learning (e.g., by video demonstrations or role play) enhanced with video feedback, and in vivo exercises. Examples of potential trained skills are maintaining eye contact, reacting more quickly to interpersonal communication, varying voice intonation, and reinforcing prosocial responses from others.

Social competence training is often carried out as a group therapy and is focused upon the management of everyday situations and the training of situation-adequate behavior. The participants learn to express their own wishes and desires, to accept at the same time the needs and wishes of the other patients, to accept proposals as well as criticism, and to behave adequately in a given situation. The group members are encouraged to express their emotions and to interact in a respectful rather than an egocentric way with the other patients and the therapist. Especially during adolescence, other common problems will be addressed, such as social roles, identity and independence, interaction with the opposite sex and specific behavior at school, at work, or in peer groups.

A number of controlled studies have demonstrated that clinically meaningful changes in behavior can occur as a result of social skills training, with improvements of up to 70% in social functioning and a shortened hospital stay. However, other evaluation studies have demonstrated that, in spite of the short-term effect of these methods, generalization and long-term effects are not convincing (Brady, 1984b). Due to this criticism and the observation that the "laboratory situation" is not comparable with real-life situations, new techniques increasingly use "in vivo" training, based on everyday tasks.

Finally, several groups have emphasized the high correlation between poor results from social competence training and cognitive deficits. They have therefore tried to integrate cognitive variables into the treatment procedure (Hoggarty et al., 1991, 1995).

These experiences have led to highly structured *manualized* therapy techniques involving video and audio learning materials as well as written instructions in order to optimize the learning situation (Lieberman & Eckman, 1989). These concepts have been used mainly in adult patients with chronic schizophrenia, and there remains insufficient experience with adolescents.

One of these integrated approaches has, however, been evaluated in young schizophrenic patients. This is called "Integrative Psychological Therapy Program for Schizophrenic Patients (IPT)" and was developed in Switzerland (Brenner et al., 1980, 1993). The program consists of five standardized therapeutic components: cognitive differentiation, social perception, verbal communication, social skills and interpersonal problem-solving. The program started originally from the classical social skills training technique, which was extended to the area of communication. It is possible to administer the program individually to patients with a different profile of schizophrenic symptoms. For example, the cognitive differentiation component can be extended in cognitive-impaired patients with the aim of stabilizing their cognitive functions, thus enabling them to optimize their achivements in the other problem areas, e.g., interpersonal problem-solving. Most of the tasks, assigned to the different therapy components, are realistic and oriented towards everyday situations, and can be offered in the form of slides and video sequences. For instance, several tasks concerning "social perception" are based on slides showing people in different emotional states and social interactions. Patients are encouraged to discuss and describe the respective situations, with the aim of achieving a more realistic assessment, learning in the process from one another.

This program, originally developed for young adults, has now been modified for adolescent schizophrenics (Kienzle et al., 1997), and seems to offer a promising approach that still needs to be evaluated systematically.

Cognitive psychotherapeutic techniques have further developed since their introduction by Beck et al. (1979), who demonstrated their effectiveness in the treatment of depression. Meanwhile, cognitive therapy has been demonstrated to be effective in children and adolescents with depressive disorder (Harrington et al., 1998). Several controlled and uncontrolled studies have extended Beck's cognitive therapy to adulthood schizophrenia, with encouraging clinical results. However, up to now there have been no large studies in children and adolescents with schizophrenia. The results from the adult studies open up a promising new field, which should be investigated in the future. Until supporting evidence is available, it still seems appropriate to extrapolate from adult studies to adolescence or even childhood, since adolescents at least are quite similar in their symptomatology to adults. Recently, several studies from the UK, Australia, and the USA, have demonstrated the efficacy of cognitive-behavioral approaches in several key areas in schizophrenia, especially therapy-resistant hallucinations and delusions. Several approaches have also addressed therapeutic efforts in the treatment of associated symptoms such as anxiety and depression.

Table 9.10 reviews the most frequently used cognitive strategies in the treatment of schizophrenia. Most of the strategies described in Table 9.10 have been used in patients with chronic schizophrenia. However, recently, several of these methods have also been investigated in first-episode schizophrenia (Jackson et al., 1998; Haddock et al., 1998).

Distraction treatment and focusing treatment have been investigated by Haddock et al. (1996) with the aim of reducing the distress and disruption caused by auditory hallucinations. In a randomized trial, 19 schizophrenic patients were allocated to either distraction or focusing treatment. *Distraction treatment* comprises several strategies designed to increase the patient's reper-

Table 9.10. Frequently used cognitive-behavioral interventions in young adults with chronic or acute schizophrenia

Cognitive strategies	Key problems/aims
Distraction treatment (Haddock et al., 1996)	Distress, disruption caused by hallucinations
Focusing treatment: focusing and exposure (Haddock et al., 1996, 1998)	Distress, disruption caused by hallucinations
Rationale responding (Kingdon & Turkington, 1994; Haddock et al., 1998)	Control over hallucination, reduction of distress
Belief modification (Chadwick & Lowe, 1990; Chadwick & Birchwood, 1994; Haddock et al., 1996)	Modification of patients' beliefs in connection with hallucinations, reduction of distress
Coping strategy enhancement (Tarrier et al., 1993)	Hallucinations, delusions
Problem-solving (Tarrier et al., 1993)	Anxiety

toire of techniques available to distract the patients from the voices. The principle of *focusing treatment* is to gradually expose the patients to the voices in a graded fashion with the aim of reducing the anxiety associated with the hallucinations, including the associated cognitions and beliefs.

Further strategies are rational responding (Kingdon & Turkington, 1994) and belief modification (Chadwick & Lowe, 1990) as well as other cognitive techniques used in the treatment of anxiety and depression. Haddock et al. (1996) demonstrated that these strategies were effective in significantly reducing the amount of time spent hallucinating and the disruption caused by the hallucination. This was measured by the Personal Questionnaire Rapid Scaling Technique (Mulhall, 1978). The effect of both techniques was quite similar; the only difference found was with regard to self-esteem which was significantly increased by focusing, whereas distraction treatment tended to decrease self-esteem.

Also, the other techniques, such as rational responding and belief modification, were successful in different samples of patients.

Chadwick and Birchwood (1994) have demonstrated the effectiveness of strategies aimed at modifying the patient's beliefs about the omnipotence and malevolence of the hallucinations. A reduction of distress associated with them was demonstrated. The same applies to rational responding with regard to control over hallucinations and reduction of distress (Kingdon & Turkington, 1994; Haddock et al., 1998).

Two different strategies (coping strategy enhancement and problem-solving) have been tested by Tarrier et al. (1993) in the treatment of persistent hallucinations and delusions in 27 patients treated with neuroleptics, with continuing symptomatology. Coping strategy enhancement included a systematic assessment of the individual's own coping strategies for dealing with the hallucinations or delusions and the main aim of the treatment was to enhance these strategies. The problem-solving approach was not mainly focused at the psychotic symptoms, but on a number of other key problems that were important for the individual patient. Both treatment techniques were effective in significantly reducing anxiety and delusions, compared with a waiting list control group, the coping strategy enhancement being superior to the problem-solving. Both treatments, however, were less effective for auditory hallucinations.

These results mainly obtained in patients with chronic schizophrenia have been replicated in a group of acute inpatients, who had recently experienced a first psychotic episode (Drury et al., 1996). This group of patients was randomly allocated to either a cognitive-behavioral treatment consisting of individual sessions, group work and family sessions, or to a conventional and rather unspecific control treatment. Both groups received the same amount of time spent on active treatment. The cognitive treatment approach was superior to conventional treatment in several respects: the time until recovery was 25 to 50% shorter, the time spent in hospital was reduced by approximately 50%, and the relapse rates were lower. This result is very encouraging because the treatment program was effective in all stages of the illness, and the number of relapses was reduced. As far as we know, there are no similar studies in adolescence; however, it seems appropriate to use this model for them at the onset of their disorder.

Recently, Haddock et al. (1998) published a preliminary report about an ongoing study using different cognitive-behavioral techniques in patients with a schizophrenic disorder of less than 2 years' duration who had experienced a first or second acute psychotic episode requiring admission to inpatient services or a day hospital. The program comprises a variety of cognitive-behavioral techniques, including the following elements: (i) assessment and engagement, (ii) formulation of key problems, (iii) intervention directed at reducing the severity and frequency of key problems, and (iv) relapse prevention. The interventions are especially targeted at reducing the severity of psychotic symptoms or at reducing associated problems such as anxiety, depression, social functioning, negative symptoms and issues related to the pharmacological treatment. If the results of this study remain convincing, the cognitive-behavioral approach may also become a standard treatment component in acute schizophrenic patients.

In conclusion, cognitive-behavioral techniques have been shown to be effective in chronic schizophrenia, resulting in reduction of distress and disruption due to hallucinations and delusions. In some studies, anxiety and depression associated with schizophrenia could also be reduced to some extent.

The use of these techniques in acute schizophrenic disorders and especially in first-episode schizophrenics looks promising, but is not yet established unequivocally. The value of these techniques in children and adolescents has to be demonstrated. However, due to the similar symptomatology in adolescent and young adult schizophrenics, results from adult studies are likely to be replicated in adolescents and even in children.

Emotional management therapy

Whereas behavioral and cognitive-oriented psychotherapeutic methods have been widely used in the treatment of schizophrenic patients, mainly in the chronic phase (recently also in earlier stages), therapeutic methods in the emotional sphere seem to be somewhat neglected. The emotional state of schizophrenic patients is, however, an important one. Approximately 20% of all schizophrenic psychoses in adolescence start with a depressive episode (Remschmidt, et al., 1973), but depressive symptoms are also extremely important over the course of the disorder. Depression in a patient entering a rehabilitation treatment program has been found to be a predictor of poor outcome at 1 year follow-up (Remschmidt, et al. 1988), a result which has since been replicated in an independent sample (Martin, 1991; Remschmidt et al., 1991).

For these and other reasons, the emotional state of schizophrenic patients should be included as an essential component in all treatment programs. This covers not only depression, but also includes the whole range of emotional functioning and responsiveness in all relevant situations.

In contrast to autistic individuals, schizophrenic patients are not impaired in their ability to identify faces (Walker et al., 1984). However, they have been found to be slower and less accurate at the recognition of emotional stimuli as compared with normal controls and depressive patients (Gaebel & Wölwer, 1992; Heimberg et al., 1992). Especially in situations characterized by stress and tension, schizophrenic patients are remarkably impaired in their ability to appraise affect (Bellack, 1996).

It is assumed that these deficits are not specific to particular emotions, but are related to information processing deficits of which attentional impairments play a central role. In spite of the difficulty of deciding which of these deficits (cognitive or emotional) is primary, it makes sense to try to address these deficits in a treatment program for schizophrenic patients. Whilst many psychological treatment programs include an emotional component, most do not primarily focus on emotional processing (Falloon, 1987; Hoggarty et al., 1995; Lieberman, 1995; Perris, 1989).

Emotional management therapy (EMT), in contrast, has been designed to help people develop and refine specific strategies for coping with the impact of distress, anxiety and dysfunction in information processing (Hodel & Brenner, 1996). According to the authors (Hodel et al., 1998), EMT consists of two subprograms that have been empirically tested and validated (Roder et al., 1997). The first includes three steps devoted to the patients' ability to describe their physiological and cognitive reaction patterns when confronted by stress, fear or excitement, and the learning and application of relaxation techniques in vivo. The second subprogram includes eight steps which address the definition and description of emotions in varying situations, the description of subjective experiences in various emotional states, and the development of coping strategies in relation to any consequent emotional distress.

The program has been administered to young schizophrenic patients and in the early stages of their psychotic disorder (Kienzle & Martinius, 1995).

In a pilot study of early schizophrenic psychosis (Hodel et al., 1998), 19 patients meeting DSM-IV criteria for schizophrenia were randomly assigned either to the EMT group or to a comparison group. The groups were matched for age and education: ten patients participated in the EMT group, nine in the comparison group. All patients were additionally on neuroleptic medication. After 4 weeks of the EMT program (11 sessions of 40–50 min for each patient), there were some significant improvements in the EMT group. These improvements were mainly in the areas of cognitive functioning; there were no significant differences between the groups in emotional well-being or social functioning. Although emotional functioning could not be demonstrated to improve, this approach seems worthy of further research. The trial undertaken involved a short therapy phase (4 weeks), and the therapy sessions might not have been intensive enough.

In conclusion, emotional management therapy has not yet been demonstrated to be an effective treatment method for young patients with schizophrenia in the subacute stage of the first episode. However, as there is no doubt that the emotional sphere is of great importance in the course of the disorder, this approach should, in our view, be continued and be thoroughly evaluated in the future.

Group programs

Group programs have been thought to be helpful in the treatment of young people with schizophrenia for a number of reasons. First, they meet the needs for communication in young people, and might therefore reduce feelings of alienation. They also demonstrate to patients that others suffer from similar problems, thus giving support to participants in group activities. Finally, as they take place with several patients in one session, they are not as time consuming as individual therapy and much more economical.

Groups therapies were originally developed to enhance self-esteem and to modify attitudes and behavior through the corrective experience of supportive group processes. Initial adaptations with a focus on special symptoms were developed in the 1970s, originating from social-cognitive theories (Bandura, 1977, 1986), and were primarily used in the treatment of anxiety states, and in order to improve assertiveness. Many of the above-mentioned psycho-therapeutic and educational techniques for the treatment of schizophrenic patients have been employed in group programs. With regard to the main focus of treatment, group programs may be divided into focused programs devoted to a special area of intervention, and integrative approaches that try to cover a wider range of problem areas with the aim of general improvement in different areas, expressed by better integration of the patients. Focused group programs have been established for improvement of skills (e.g., social skills training, problem-solving, communication) and education (e.g., information about illness and treatment, management of medication and relapses). Integrative approaches include different areas of functioning that are typically impaired in schizophrenic patients. For instance, the above-described "Integrative Psychological Therapy Program for Schizophrenic Patients (IPT)" (Brenner et al., 1980; Brenner et al., 1993) has been applied as a group program.

Since schizophrenic patients have impairments in focusing attention and are often highly sensitive to social overstimulation, group programs have to be well structured and supportive. Mainly insight-oriented and conflict-enhancing group therapies are not appropriate (Leszcz et al., 1985; Schooler & Spohn, 1982). Especially in acute psychotic states, the use of group therapies has been questioned and even considered harmful (Ciompi, 1983; Kanas et al., 1980).

There are not many group programs for adolescents and young adults that focus on the early stages of the schizophrenic disorder. A recent study used an integrated group approach and included a group of 34 patients with first schizophrenic episode aged 16 to 30 years. This group was compared to 61 other patients who received a conventional treatment. There were no significant differences on any outcome measure between the two groups (Albiston et al., 1998).

Family-oriented measures (see also Chapter 8)

It is self-evident that the families of children and adolescents with schizophrenic psychoses have to be included in the planning and concept of therapy. However, empirical research has shown that ambitious family therapy concepts which have been propagated in the last two decades have not reaped the benefits hoped for. It is now quite clear that the typical "psychotic family" has no more basis in reality than the "schizophrenogenic mother." However, studies using the concept of expressed emotions have shown that emotional factors within the family play an important role in relapses of the disorder. Therefore, in every child and adolescent with schizophrenia, one has to decide on the extent to which the family should be integrated into the therapeutic process. This depends on the patient, the disorder, the structure and stability of the family, as well as on the therapist's experience (Remschmidt, 1993a).

Family interventions in childhood or adolescent onset schizophrenia comprise a combination of psychoeducational and behavioral approaches with practical support to the patient and the family and an attempt to reduce high levels of "expressed emotions" by the family members, especially criticism and hostility. From adult psychiatry settings, there is evidence that reducing the amount of expressed emotion is associated with a reduction of subsequent relapse rates and better social functioning (Dixon & Lehmann, 1995; Penn & Mueser, 1996). It is, however, not yet clear if the same efficacy can be achieved in families with a schizophrenic child or adolescent. There is some evidence that the situation in these families may be somewhat different. Attempts to replicate the findings from adult psychiatry have not so far been successful and studies have failed to replicate the concept of expressed emotions in children (Asarnow et al., 1994a). Alternative strategies will therefore have to be developed in these families (Asarnow et al., 1994b).

From these considerations, the question arises as to whether so-called expressed emotions are actually an epiphenomenon which emerges during the course of the disorder. Most studies concerning expressed emotions in schizophrenia have been carried out in patients suffering from chronic schizophrenia, and the impressive results in terms of reduced rates of relapses apply only to this group.

In our department, family work is carried out in every case and starts at admission of the patient or even beforehand on an outpatient basis. Three levels of intervention have been proved to be useful (see Table 9.11).

Family counseling and psychoeducational approaches

The main aim of this type of intervention is the development of a stable therapeutic alliance. This comprises detailed information about the disorder, including etiology, measures of treatment, course and prognosis. Special emphasis has to be laid on medication, including the most important effects and side effects of the different compounds used.

It is very important to minimize information deficits in the parents as well as the patients and also to reduce an underlying feelings of guilt in the parents. Family counseling is a continuous process and has to include feedback by the parents which enables the therapist to tailor all information to their and the patient's needs.

Typical methods to achieve these goals are the gradual appropriate provision of information about the disorder, which will reduce insecurity and give the family a continuous positive feedback if they adequately adhere to the recommendations given.

In some clinical settings, special information sheets for the parents are used, and frequently questions by the parents are collected and answered by experienced professionals. By collecting this material, a sound body of knowledge can be shared with the families, which gives a feeling of security to the families, the therapist and the whole team.

Supportive and structural family therapy

The main aim of this level of family intervention is the neutralization and control of symptoms. This means that secondary problems, conflicts and vicious circles, which frequently develop in the course of psychotic disorder, need to be interrupted. In this process, individual symptomatology is disconnected as far as possible from the family interactions. While the first level (family counseling) was carried out individually with the parents on the one side, and with the patient on the other, supportive and structural family therapy is carried out during joint sessions in which both the parents and the patient actively take part, sometimes also with siblings and other family members. This second level of family intervention is only possible when a significant reduction of symptoms has already taken place and good co-operation of the family has

Table 9.11. Co-operation with families of children and adolescents with psychotic disorders

Level	Intervention	Focal problem	Aims	Typical methods
I	Family counseling	Information deficits, discouragement, frustation, feelings of insecurity, vague feelings of guilt	Development of stable therapeutic alliance	Orientation and security through information; positive connotation
II	Supporting and structuring family therapy	Escalating circles of interaction between patient's symptoms and family involvement	Neutralization and control of symptoms, disconnection of causal links between family interaction and patient's symptoms (interruption of secondary dynamics)	Clear agreements and determinations, behavior contracts ("direct" interventions)
III	Extended, development-oriented family therapy	Relationship patterns and family conflicts which inhibit development	Extension of scope of decisions and actions, realization of developmental options	Reframing, paradox and provocative methods ("indirect" methods), conflict negotiation, non-verbal and actional methods

Adapted from Mattejat (1989, 1997); Remschmidt (1993a).

been achieved. The joint sessions are arranged more frequently prior to home visits or especially before discharge. As far as the methodology is concerned, clear agreements and contracts are used in order to make sure that the family follows the recommendations discussed during the joint family sessions.

Naturally, difficulties commonly emerge during the process of family intervention, irrespective of the level on which they are carried out. It is therefore useful to include behavioral therapeutic methods in order to facilitate certain measures within the family. For example, non-compliance with regard to medication or aggressive outbursts are sometimes important problems that have to be dealt with in the therapeutic regime. Clearly defined tasks with regard to these issues can agreed upon, and their fulfilment verified at the next session.

Extended development-oriented family therapy

This third level of family intervention is carried out in only a minority of families with a psychotic child or adolescent. The focus is laid on the patterns of relationships between the family members and typical family conflicts which inhibit the patient's development. The main aims are concentrated upon the patient's growing independence and separation from the family. It is very important to facilitate growing confidence in the patient's abilities to enable the parents to release their child from being viewed as a patient and to concede greater responsibility to him or her.

These are problems which apply to all families and not especially to families of psychotic patients. However, due to the severity of the disorder, many parents tend to become overinvolved, and have difficulties with permitting an appropriate amount of freedom and responsibility to their child in an age- and development-appropriate manner. In such cases, patterns of family interactions and their convictions can be shifted by redefinition of certain problems, and by concrete proposals for the solution of a given problem. This therapeutic approach is a complicated one, and requires sensitivity and care from the therapist who must continuously check whether his interventions are over-straining the family going beyond the limits of their capacity. The methods used to achieve these goals may include paradoxical interventions, reframing, and conflict negotiation. Non-verbal methods such as role play and psycho-drama have also been found to be useful.

In our experience, such therapy programs can reduce the patients' level of emotional stress to some extent. In addition, depot-neuroleptic medication may reduce the patients' sensitivity to environmental stress.

The description of this program has mainly concentrated on those cases in whom reintegration into their families after inpatient treatment was possible. However, in about 30 to 40% of children and adolescents with schizophrenia, this is not possible (Remschmidt, 1993b). For this group, a special rehabilitation programme is necessary. Naturally, however, family measures as outlined above, are extremely important in this program as well, and follow the same lines.

Specific measures of rehabilitation

Indications and general principles

Residential rehabilitation for adolescents with schizophrenia may be indicated because of either the nature or the course of the illness. In particular, it may be advisable if there are marked negative symptoms after treatment of the acute episode or when troublesome residual symptoms render reintegration of the adolescent into the family impossible. Alternatively, there may be factors within the family, such as poor interfamilial relationships, high expressed emotion or overprotection, which make a prolonged phase of rehabilitation desirable. Finally, residential rehabilitation is indicated when there are specific educational issues, for example, to enable the adolescent to achieve a recognized level of educational achievement, such as an academic or vocational qualification. The rehabilitation of adolescents with psychotic illnesses involves the coordination of a number of interrelated measures which should be included in a comprehensive rehabilitation program. Such a program has been developed in connection with the Department of Child and Adolescent Psychiatry of the Philipps-University of Marburg at the rehabilitation centre "Leppermühle" near Marburg (Martin & Remschmidt, 1983; Martin, 1991). This rehabilitation program is of 2 years' duration and includes the following components (Martin, 1991):

(i)   A well-structured educational facility with expertise in dealing with the particular special needs of these adolescents is required. It should be appropriately staffed with skilled carers, social workers and teachers, and should offer not only adequate care and supervision but also the opportunity of a range of living options from a staffed therapeutic community setting to smaller, supervised units integrated into the local community.

(ii)   An integral component of the rehabilitation process should be helping the adolescents to realize their educational capacity, with the acquisition of relevant qualifications. This may involve individual tuition in order to achieve basic academic qualifications, or attendance at local schools or colleges for higher academic or vocational qualifications. The "Schule für Kranke" (School for Sick Children) is a special school for physically and/or mentally handicapped adolescents. It offers an additional educational year to the equivalent normal schools, and as a result of the high teacher:pupil ratio, specially trained teachers and small class size, allows a degree of flexibility which permits each child to work at his/her own pace.

(iii) Individual supportive psychotherapy and additional group work involving social skills training are usually indicated.

(iv) Occupational therapy is just as important as academic rehabilitation and, for older adolescents, this should involve integration into appropriate work activities. This is generally undertaken gradually, such that periods of supported work experience lead to increasing confidence and competence in the workplace. The aim is to enable the adolescent to be able to cope with the pressures involved in an eight hour working day. As more time is spent in work-related activities, proficiency increases and the adolescent learns and perfects a broader range of skills. The long-term aim is that a placement is found in an industrial firm or business, or in a training establishment which offers the opportunity to train in a specific trade.

(v) Finally, medication should be individually tailored in order to minimize the risk of relapse.

These general principles have been realized in an integrated rehabilitation programme which is described in the next section of this chapter.

Practical aspects and organization
Background

The development of a residential rehabilitation program for young schizophrenics was made possible through co-operation with a well-established body responsible for the provision of residential institutions, the "Association for the care and welfare of young people" based in Giessen. The institutions run by this association (a psychotherapeutic unit for adolescents with neurotic or psychosomatic illnesses in Giessen and a children's home in Busek) had always enjoyed a constructive working relationship with the University Department of Child and Adolescent Psychiatry at the Philipps-University in Marburg. With our support, the children's home "Leppermühle" was developed into a therapeutic psychiatric facility, which offers residential rehabilitation to children and adolescents suffering from schizophrenia, epilepsy, autism and other severe psychiatric disturbances. Thus the educational model on which the children's home was based was modified to a youth authority funded, social psychiatry orientated facility. Today, the "Leppermühle" comprises a number of mixed sex living units, each with approximately ten adolescents, an attached school and a well-established occupational and recreational therapeutic section. The medical and psychotherapeutic input is provided by two doctors and three psychologists under the supervision of a consultant psychiatrist from the

Department of Child and Adolescent Psychiatry of the Philipps-University, Marburg.

Day-to-day running of the rehabilitation program

There are four carers responsible for each residential group of about ten adolescents. Within this basic structure, individual programs are developed to help the adolescents become as independent as possible in areas such as dealing with money, shopping for clothes, cooking, use of public transport, etc. In addition, they are encouraged to make their own arrangements for meeting up with friends, participate in planning trips and holidays and deal with officials or public authorities when necessary. Maintenance of contact with their family of origin is considered both important and desirable by the unit. Adolescents are also encouraged to participate in recreational activities with their own residential group such as sport, trips to the nearby town of Giessen and other local cultural or church-related activities.

An integral component of rehabilitation for those adolescents still of school age is to realize their full academic potential. The attached school offers the opportunity to complete courses leading to three different qualifications up to, and including, basic and advanced academic qualifications. In addition, when appropriate, adolescents can attend a variety of schools or colleges in Giessen to obtain higher academic or vocational qualifications in a large range of subjects. The school day is normally from 8.00 to 12.00, Monday to Friday, with additional classes in the last year(s) from 13.00 to 15.30. After completing their schooling, most adolescents find it difficult to move on immediately to an apprenticeship or training and for this reason the unit has developed an extensive range of work experience and occupational therapy options.

These include workshops for carpentry and metalwork, a garden area and a training kitchen where experience can be gained in cookery and housekeeping. Depending on levels of stamina, up to 8 hours a day, 5 days a week can be spent on these activities. For those unable to cope with long stretches at work, an alternative individual program is drawn up, which may involve less demanding individual sessions until more intensive work experience is possible. After a period of stable full-time work experience, adolescents are encouraged to transfer to a formal training or apprenticeship outside the Unit. The organization and coordination of these measures is set out in Fig. 9.7. All patients have individual supportive psychotherapy sessions, and the majority require maintenance drug therapy. The group therapy method used is based on that described by Brenner et al. (1980, 1987). Contact with the family of origin is encouraged, but depends, of course, to some degree on levels of co-operation. Individual

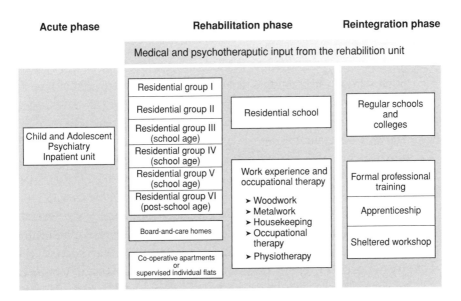

Fig. 9.7. Structure and organization of the rehabilitation program at the Leppermühle.

meetings with parents are offered at regular intervals, and they are also encouraged to attend the so-called "parent afternoons" to which all parents from a residential group are invited.

As a result of the high staffing levels in the Unit, it is often possible to deal with mild relapses in the Unit itself. It must be emphasized, however, that without the support of, and close contact with, the clinic, in particular, the ability to admit a patient immediately when required, the work at the Leppermühle would be unthinkable. Short or relatively short hospital admissions do not break the routine of the rehabilitation process, and after the treatment of the acute crisis or relapse readmission to the Unit is invariably possible.

Evaluation

This rehabilitation program and parts of it have been evaluated by several studies. We describe here one of the most detailed studies of 88 adolescents (50 males and 38 females), aged 12 to 21 (suffering from schizophrenic psychoses and participating in the above described rehabilitation program) who were included in a 1-year longitudinal study, during which each patient was examined at 3-month intervals by means of a standardized test battery, individual standardized mental state examination, and several rating scales. All patients were in the rehabilitation programme of the "Leppermühle" described above. This group of patients included schizophrenic adolescents, who could not be discharged after inpatient treatment to their families, because their condition had become chronic. The subtypes of schizophrenia according to ICD-9 were as follows: one patient had a diagnosis of "schizophrenia simplex" (295.0), 23 suffered from a hebephrenic type (295.1), 47 from the paranoid type (295.3), and 17 from a schizo-affective type (295.7). 12 patients (15.6%) out of the 77 from whom reliable data were available had a schizophrenic mother and 8 of 70 (11.4%) a schizophrenic father. A total of 14 patients of 45 (31%) had other schizophrenic relatives. For the remainder of the patients, reliable data from family histories were not available.

There was a slight dominance of the lower levels of intelligence.

All patients ($N = 88$) were investigated by a test battery and several other methods, including self-rating scales and psychopathological examination, and underwent special ratings with respect to the rehabilitation process. Table 9.12 gives an overview of the areas of investigation and the instruments that were employed. As the table demonstrates, four areas of investigation were used during the study:

(i)   investigation of cognitive functions by objective testing;
(ii)   subjective measures as the state of mental health by means of self-rating scales;
(iii) an independent psychopathological investigation by a psychiatrist blind to the results of the other measures;
(iv) measures concerning the course of rehabilitation, including the level of psycho-social functioning and a special behavior rating scale with subscales on practical abilities, social abilities, emotional behaviour, and unusual psychopathological disturbances.

All the measures listed in Table 9.12 were administered at the beginning of the study to all 88 patients. In a subsample of 74 patients, all of the measures, except the Global Assessment Scale, were administered at intervals of 3 months (i.e., four times) until the end of the first year of the rehabilitation program. At that time, for each patient the Global Assessment Scale (Shaffer et al., 1983; German version by Steinhausen, 1985) was administered independently.

Results of the cross-sectional analysis

The cross-sectional analysis including all 88 patients produced the following results. As a group, schizophrenic patients revealed remarkable deficiencies concerning attention and language-independent intelligence as compared with normal controls. This did not apply to language-dependent intelligence or to memory. There were also notable differences in all the self-rating scales shown in Table 9.12. All these differences in comparison with normal controls were highly significant. However, there were only two parameters that differenti-

Table 9.12. Areas of investigation and instruments used

Areas of investigation	Tests and scales
Cognitive functioning (objective testing)	
Attention/concentration	Attention test d2 (Brickenkamp, 1975)
Memory	Memory subtest of the WAIS (Wechsler, 1964)
Intelligence (language-independent)	Achievement test, subscale 3 (Horn, 1983)
Intelligence (language-dependent)	Achievement test, subscale 6 (Horn, 1983)
Subjective state of mental health	
Paranoia self-rating scale	Paranoia depression inventory, Paranoia scale (PDS-P) (von Zerssen, 1976a)
Depression self-rating scale	Paranoia depression inventory, Depression scale (PDS-D) (Von Zerssen, 1976a)
Somatic complaints self-rating scale	List of complaints (Von Zerssen, 1976b)
Uncharacteristic deficits (schizophrenic basic disturbance)	Frankfurt complaints questionnaire (Süllwold, 1977)
Psychopathology (independent rating)	
Thought disorders	Independent psychopathological investigation thinking disorders scale
Affective disorders	Independent psychopathological investigation affective disorders scale
Course of rehabilitation (independent rating)	
Level of psychosocial functioning	Global assessment scale for children and adolescents (Shaffer et al., 1983; Steinhausen, 1985)
Behavior rating scale	Behavior rating scale of care workers (EFB-P) (Rühl, 1988)

ated between the three subtypes of schizophrenia (paranoid, hebephrenic, schizo-affective). These were activation and motivation in the independent psychopathological investigation and practical abilities in the behavior rating scale for care workers. The subgroups of hebephrenic patients revealed the most pronounced deficiencies in both variables. A factor analysis was carried out, according to the maximum-likelihood method involving five scales (attention test, language-independent intelligence, paranoia scale, depression scale, and Frankfurt complaints questionnaire). The result was a two-factor solution, explaining 65% of the total variance. Factor 1 showed high positive loadings to the variables paranoid tendencies, depression, and uncharacteristic deficits in the Frankfurt complaints questionnaire. This factor could be interpreted as "subjective psychopathological symptoms and complaints." Factor 2 was characterized by high loadings to the variables attention and language-independent intelligence. This factor could be interpreted as "impaired cognitive abilities."

Results of the longitudinal analyses

Longitudinal analyses was carried out in 64 patients who had been followed up for one year, the investigation taking place four times at intervals of 3 months. The following results were obtained.

There was a significant improvement in attention, language-independent intelligence, and memory over time.

An improvement of the subjective psychopathological symptoms could also be observed.

The same improvement was also present for psychopathological symptoms and practical abilities as rated by the care workers during the course of the rehabilitation programme.

However, there was again *no difference* concerning the measures with respect to the three subgroups of schizophrenia (paranoid, hebephrenic and schizoaffective).

Results concerning subgroups

In order to derive subgroups as a special method, a latent-class analysis (LCA; Lazarsfeld & Henry, 1968) was administered, which allowed the derivation of independent groups. For this analysis, four variables were chosen, which had been described as relevant. The four variables were: attention score, language-independent intelligence, depression score, and paranoia score. As Fig. 9.8 shows, the LCA results in a clear hierarchy of the four variables. The depression score was decisive for the two classes arising as result of this analysis. Class 1 was characterized by: low depression score, low paranoid tendencies, good achievement in the attention test, and high scores concerning language-independent intelligence. Beyond these differences, the first group also differed from the second one with respect to many other variables such as: older age at start of the rehabilitation program, higher education level, greater language-dependent intelligence, lower scores of subjective complaints, and higher scores in the behavior rating scale with respect to practical and social abilities.

Class 2 was characterized by the complementary features: high depression score, greater paranoid tendencies, disturbances of attention, and impairment of language-independent intelligence. Beyond these differences, there were also

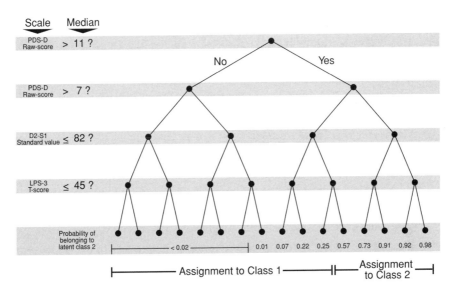

Fig. 9.8. Subgroups of schizophrenic patients derived from a latent class analysis: hierarchy of the scales PDS-D, PDS-P, D2-S1 and LPS-3. Probability of belonging to the latent classes 1 or 2. The figure demonstrates the importance of the different scales for the assignment to the LCA-classes.

additional characteristics, such as more subjective complaints and higher scores concerning psychopathological symptoms.

Results on prediction

Finally, an attempt was made to predict the success of the program after 1 year by variables present at the beginning of the rehabilitation program. For that purpose, a special type of discriminant analysis, called classification and regression trees (CART) was administered (Breiman et al., 1984). As a criterion variable, the Global Assessment score was used, and subdivided dichotomously into two categories: 70–100 points reflected a good prognosis, and 0–69 points a poor or intermediate prognosis. All other variables (cognitive variables, self-rating scales, psychopathological variables, and variables of the behavior rating scale) were used to predict the course of the rehabilitation program after 1 year as measured by the Global Assessment Scale. The depression score (PDS-D) was again of decisive importance for the subclassification of the two groups. According to this method, patients with a good prognosis (scores over 70) could be predicted in all cases ($n = 10$, 100%), whereas an intermediate or poor prognosis could be predicted only in 74% ($n = 40$). As the CART program has an inbuilt cross-validation, it was possible to check the probability of classification by this procedure. Under the conditions of the cross-validation, 80% of those with good prognosis could be predicted correctly, and 72 with intermediate prognosis (Remschmidt et al., 1991). The results are summarized here:

(i)   Schizophrenic adolescents attending a rehabilitation program who are characterized by deficits in cognitive functioning, subjective complaints and psychopathological symptoms seem to profit from a structured 1-year rehabilitation program. Most of these deficiencies improved considerably.

(ii) However, this improvement does not occur in all patients. It applies to a subgroup of schizophrenic patients characterized by higher cognitive abilities and less somatic and psychiatric symptoms. Interestingly, this differentiation is independent of the classical subtypes of schizophrenia (hebephrenic, paranoid and schizo-affective).

The status at the end of the 1-year rehabilitation program could best be predicted by the depression score at the beginning of the rehabilitation program, which is in line with a result of an earlier study using an independent sample (Remschmidt et al., 1988). Further studies should therefore examine emotional parameters carefully and not only the cognitive ones.

A comprehensive treatment and rehabilitation program

In this last part of the treatment chapter, we describe a comprehensive treatment and rehabilitation program, which has been developed over a period of 20 years in the department of child and adolescent psychiatry of the Philipps-University of Marburg, and has been administered meanwhile to more than 500 children and adolescents with schizophrenic disorders.

Table 9.13 gives an outline of the program and demonstrates that the program includes four phases of treatment, respectively, rehabilitation, the first two being carried out in the clinical department and phases 3 and 4 taking place in an associated rehabilitation centre. The basic philosophy of this program is the component approach to therapy and rehabilitation. This approach means that treatment and rehabilitation is based on different components, individually tailored to each patient and taking into account the stage of the disorder, age and developmental stage, the cognitive level, the personality, the family and psychosocial situation. Especially in children and adolescents, the school situation and, if the patient has already finished school, the professional and vocational situation is of great importance. In all children and adolescents, it has to be emphasized that they should, where possible, finish school and complete a vocational training. The component model implies further a dynamic structure, which means that the different components of treatment and rehabilitation can be changed, prolonged or shortened according to each

Table 9.13. A comprehensive treatment and rehabilitation program

Inpatient treatment of acute psychotic state	Inpatient treatment of partially remitted psychotic states	Rehabilitation (I)	Rehabilitation (II)
Neuroleptics	Neuroleptics	Neuroleptics	Neuroleptics
Psychoeducation including counseling and family involvement	Social skills training	Schooling	Schooling or supported
	Interpersonal problem solving	Work skills	employment and job
	schooling	Social skills training	coaching
Supportive psychotherapy	Attentional skills training	Interpersonal problem solving	Psychotherapy
Occupational therapy	Verbal concept exercises	Family-based interventions	Crisis management Family counseling
Group activities	Family-based interventions	Individual psychotherapy	Training in community living
Adaptive and stress management skills	Home visits		
Focus:	*Focus:*	*Focus:*	*Focus:*
Neutralization and control of symptoms	Treatment of cognitive disturbances and problems in psychosocial adjustment; prevention of withdrawal/negative symptoms	Goal setting; coping strategies, prevention of relapse	Independence; psychosocial reintegration; to achieve symptomatic and social recovery

patient's individual needs and to the possibilities of co-operation with his family or with his peer group.

Inpatient treatment phases

Most clinicians agree that at least acute states of schizophrenic disorders require inpatient treatment which can be continued on a daypatient and later sometimes an outpatient basis. Access to inpatient beds is undoubtedly needed (Jaffa, 1995). As demonstrated in Table 9.13, treatment in the acute phase of a psychotic disorder is based on several components, including neuroleptic medication, psychoeducation including family counseling and other different

254 H. Remschmidt et al.

measures individually tailored to each patient's needs and to the current situation of the disorder. These comprise supportive psychotherapy, occupational therapy, group activities and the training of everyday skills. The practicalities of administering components may differ from patient to patient; however, the principles are the same. The major focus in this *first acute phase* is on neutralization and control of the acute psychotic symptoms. In achieving this goal, it is important that the different components of the program are sensibly coordinated and that the various professionals involved work collaboratively rather than competitively. Working together with the family helps to minimize any feelings of isolation or sense of being abandoned which the patient may feel. From the onset of inpatient treatment, careful and detailed information should be provided to parents and other family members as well as to the patient himself (as far his/her mental state allows). This has to be done very carefully in order to avoid the patient incorporating this information into his delusional system. Detailed information should usually only be offered to the patient once the acute symptomatology has regressed and they have achieved a partial remission. This usually takes 8 to 10 weeks, by which time the patient has reached the second phase of inpatient treatment, namely the phase of remission or partial remission.

In this *second phase*, the neuroleptic treatment is continued. Often, medication is switched from a classical to an atypical neuroleptic, because of the reduced side adverse effects and partially because of the effect against negative symptoms. The presence of negative symptoms often only becomes apparent after the acute positive symptoms have been treated successfully. In a number of patients, the negative symptoms are dominated by the positive ones and are therefore overlooked during the acute stage.

The second inpatient treatment phase is based predominantly on the components which help the patient's reintegration in an age- and developmental stage-appropriate way. This means that a major focus is laid on schooling, social skills training, attention and concentration, problem-solving skills and individual coping strategies that can be used in daily activities. At the same time, family-based interventions become very important in all cases where the patient was living in a family before inpatient treatment. In other cases, the social reference group (e.g., care workers, if the patient had been living in a residential home) have to be included and home visits are recommended in order to provide the patient with reassurance and security.

The major focus of this second inpatient treatment is concentrated on cognitive and emotional problems, improvement of social skills and the treatment of negative symptoms (if present). In order to achieve these goals, the clinical setting must have adequate school and vocational facilities as well as facilities for occupational therapy, work therapy, recreation activities, and sports.

Ideally, the patient's discharge should be possible after the second inpatient treatment phase which lasts, on average, between 6 and 8 weeks. If a remission has been achieved in this phase, the neuroleptic medication is frequently changed to a depot neuroleptic compound in order to prevent a relapse of a psychotic episode. This depot neuroleptic treatment should be continued for 2 years, and outpatient consultations should be carried out at 3 monthly intervals in order to review the patient's symptoms, to provide counseling for the patient and the parents with regard to everyday problems, and finally to detect a possible relapse at the earliest point in time.

If a remission was not achieved during the two inpatient treatment phases and reintegration into the family is not possible, a rehabilitation program should be instituted.

Rehabilitation phases

The rehabilitation phases take place outside of a clinical department in a specialized rehabilitation centre, as described in Chapter 4. Altogether, the two rehabilitation phases take 2 years, aiming at stepwise growing independence.

During the first phase in the rehabilitation program, which is the third phase in the whole treatment program, much emphasis is laid on the areas of schooling, working skills, social skills training, and interpersonal problem-solving. As far as school is concerned, all patients who have not yet finished school are offered the possibility to attend the appropriate school class in the school attached to the rehabilitation center. Experienced and qualified teachers are able to tailor the school program to the needs and abilities of the individual patient. Also, the time which the patient spends at school can be adapted individually to his/her capabilities within a plan which allows the individual to gradually extend the time attended and to increase the difficulties of the tasks. At the same time, individual psychotherapy is continued, based on supportive strategies and cognitive-behavioral interventions. Within these approaches, the therapist tries to discover coping strategies that the patient has successfully used in the past. These very often form the nucleus of newly developed coping strategies for everyday problems and future tasks.

During this first phase of rehabilitation which usually has a duration of up to 1 year, the patient is living together with eight or nine other patients within the rehabilitation centre in a family-like structured apartment. The patient usually has a single room or sometimes shares a room with one other patient. There is a structured program for leisure time and weekends, if they are to be spent in the institution. The major goal of this first phase of rehabilitation is the reintegration of the patient within the institution, the development of coping strategies and the prevention of relapses.

The second rehabilitation phase follows the same principles, but brings a major change for the patient. The patient leaves the institution and moves into an apartment outside in the community, together with up to four other patients, still under supervision of the care workers, social workers, doctors and psychologists from the rehabilitation center. In most cases, the patient still attends the rehabilitation center facilities (e.g., school, work therapy, vocational activities, etc.). Some patients, however, are able to attend schools outside the institution in the community or start work within the community. During this second phase of rehabilitation, which usually also lasts for 1 year, neuroleptic treatment as well as a supportive psychotherapy is continued, but the patient is permitted much more independence and can spend leisure time outside the living group in the community without major restrictions. Due to the psychoeducational approach, the patient should now be well informed about the nature of the disorder, about the medication and possible adverse effects and should be able to recognize first symptoms of a relapse. At the same time, contact with the family is encouraged, with family work continuing during both rehabilitation phases in a way appropriate to the individual patient. There are, however, some cases where this is not encouraged because of extreme family crises and the high emotional stress for the patient.

In this second phase of rehabilitation, it is also possible for the patient to have a single apartment and to be more or less completely independent except for the agreement to continue consultations from time to time or to accept visits from the rehabilitation center. The major goal of this second phase of rehabilitation is independence, self-sufficiency, psychosocial reintegration, and the continuation of school and professional work without significant support from the rehabilitation center.

REFERENCES

Albiston, D.J., Francey, S.M., & Harrigan, S.M. (1998). Group programmes for recovery from early psychoses. *British Journal of Psychiatry*, **172** (Suppl. 33), 117–21.

American Psychiatric Association (1990). Task Force on ECT . The practice of ECT, Recommendations for treatment, training and privileging. *Convulsive Therapy*, **6**, 85–120.

Arima, T., Samura, N., Nomura, Y., & Segawa, T. (1986). Comparison of effects of tiapride and sulpiride on D-1, D-2, D-3, and D-4 subtypes of dopamine receptors in rat striatal and bovine caudate nucleus membranes. *Japanese Journal of Pharmacology*, **41**, 419–23.

Armenteros, J.L., Whitaker, A.H., Welikson, M., Stedge, D.J., & Gorman, J. (1997). Risperidone in adolescents with schizophrenia: an open pilot study. *Journal of the American Academy of Child and Adolescent Psychiatry*, **36**, 694–700.

Arvanitis, L.A. & Miller, B.G. (1997). Multiple fixed doses of "Seroquel" (quetiapine) in patients with acute exacerbation of schiziophrenia: a comparison with haloperidol and placebo. The Seroquel Trial 13 Study Group. *Biological Psychiatry*, **42**, 233–46.

Asarnow, J.R., Tompson, N.D., & Goldstein, M.J. (1994a). Childhood-onset schizophrenia: a follow-up study. *Schizophrenia Bulletin*, **20**, 599–617.

Asarnow, J.R., Tompson, N.D., Hamilton, E.B., Goldstein, M.J., & Guthrie, D. (1994b). Family expressed emotion, childhood-onset depression, and childhood-onset schizophrenia spectrum disorder: is expressed emotion a non-specific correlate of child psychopathology or a specific risk factor for depression? *Journal of Abnormal Child Psychology*, **22**, 129–46.

Baldessarini, R.J. (1996). Drugs and the treatment of psychiatric disorders. In *Goodman and Gilman's the Pharmacological Basis of Therapeutics*, 9th edn, ed. A.G. Gilman, T.W. Rall, A.S. Nies, & P. Taylor, pp. 404–6. New York: McGraw-Hill.

Bandelow, B., Grohmann, R., & Rüther, E. (1993). Unerwünschte Begleitwirkungen der Neuroleptika und ihre Behandlung. In *Therapie psychiatrischer Erkrankungen*, ed. H.J. Möller, pp. 166–83. Stuttgart: Enke.

Bandura A. (1977). *Social Learning Theory*. Englewood Cliffs, NJ: Prentice-Hall.

Bandura, A. (1986). *Social Foundations of Thought and Action*. Englewood Cliffs, NJ: Prentice-Hall.

Bauer, D. & Gärtner, H.J. (1983). Wirkung der Neuroleptika auf die Leberfunktion, das blutbildende System, den Blutdruck und die Temperaturregulation. Ein Vergleich zwischen Clozapin, Perazin und Haloperidol anhand von Krankenblattauswertungen. *Pharmacopsychiatria*, **16**, 23–9.

Beasley, C.M., Tollefson, G.D., & Tran, P.V. (1997). Efficacy of olanzapine: an overview of pivotal clinical trials. *Journal of Clinical Psychiatry*, **58** (Suppl. 10), 7–12.

Beck, A.T., Rush, A.J., Shaw, B.F., & Emery, G. (1979). *Cognitive Therapy of Depression*. New York: Guilford Press.

Bellack, A.S. (1996). Defizitäres Sozialverhalten und Training sozialer Fertigkeiten, Neue Entwicklungen und Trends. In *Integrative Therapie der Schizophrenie*, ed. W. Böker & H.D. Brenner, pp. 191–202. Bern: Huber.

Benfenati, F., Bernardi, P., Cortelli, P., Capelli, M., Adani, C., Calza, L., & Agnati, L.F. (1981). Possible mixed agonist–antagonist activity of D-sulpride at dopamine receptor level in man. *Neuroscience Letters*, **26**, 289–95.

Benkert, O. & Hippius, H. (1996). *Psychiatrische Pharmakotherapie*. Berlin: Springer.

Berner, P. & Schönbeck, G. (1987). Biologische Behandlungsmethoden. In *Psychiatrie der Gegenwart*, vol. 4, ed. H.P. Kisker, H. Lauter, J.E. Meyer, P. Müller, & E. Strömgren, pp. 237–84. Berlin: Springer.

Bezchlibnyk-Butler, K.Z. & Jeffries, J.J. (eds.) (1991). *Clinical Handbook of Psychotropic Drugs*. Toronto: Hogrefe and Huber.

Bleeham, T. (1993). *Leponex*® – Clozaril® (Clozapine) – Literature Review, Basel: Sandoz Pharma Ltd.

Bondolfi, G., Dufour, H., Patris, M., May, J.P., Billeter, U., Eap, C.B., & Baumann, P. (1998). Risperidone versus clozapine in treatment-resistant chronic schizophrenia: a randomized double-blind study. The Risperidone Study Group. *American Journal of Psychiatry*, **155**, 499–504.

Brady, J.P. (1984a). Social skills training for psychiatric patients. I. Concepts, methods and clinical results. *American Journal of Psychiatry*, **141**, 333–40.

Brady, J.P. (1984b). Social skills training for psychiatric patients. II. Clinical outcome-studies *American Journal of Psychiatry*, **141**, 491–8.

Brannan, M.D., Riggs, J.J., Hageman, W.E., & Pruss, T.P. (1980). A comparison of the cardiovascular effects of haloperidol, thioridazine and chlorpromazine HCl. *Archives Internationales de Pharmacodynamie et de Therapie*, **244**, 48–57.

Breese, G.R., Criswell, H.E., & Mueller, R.A. (1990). Evidence that lack of brain dopamine during development can increase the susceptibility for aggression and self-injurious behavior by influencing D1-dopamine receptor function. *Progress in Neuro-Psychopharmacology and Biological Psychiatry*, **145** (Suppl.), 65–80.

Breiman, L., Friedman, J., Olshen, A., & Stone, G.J. (1984). *CART: Classification and regression trees*. Belmont: Wadsworth.

Brenner, H.D., Stramke, W.G., Mewes, J., Liese, F., & Seeger, G. (1980). Erfahrungen mit einem spezifischen Therapieprogramm zum Training kognitiver und kommunikativer Fähigkeiten in der Rehabilitation chronisch schizophrener Patienten. *Nervenarzt*, **51**, 106–12.

Brenner, H.D., Hodel, B., Kube, G., & Roder, V. (1987). Kognitive Therapie bei Schizophrenen: Problemanalyse und empirische Ergebnisse. *Nervenarzt*, **58**, 72–83.

Brenner, H.D., Roder, V., & Merlo, M.C.G. (1993). Verhaltenstherapeutische Verfahren bei schizophrenen Erkrankungen. In *Therapie psychiatrischer Erkrankungen*, ed. H-J. Möller, pp. 222–30. Stuttgart: Enke.

Brickenkamp, R. (1975). *Test d2. Aufmerksamkeits-Belastungs-Test*, Göttingen: Hogrefe.

Bymaster, F.P., Calligaro, D.O., Falcone, J.F., Marsh, R.D., Moore, N.A., Tye, N.C., Seeman, P., & Wong, D.T. (1996). Radioceptor binding profile of the atypical antipsychotic olanzapine. *Neuropsychopharmacology*, **14**, 87–95.

Cardoni, A.A. (1995). Risperidone: review and assessment of its role in the treatment of schizophrenia. *Annals of Pharmacotherapy*, **29**, 610–18.

Carman, J., Peuskens, J. & Vangeneugden, A. (1995). Risperidone in the treatment of negative symptoms of schizophrenia: a meta-analysis. *International Clinical Psychopharmacology*, **10**, 207–13.

Casey, D.E. (1997). The relationship of pharmacology to side effects. *Journal of Clinical Psychiatry*, **58**, 55–62.

Chadwick, P. & Lowe, F. (1990). The measurement and modification of delusional beliefs. *Journal of Consulting and Clinical Psychology*, **58**, 225–32.

Chadwick, P. & Birchwood, M. (1994). The omnipotence of voices: cognitive approach to auditory hallucinations. *British Journal of Psychiatry*, **164**, 190–201.

Chouinard, G., Annable, L., & Steinberg, S. (1986). A controlled clinical trial of fluspirilene, a long-acting injectable neuroleptic, in schizophrenics patients with acute exacerbation. *Journal of Clinical Psychopharmacology*, **6**, 21–6.

Chouza, C., Romero, S., Lorenzo, J., Camano, J.L., Fontana, A.P., Alterwain, P., Cibils, D., Gaudiano, J., Feres, S., & Solana, J. (1982). Traitement des dyskinesies par le tiapride. *Semaine des Hopitaux*, **58**, 725–33.

Ciompi, L. (1983). How to improve the treatment of schizophrenia: a multicausal concept and its theoretical components. In *Psychosocial Intervention in Schizophrenia*, An International View, ed. H. Stierlin, L. Wynne, & M. Wirschung, pp. 53–66. New York: Springer-Verlag.

Clark, A.F. & Lewis, S.W. (1998). Practitioner review: treatment of schizophrenia in childhood and adolescence. *Journal of Child Psychology and Psychiatry*, **39**, 1071–81.

Claus, A., Bollen, J., De Cuyper, H., Eneman, M., Malfroid, M., Peuskens, J., & Heylen, S. (1992). Risperidone versus haloperidol in the treatment of chronic schizophrenic inpatients: a multicentre double-blind comparitive study. *Acta Psychiatrica Scandinavica*, **85**, 295–305.

Cohen, D., Paillere-Martinot, M.L., & Basquin, M. (1997). Use of electroconvulsive therapy in adolescents. *Convulsive Therapy*, **13**, 25–31.

Colonna, L. (1994). Antideficit properties of neuroleptics. *Acta Psychiatrica Scandinavica*, **89** (Suppl. 380), 77–82.

Coward, D.M. (1992). General pharmacology of clozapine. *British Journal of Psychiatry*, **160** (Suppl. 17), 5–11.

Dahl, S. & Refsum, H. (1976). Effects of levomepromazine, chlorpromazine and their sulfoxides on isolated rat atria. *European Journal of Pharmacology*, **37**, 241–8.

Degner, D. & Rüther, E. (1998). "Atypische" Neuroleptika in der Schizophreniebehandlung. *Nervenheilkunde*, **17**, 472–9.

Delay, J., Deniker, P., & Harl, J. (1952). Utilization therapeutique psychiatrique d'une phenothiazine d'action centrale elective (4560 RP). *Annales Medico-Psychologiques* (Paris), **110**, 112–17.

Demisch, K. & Staib, A.H. (1994). Behandlung psychopathologischer Syndrome. In *Klinische Pharmakologie*, ed. N. Rietbrock, A.H. Staib & D. Lowe, pp. 286–302. Darmstadt: Steinkopff.

Desilva, P.H., Darvish, A.H., McDonald, S.M., Cronin, M.K., & Clark, K. (1995). The efficacy of prophylactic ondansetron, droperidol, perphenazine and metaclopramide in the prevention of nausea and vomiting after major gynecologic surgery. *Anesthesia and Analgesia*, **81**, 139–43.

Deutsche Gesellschaft für Kinder- und Jugendpsychiatrie (ed.) (1994). Zur Behandlung schizophrener Psychosen des Kindes- und Jugendalters mit Clozapin (Leponex). Konsensus-Konferenz vom 4. März 1994. *Zeitschrift für Kinder- und Jugendpsychiatrie*, **22**, 325–7.

DiFrancesco, G.F. (1994). Are the cardiovascular effects and "5-HT syndrome" induced by MDL 73 975 and flesinoxan in the dog mediated by the 5-HT1A receptors? *European Journal of Pharmacology*, **262**, 205–15.

Dixon, L.B. & Lehmann, A.F. (1995). Family interventions for schizophrenia. *Schizophrenia Bulletin*, **21**, 631–43.

Drury, V., Birchwood, M., Cochrane, R., & Macmillan, F. (1996). Cognitive therapy and recovery from acute psychosis. I. Impact on symptoms. *British Journal of Psychiatry*, **169**, 593–601.

Dubovsky, S.L. (1987). Psychopharmacologic treatment in neuropsychiatry. In *Textbook of Neuropsychiatry*, ed. R.E. Hales & S.C. Yudofsky, pp. 411–38. Washington DC: The American Psychiatric Press.

Ebert, D. (1997). Quetiapin – ein atypisches Neuroleptikum. *Fundamenta Psychiatrica*, **11**, 79–84.

Egan, M.F., Apud, J., & Wyatt, R.J. (1997). Treatment of tardive dyskinesia. *Schizophrenia Bulletin*, **23**, 583–609.

Ekblom, B. & Haggstrom, J.E. (1974). Clozapine (Leponex) compared with chlorpromazine: a double-blind evaluation of pharmacological and clinical properties. *Current Therapy Research*, **16**, 945–57.

Falloon, I.J.R. (1987). Cognitive and behavioural interventions in the self-control of schizophrenia. In *Psychosocial Treatment of Schizophrenia*, ed. J.S. Strauss, W. Böker, & H.D. Brenner, pp. 180–90. Toronto: Huber.

Fleischhacker, W.W., Barnas, C., Stuppack, C.H., Sperner-Unterweger, B., Miller, C., & Hinterhuber, H. (1991). Zotepin vs. Haloperidol bei paranoider Schizophrenie: eine Doppelblindstudie. *Fortschritte der Neurologie-Psychiatrie*, **59** (Suppl. 1), 10–13.

Fleischhauer, J. (1978). Beziehung zwischen Dosishöhe und Behandlungsergebnis. Doppelblinduntersuchung mit Pimozid in zwei Dosierungen. *Arzneimittelforschung*, **28**, 1491–2.

Flynn, S.W., Mac Ewan, G.W., Altman, S., Kopala, L.C., Fredrikson, D.H., Smith, G.N., & Honer, W.G. (1998). An open comparison of clozapine and risperidone in treatment-resistant schizophrenia. *Pharmacopsychiatry*, **31**, 25–9.

Fox, S.H., Moser, B., & Brotchie, J.M. (1998). Behavioral effects of 5-HT2C receptor antagonism in the substantia nigra zona reticularis of the 6-hydroxydopamine-lesioned rat model of Parkinson's disease. *Experimental Neurology*, **151**, 35–49.

Frangos, H., Zissis, N.P., Leontopoulos, I., Diamantas, N., Tsitouridis, S., Gavriil, I., & Tsolis, K. (1978). Double-blind therapeutic evaluation of fluspirilene compared with fluphenazine decanoate in chronic schizophrenics. *Acta Psychiatrica Scandinavica*, **57**, 436–46.

Fulop, G., Phillips, R.A., Shapiro, A.K., Gomes, J.A., Shapiro, E., & Nordlie, J.W. (1987). ECG changes during haloperidol and pimozide treatment of Tourette's disorder. *American Journal of Psychiatry*, **144**, 673–5.

Gaebel, W. & Wölwer, W. (1992). Facial expression and emotional face recognition in schizophrenia and depression. *European Archives of Psychiatry and Clinical Neuroscience*, **242**, 36–52.

Gardner, D.M. (1997). Olanzapine. *Child and Adolescent Psychopharmacology News*, **2**, 1–5.

Gattera, J.A., Charles, B.G., Williams, G.M., Cavenagh, J.D., Smithurst, B.A., & Luchjenbroers, J. (1994). A Retrospective study of risk factors of akathisia in terminally ill patients. *Journal of Pain and Symptom Management*, **9**, 454–61.

Gerhardt, S., Gerber, R., & Liebman, J.M. (1985). SCH 23390 dissociated from conventional neuroleptics in apomorphine climbing and primate acute dyskinesia models. *Life Sciences*, **37**, 2355–63.

Gerlach, J. & Casey, D.E. (1984). Sulpiride in tardive dyskinesia. *Acta Psychiatrica Scandinavica*, **69** (Suppl. 311), 93–102.

Ghaziuddin, N. (1998). Use of electroconvulsive therapy in childhood psychiatric disorders. *Child and Adolescent Psychopharmacology News*, **3**(2), 1–8.

Ghaziuddin, N., King, C.A., Naylor, M.W., Ghaziuddin, M., Chaudhary, C., Giordani, B., DeQuardo, J.R., Tandon, R., & Greden, J.F. (1996). Electroconvulsive treatment in adolescents with pharmacotherapy refractory depression. *Journal of Child and Adolescent Psychopharmacology*, **6**, 259–71.

Göthert, M., Bönisch, H., Schlicker, E., & Helmchen, H. (1996). Psychopharmaka. Pharmakotherapie psychischer Erkrankungen. In *Pharmakologie und Toxikologie*, ed. W. Forth, D. Henschler, W. Rummel, & K. Starke, pp. 285–317. Heidelberg: Spektrum Akademischer Verlag.

Haddock, G., Bentall, R.P., & Slade, P.D. (1996). Focussing vs. distraction approaches in the treatment of persistant auditory hallucinations. In *Behavioural intervention with psychotic disorders*, ed. G. Haddock & P.D. Slade. London: Routledge.

Haddock, G., Morrison, A.P., Hopkins, R., Lewis, S., & Tarrier, N. (1998). Individual cognitive-behavioural interventions in early psychoses. *British Journal of Psychiatry*, **172** (Suppl. 33), 93–100.

Harrington, R., Whittacker, J., Shoebridge, P., & Campbell, F. (1998). Systematic review of efficacy of cognitive behaviour therapies in childhood and adolescent depressive disorder. *British Medical Journal*, **316**, 1559–63.

Heimberg, C., Gur, R., & Erwin, R.J. (1992). Facial emotion discrimination: III. Behavioural findings in schizophrenia. *Psychiatry Research*, **42**, 253–65.

Heuyer, G., Dauphin, F., & Lebovici, S. (1947/48). La Pratique de l'electrochoc chez l'enfant. *Zeitschrift für Kinderpsychiatrie*, **14**, 60–4.

Hirsch, S.R. (1994). Seroquel: an example of an atypical antipsychotic drug. *Neuropsychopharmacology*, **10** (Suppl. 3), 371S.

Hodel, B. & Brenner, H.D. (1996). Ein Trainingsprogramm zur Bewältigung von maladaptiven Emotionen bei schizophrenen Erkrankungen. Erste Ergebnisse und Erfahrungen. *Nervenarzt*, **67**, 564–71.

Hodel, B., Brenner, H.D., Merlo, M.C.G., & Teuber, J.F. (1998). Emotional management therapy in early psychosis. *British Journal of Psychiatry*, **172** (Suppl. 33), 128–33.

Hoggarty, G.E., Anderson, C.M., Kornblith, S.J., Greenwald, D.P., Ulrich, R.F., & Carter, M. (1991). Family psychoeducation, social skills training and maintenance chemotherapy in the aftercare of schizophrenia. II. Two-year effects of a controlled study on relapse and adjustment. *Archives of General Psychiatry*, **48**, 340–7.

Hoggarty, G.E., Kornblith, S.J., Greenwald, D., DiBarry, A.L., Cooley, S., Flesher, S., Reiss, D., Carter, M., & Ulrich, R. (1995). Personal therapy: a disorder-relevant psychotherapy for schizophrenia. *Schizophrenia Bulletin*, **21**, 379–93.

Hori, M., Suzuki, T., Sasaki, M., Shiraishi, H., & Koizumi, J. (1992). Convulsive seizures in schizophrenic patients induced by zotepine administration. *Japanese Journal of Psychiatry and Neurology*, **46**, 161–7.

Horn, W. (1983). *Leistungsprüfsystem LPS*, 2nd edn. Göttingen: Hogrefe.

Irjala, J., Koskinen, P., Scheinin, M., Kanto, J., & Scheinin, H. (1996). Biochemical and clinical assessment of histamine blockade. *International Journal of Clinical Pharmacology and Therapeutics*, **34**, 269–73.

Jackson, H., McGorry, P., Edwards, J., Ulbert, C., Henry, L., Frency, S., Maude, D., Cocks, J., Power, P., Harrigan, S., & Dudgeon, P. (1998). Cognitively-oriented psychotherapy for early psychoses (COPE). *British Journal of Psychiatry*, **172** (Suppl. 33), 93–100.

Jaffa, T. (1995). Adolescent psychiatry services. *British Journal of Psychiatry*, **166**, 306–10.

Janssen, P.A. & Awouters, F.H.L. (1995). *Antipsychotic Agents. In Principles of Pharmacology*, ed. P.L. Munson , R.A. Mueller, & G.R. Breese, pp. 289–308. New York: Chapman and Hall.

Kahn, R.S., Davidson, M., Siever, L., Gabriel, S., Apter, S., & Davis, K.L. (1993). Serotonin function and treatment response to clozapine in schizophrenic patients. *American Journal of Psychiatry*, **150**, 1337–42.

Kanas, N., Rogers, M., Kreth, E., Patterson, L., & Campbell, R. (1980). The effectiveness of group psychotherapy during the first three weeks of hospitalization: a controlled study. *Journal of Nervous and Mental Disease*, **168**, 487–92.

Kane, J., Honigfield, G., Singer, J. et al. (1988). Cloozapine for the treatment-resistant schizophrenic. *Archives in General Psychiatry*, **45**, 789–96.

Kaplan, H.I., Sadock, B.J., & Grebb, J.A. (1994). *Synopsis of Psychiatry*, Kaplan and Sadock's 6th edn. Baltimore, MD: Williams and Wilkins.

Kienzle, N. & Martinius, J. (1995). Modifikationen und Adaptationen des IPT für die Anwendung bei schizophrenen Jugendlichen. In *Integriertes psychologisches Therapieprogramm für schizophrene Patienten (IPT)*, ed. V. Roder, H.D. Brenner, N. Kienzle, & B. Hodel, pp. 171–82. Weinheim: Psychologie-Verlagsunion.

Kienzle, N., Braun-Scharm, H., & Hemme, M. (1997). Kognitive, psychoedukative und familientherapeutische Therapiebausteine in der stationären jugendpsychiatrischen Versorgung. In *Die Behandlung schizophrener Menschen. Integrative Therapiemodelle und ihre Wirksamkeit*, ed. V. Dittmar, H.E. Klein, & D. Schön, pp. 139–52. Regensburg: Roderer.

Kingdon, D.G. & Turkington, D. (1994). *Cognitive Behaviour Therapy of Schizophrenia*. New York: Guilford Press.

Kornhuber, J. & Weller, M. (1994). Aktueller Stand der biochemischen Hypothesen zur Pathogenese der Schizophrenie. *Nervenarzt*, **65**, 741–54.

Kretschmar, R. & Stille, G. (1995). Psychopharmaka. In *Pharmakologie und Toxikologie*, ed. C.J. Estler, pp. 193–201. Stuttgart: Schattauer.

Kumra, S., Frazier, J.A., Jacobsen, L.K., McKenna, K., Gordon, C.T., Lenane, M.C., Hamburger, S.D., Smith, A.K., Albus, K.E., Alaghband-Rad, J., & Rapoport, J.L. (1996). Childhood-onset schizophrenia: a double-blind clozapine-haloperidol comparison. *Archives of General Psychiatry*, **53**, 1090–7.

Kumra, S., Jacobsen, L.K., Lenane, M., Karp, B.I., Frazier, J.A., Smith, A.K., Bedwell, J., Lee, P., Malanga, C.J., Hamburger, S., & Rapoport, J.L. (1998). Childhood onset schizophrenia: an open label study of olanzapine in adolescents. *Journal of the American Academy of Child and Adolescent Psychiatry*, **37**, 377–85.

Kutcher, S. (1998). The identification management of akathisia. *Child and Adolescent Psychophar-*

macology News, **3**, 11–12.

Kutcher, S. & Robertson, H.A. (1995). Electroconvulsive therapy in treatment resistant bipolar youth. *Journal of Child and Adolescent Psychopharmacology*, **5**, 167–75.

Kutcher, S., Williamson, P., MacKenzie, S., Marton, P., & Ehrlich, M. (1989). Successful clonazepam treatment of neuroleptic-induced akathisia in an older adolescent. A double-blind placebo-controlled study. *Journal of Clinical Psychopharmacology*, **9**, 403–6.

Lazarsfeld, P.F. & Henry, N.W. (1968). *Latent structure analysis*. Boston: Houghton Mifflin.

Leszcz, M., Yalom, I.D., & Norden, M. (1985). The value of inpatient group psychotherapy, patients' perceptions. *International Journal of Group Psychotherapy*, **35**, 411–33.

Leysen, J.E., Gommeren, W., Eens, A., de Chaffroy de Courcelles, D., Stoof, J.C., & Janssen, P.A.J. (1988). Biochemical profiles of risperidone, a new antipsychotic. *Journal of Pharmacology and Experimental Therapeutics*, **247**, 661–70.

Lieberman, R.P. (1995). *Social and Independent Living Skills: The Community Re-entry Programme*. Los Angeles, CA: UCLA Department of Psychiatry.

Lieberman, R.P. & Eckman, T.A. (1989). Zur Vermittlung von Trainingsprogrammen für soziale Fertigkeiten an psychiatrischen Einrichtungen: Möglichkeiten der praktischen Umsetzung eines neuen Rehabilitationsansatzes. In *Schizophrenie als systemische Störung. Die Bedeutung intermediärer Prozesse für Theorie und Therapie*, eds. W. Böker & H.D. Brenner, pp. 256–67. Bern: Huber.

Marder, S.R. & Meibach, R.C. (1994). Risperidone in the treatment of schizophrenia. *American Journal of Psychiatry*, **15**, 925–35.

Marder, S.R. & Meibach, R.C. (1994). Risperidone in the treatment of schizophrenia. *American Journal of Psychiatry*, **154**, 825–35.

Martin, M. (1991). *Der Verlauf der Schizophrenie im Jugendalter unter Rehabilitationsbedingungen*. Stuttgart: Enke.

Martin, M. & Remschmidt, H. (1983). Ein Nachsorge- und Rehabilitationsprojekt für jugendliche Schizophrene. *Zeitschrift für Kinder- und Jugendpsychiatrie*, **11**, 234–42.

Mattejat, F. (1989). Familientherapie bei psychotischen Jugendlichen. Lecture presented at the University of Innsbruck.

Mattejat, F. (1997). Familientherapie, In *Psychotherapie im Kindes- und Jugendalter*, ed. H. Remschmidt, pp. 148–74. Stuttgart: Thieme.

Miller, L.G. & Jankovic, J. (1990). Neurological approach to drug-induced movement disorders: a study of 125 patients. *Southern Medical Journal*, **83**, 525–32.

Moise, F.N. & Petrides, G. (1996). Case study: electroconvulsive therapy in adolescents. *Journal of the American Academy of Child and Adolescent Psychiatry*, **35**, 3.

Möller, H.J., Kissling, W., Stoll, K.D., & Wendt, G. (1989). *Psychopharmakotherapie*. Stuttgart: Kohlhammer.

Mulhall, D.J. (1978). *Manual for the personal questionnaire rapid scaling technique*. Windsor: NFER Publishing Company.

Neale, J.M. & Oltmanns, T.F. (1980). *Schizophrenia*. New York: John Wiley.

Nissen, G., Fritze, J., & Trott, G.E. (1998). *Psychopharmaka im Kindes- und Jugendalter*. Stuttgart: Gustav Fischer.

Palayodan, A. (1983). Tiapride et alcoholisme. *Semaine Des Hopitaux*, **59**, 1184–6.

Parmar, R. (1993). Attitudes of child psychiatrists to electroconvulsive therapy. *Psychiatry Bulletin*, **17**, 12–13.

Peacock, L., Solgaard, T., Lublin, H., & Gerlach, J. (1996). Clozapine versus typical antipsychotics. A retro- and prospective study of extrapyramidal side effects. *Psychopharmacology* (Berlin), **124**, 11–96.

Penn, D.L. & Mueser, K.T. (1996). Research update on the psychosocial treatment of schizophrenia. *American Journal of Psychiatry*, **153**, 607–17.

Perris, C. (1989). *Cognitive Therapy with Schizophrenic Patients*. New York: Guilford.

Petit, M., Raniwalla, J., Tweed, J., Leutenegger, E., Dollfus, S., & Kelly, F. (1996). A comparison of an atypical and typical antipsychotic, zotepine versus haloperidol in patients with acute exacerbation of schizophrenia: a parallel-group double-blind trial. *Psychopharmacology Bulletin*, **32**, 81–7.

Porsolt, R.D. & Jalfre, M. (1981). Neuroleptic-induced acute dyskinesia in rhesus monkeys. *Psychopharmacology* (Berlin), **75**, 16–21.

Rang, H.P. & Dale, M.M. (1991). *Pharmacology*. Edinburgh: Churchill Livingston.

Ravn, J., Scharff, A., & Aaskoven, O. (1980). 20 Jahre Erfahrung mit Chlorprothixen. *Pharmakopsychiatrie, Neuro-Psychopharmakologie*, **13**, 34–40.

Remington, G. (1997). Selecting a neuroleptic and the role of side effects. *Child and Adolescent Psychopharmacology News*, **2**, 1–5.

Remington, G. & Kapur, S. (1996). Neuroleptic-induced extrapyramidal symptoms and the role of combined serotonin-dopamine antagonism. *Journal of Clinical Psychiatry Monographs*, **14**, 14–24.

Remschmidt, H. (1992). *Psychiatrie der Adoleszenz*. Stuttgart: Thieme Verlag.

Remschmidt, H. (1993a). Schizophrenic psychoses in children and adolescents. *Triangle*, **32**, 15–24.

Remschmidt, H. (1993b). Childhood and adolescent schizophrenia. *Current Opinion in Psychiatry*, **6**, 470–9.

Remschmidt, H., Brechtel, B., & Mewe, F. (1973). Zum Krankheitsverlauf und zur Persönlichkeitsstruktur von Kindern und Jugendlichen mit endogen-phasischen Psychosen und reaktive Depressionen. *Acta Paedopsychiatrica*, **40**, 2–17.

Remschmidt, H., Martin, M., Albrecht, G., Gerlach, G., & Rühl, D. (1988). Der Voraussagewert des Initialbefundes für den mittelfristigen Rehabilitationsverlauf bei jugendlichen Schizophrenen. *Nervenarzt*, **59**, 471–6.

Remschmidt, H., Martin, M., Schulz, E., Gutenbrunner, C., & Fleischhaker, C. (1991). The concept of positive and negative schizophrenia in child and adolescent psychiatry. In *Negative and positive schizophrenia*, ed. A. Marneros, N.C. Andreasen, & and M.T. Tsuang, pp. 219–42. Berlin-Heidelberg: Springer.

Remschmidt, H., Schulz, E., Martin, M., Warnke, A., & Trott, G-E. (1994a). Childhood-onset schizophrenia: history of the concept and recent studies. *Schizophrenia Bulletin*, **20**, 727–45.

Remschmidt, H., Schulz, E. & Martin, M. (1994b). An open trial of clozapine in thirty-six adolescents with schizophrenia. *Journal of Child and Adolescent Psychopharmacology*, **4**, 31–41.

Remschmidt, H., Martin, M., Schulz, E., & Trott, G.E. (1995). Etiology of schizophrenia: perspectives from childhood psychoses. In *Psychotic Continuum*, ed. A. Maneros, N.C. Andreasen, & M.T. Tsuang, pp. 67–85. Berlin: Springer.

Remschmidt, H., Schulz, E., & Herpertz-Dahlmann, B. (1996). Schizophrenia psychoses in childhood and adolescence: a guide to diagnosis and drug choice. *CNS Drugs*, **6**, 100–12.

Remschmidt, H., Fleischhaker, C., & Schulz, E. (1999). Clozapine treatment in childhood and adolescent onset schizophrenia. *Child and Adolescent Psychopharmacology News*, **8**, 324–7.

Rey, J.M. & Walter, G. (1997). Half a century of ECT use in young people. *American Journal of Psychiatry*, **154**, 595–602.

Roder, V., Brenner, H.D., Kienzle, N., & Hodel, B. (1997). Integriertes psychologisches Therapieprogramm für schizophrene Patienten (IPT). *Materialien für die psychosoziale Praxis*, 4th edn. Weinheim: Beltz.

Rühl, D. (1988). *Untersuchungen zur Basisstörung schizophrener Jugendlicher*, Doctoral dissertation, University of Marburg.

Sandor, P., Musisi, S., Moldofsky, H., & Lang, A. (1990). Tourette syndrome; a follow-up study. *Journal of Clinical Psychopharmacology*, **10**, 197–9.

Schmidt, L.G., Grohmann, R., Helmchen, H., Langscheid-Schmidt, K., Müller-Oerlinghausen, B., Poser, W., Rüther, E., Scherer, J., Strauss, A., & Wolf, B. (1984). Adverse drug reactions. An epidemiological study at psychiatric hospitals. *Acta Psychiatrica Scandinavica*, **70**, 77–89.

Schneekloth, T.D., Rummans, T.A., & Logan, K.M. (1993). Electroconvulsive therapy in adolescents. *Convulsive Therapy*, **9**, 158–66.

Schönhofer, P.S. & Schwabe, U. (1992). Therapeutischer Einsatz von Psychopharmaka. In *Pharmakotherapie. Klinische Pharmakologie*, ed. G. Fülgraff & D. Palm, pp. 242. Stuttgart: Gustav Fischer Verlag.

Schooler, C. & Spohn, H.E. (1982). Social dysfunction and treatment failure in schizophrenia. *Schizophrenia Bulletin*, **8**, 85–98.

Schotte, A., Bonaventura, P., Janssen, P.F., & Leysen, J.E. (1995). In vitro receptor binding and in vivo receptor occupancy in rat and guinea pig brain: risperidone compared with antipsychotic hitherto used. *Japanese Journal of Pharmacology*, **69**, 399–412.

Schulz, E., Fleischhaker, C., & Remschmidt, H. (1996). Correlated changes in symptoms and neurotransmitter indices during maintenance treatment with clozapine or conventional neuroleptics in adolescents and young adulthood schizophrenia. *Journal of Child and Adolescent Psychopharmacology*, 6, 119–31.

Schulz, E., Fleischhaker, C., Clement, H.W., & Remschmidt, H. (1997). Blood biogenic amines during clozapine treatment of early-onset schizophrenia. *Journal of Neural Transmission*, **104**, 1077–89.

Seeman, P. (1993). *Receptor Tables*, vol. 2: *Drug Dissociation Constants for Neuroreceptors and Transporters*. Toronto: SZ Research.

Shaffer, D., Gould, M.S., Brasic, J., Ambrosini, P., Fisher, P., Bird, H., & Aluwahlia, S. (1983). A children's global assessment scale (CGAS). *Archives of General Psychiatry*, **40**, 1228–31.

Sokoloff, P., Giros, B., Martres, M.P., Andrieux, M., Besancon, R., Pilon, C., & Bouthenet, M.L. (1992). Localisation and function of the D-3 dopamine receptor. *Arzneimittelforschung*, **42**, 224–30.

Steinhausen, H.C. (1985). Eine Skala zur Beurteilung psychisch gestörter Kinder und Jugend-dlicher. *Zeitschrift für Kinder- und Jugendpsychiatrie*, **13**, 230–40.

Strober, M., Rao, U., DeAntonio, M., Liston, E., State, M., Amaya-Jackson, L., & Latz, S. (1998). Effects of ECT in adolescents with severe endogenous depression resistant to pharmacotherapy. *Biological Psychiatry*, **43**, 335–8.

Süllwold, L. (1977). *Symptome schizophrener Erkrankungen. Uncharakteristische Basisstörungen.* Berlin: Springer.

Sweet, C. (1975). Drug-induced dystonia. *American Journal of Psychiatry*, **132**, 532–4.

Tarrier, M., Beckett, R., Harwood, S., Baker, A., Yusupoff, L., & Ugarteburu, I. (1993). A trial of two cognitive-behavioural methods of treating drug-resistant residual psychotic symptoms in schizophrenic patients: I. Outcome. *British Journal of Psychiatry*, **162**, 524–32.

Tolbert, H.A. (1996). Psychoses in children and adolescents, a review. *Journal of Clinical Psychiatry*, **57** (Suppl 3); 4–8, discussion 46–7.

Tollefson, G.D., Beasely, C.M., Tran, P.V. et al. (1994). Olanzapine: a novel antipsychotic with a broad spectrum profile. Society of Biological Psychiatry, Philadelphia, PA, 19–21 May 1994.

Toren, P., Laor, N., & Weizman, A. (1998). Use of atypical neuroleptics in child and adolescent psychiatry. *Journal of Clinical Psychiatry*, **59**, 644–56.

Uchida, S., Honda, F., Otsuka, M., Satoh, Y., Mori, J., Ono, T., & Hitomi, M. (1979). Pharmacological study of [2-Chloro-11-(2-dimethylaminoethoxy)dibenzo[b,f]thiepine] (Zotepine), a new neuroleptic drug. *Arzneimittelforschung*, **29**, 1588–94.

Van Rossum, J.M. (1966). The significance of dopamine receptor blockade for the mechanism of action of neuroleptic drugs. *Archives of International Pharmacodynamic Therapy*, **160**, 492–4.

Van Tol, H.H.M., Bunzow, J.R., Guan, H.C., Sunahara, R.K., Seeman, P., Niznik, H.R., & Civelli, O. (1991). Cloning of the gene for a human dopamine D-4 receptor with high affinity for the antipsychotic clozapine. *Nature*, **350**, 610–14.

Von Bardeleben, U., Benkert, O., & Holsboer, F. (1987). Clinical and neuroendocrine effects of zotepine – a new neuroleptic drug. *Pharmacopsychiatry*, **20**, 28–34.

Von Zerssen, D. (1976a). *Paranoid-Depressivitäts-Skala (PDS)*. Weinheim: Beltz.

Von Zerssen, D. (1976b). *Beschwerde-Liste (BL)*, Weinheim: Beltz.

Walker, E., McGuire, M., & Bettes, B. (1984). Recognition and identification of facial stimuli by schizophrenics and patients with affective disorders. *British Journal of Clinical Psychology*, **23**, 37–44.

Wallace, Ch., Nelson, C.J., Lieberman, R.P., Aitchison, R.A., Lukoff, D., Elder, J.P., & Ferris, Ch. (1980). A review and critique of social training with schizophrenic patients. *Schizophrenia Bulletin*, **6**, 42–63.

Walter, G. & Rey, J.M. (1997). An epidemiological study of the use of ECT in adolescents. *Journal of the American Academy of Child and Adolescent Psychiatry*, **36**, 809–15.

Wechsler, D. (1964). *Die Messung der Intelligenz Erwachsener. Textband zum Hamburg–Wechsler-Intelligenztest für Erwachsene (HAWIE)*, 3rd edn. Bern: Huber.

Young, C.R., Bowers, M.B., & Mazure, C.M. (1998). Management of the adverse effects of clozapine. *Schizophrenia Bulletin*, **24**, 381–90.

Zahn, T.P. & Pickar, D. (1993). Autonomic effects of clozapine in schizophrenia, comparison with placebo and fluphenazine. *Biological Psychiatry*, **34**, 3–12.

10

Course and prognosis

Sally Nicola Merry and John Scott Werry

Introduction

This chapter is about course and outcome. *Course* is the pattern of illness over some length of time, while *outcome* refers to the end state at some distant point and may be short, medium or long term. While clearly there will may be some link between course and outcome, this is by no means always the case. For example, in theory, those who have a single psychotic episode may have a poor outcome while those that have many may do quite well. Some may have a slow deterioration and other a relatively rapid. Some may have many symptoms and some few. For this reason, course and outcome will be discussed separately. In the interests of clarity, premorbid state and onset have been separated out from course.

Overview

While exact figures are not known, it has been estimated that schizophrenia begins before the age of 10 in 3.5% of cases, with another 2.7% beginning between the ages of 10 and 15 (Asarnow, 1994), so that around 5–6% of cases may start before age 16.

While there are many studies of diverse aspects of schizophrenia, there are relatively few of child and adolescent schizophrenia and studies of longer term outcome in the younger age group are particularly scarce. For example, in the recent special issue of the *Schizophrenia Bulletin* (1994) on child and adolescent onset schizophrenia, only two studies systematically addressed longer-term outcome.

Knowledge about course and outcome in adults is more extensive, and has been summarized in a number of reviews (e.g., Westermeyer & Harrow, 1988; Marengo, 1994). These have shown that outcome today is better than that reported in the Kraepelinian period, with complete remission in about a quarter of patients. However, most patients with schizophrenia still experience persisting or episodic symptoms and difficulties in work and social settings that occur throughout their lives. It appears that deterioration is an early phenomenon with much of the disability being established in the first 5 years, and possibly the first 2. After this, many patients reach a plateau and may even improve thereafter.

The course of the illness, however, may follow very different patterns for different patients. Early or insidious onset, male sex, poor premorbid adjustment, family history of schizophrenia, poor academic record, family disruption, institutionalization, longer time to first treatment, disorganized or undifferentiated subtype, and living in a developed country all appear to affect course and outcome adversely (Strauss & Carpenter, 1974; Westermeyer & Harrow, 1988; Werry et al., 1991; Johnstone et al., 1995; Maziade et al., 1996b).

Methodological issues

Reviews, especially that by Westermeyer and Harrow (1988), have also addressed the methodological problems in outcome studies which are recognized to be among the most difficult to pursue and execute. One of the more important issues is that of diagnosis. The early definition by Kraepelin included a characteristically deteriorating course embodied in the term dementia praecox. Bleuler changed the name of the disorder to "the schizophrenias" in part to reflect his view that the disorder(s) had a less inexorably bad outcome. Under the influence of the new psychoanalytic theory, he also saw outcome as much more of an interaction between disease and personality. In America in the late 1940s and 1950s, this led to schizophrenia and other psychoses being regarded as the extreme end of a continuum of severity of psychopathology, manifest in such terms as "borderline states," rather than qualitatively distinct disorders. Clear differences in the use of the term schizophrenia between America and Great Britain and other parts of Europe emerged.

In the 1980s, in a taxonomic revolution, there was a clear return to near Kraeplinian criteria in DSM-III, with not only a reiteration of the distinct disease notion and of "first-ranked symptoms" of Schneider, but also the inclusion of a chronic or recurrent course of the illness as an integral part of the definition of schizophrenia.

The matter is even more complicated when the issue of early onset schizophrenia is considered, as there has been uncertainty about whether to apply adult diagnostic criteria to children or indeed whether it is the same disorder as in adults. Over the years, different views have predominated, with adult criteria being applied prior to the 1960s (Eisenberg, 1957) and again from the 1980s, although even studies before the 1960s summarized by Eisenberg (1957), include cases that would not be considered early onset schizophrenia today. In the intervening period of DSM -II and ICD-8, criteria were extremely broad, and included autism and other pervasive developmental disorders under child-hood schizophrenia, rather more consistent with the American view of psychoses as a matter of severity not specificity (Werry, 1992). DSM-III and ICD-9 marked a return to Kraepelinian criteria.

A problem discussed in more detail below, is that early onset is often insidious or set against the backdrop of major developmental and/or personality abnormality, so that the differentiation between what in adults is called schizotypal disorder and frank schizophrenia is often quite difficult (Werry, 1992).

Another major diagnostic difficulty in children and adolescents, is that studies show that it can be very difficult to differentiate from bipolar disorder and schizo-affective disorder in the early stages (Werry et al., 1991; Cawthron et al., 1994). Until recently, this error favored misdiagnosing bipolar disorder as schizophrenia (Werry et al., 1991). Since, in general, bipolar disorder carries a different (better) prognosis than schizophrenia, this problem may erroneously improve apparent outcome. Further, some of the follow-up studies cover follow-up of psychosis rather than schizophrenia, and the data for specific diagnoses may be limited.

Other methodological problems include the varying outcome characteristics and predictor variables, and the kind, or more often the lack, of comparison groups. Description of long-term course is extremely variable even in studies of adults and scant in childhood schizophrenia.

Finally, longitudinal studies bring well-known problems of their own (Westermeyer & Harrow, 1988) such as subject attrition and varying follow-up intervals. Most studies are retrospective and utilize not research protocols but clinical charts to establish diagnostic and predictor criteria. This leads to problems of variability, incompleteness and unknown reliability of initial data capture.

Developmental considerations

As repeatedly noted in this monograph, developmental characteristics are most important in considering schizophrenia in children and adolescents. The most visible marker of this is age, which has both biological and chronological aspects. It has been characteristic of American studies to refer to schizophrenia beginning before age 13 as "prepubertal," which is incorrect in view of the wide age range of onset of puberty and could impede studies, especially biological ones. Even the terms child or adolescent schizophrenia are imprecise since the World Health Organization now suggests that childhood ends at age 10 and adolescence at 24!

Some have suggested (Werry et al., 1991) that schizophrenia in this group should be called "early onset" schizophrenia (EOS) if occurring before the age of 18 and "very early onset" schizophrenia (VEOS) if onset is before the age of 13. For the purposes of this discussion, we shall define "adolescent" as aged 13–17 and "childhood schizophrenia" to refer to schizophrenia which starts before the age of 13.

There is conflict about how early it is possible to diagnose schizophrenia in childhood. Eggers and Bunk (1997) argue that it is difficult before the age of 5 or 6 and that some symptoms, such as delusions, are difficult to diagnose before age 9. However, others dispute this difficulty and there are case reports of children as young as 3 years of age (Werry, 1992). Be that as it may, the age range covered by childhood and adolescent schizophrenia is one of rapid, huge and conspicuous physical, personal and social change and differentiation. It is important to consider how these changes might affect symptoms, course and outcome. It is clear that many of the critical symptoms of schizophrenia, such as first ranked delusions, hallucinations and passivity phenomena require a degree of cognitive maturity if they are to be recognized and described by the person affected. Developmental differences such as poorly formulated and unsophisticated delusions, age-related changes in the presentation of thought disorders such as higher rates of loose associations and illogical thinking in younger children (Caplan, 1994), and relative commonness of visual hallucinations have been noted (Werry, 1992).

It is usually supposed that early onset schizophrenia carries a particularly poor prognosis, although evidence for this has not necessarily been strong and is confounded by some of the difficulties outlined above. Schizophrenia can be a devastating disorder with intellectual and emotional impoverishment in adults. It is likely to be all the more severe when it strikes before these important functions have had time to mature. It has also been postulated, with some supporting evidence (Werry et al., 1991; Werry et al., 1994) that the early onset form of schizophrenia is a more virulent form of the disease with a stronger biological predisposition (for example, as shown by the twofold increase in aggregation of first-degree relatives in childhood onset schizophrenia (Asarnow, 1994; Strandberg et al., 1994)). In contrast, one study of a large group of patients with schizophrenia has shown that good outcome is associated with strong family history or central nervous system injury, while poor outcome is related to negative symptoms, in turn correlated with early onset, male sex and poor academic record. The authors note that family history was often unavailable in the poor outcome group, possibly due to greater fragmentation of families, so that statements about the impact of family history were difficult to make (Johnstone et al., 1995). At a biological level, there is also the question of the effect of differing maturation of systems such as the dopaminergic (Weinberger, 1987) on the effect of treatment and on outcome in general. Weinberger has argued that the rapid rise of schizophrenia in adolescence and early adulthood and its decay in incidence thereafter, represents an interaction between the maturation of the dopaminergic systems during that period and the intense psychosocial stresses of adolescence.

In summary, much of the source of developmental effects remains unknown, but it seems likely that the effects are profound and will affect outcome.

Studies in adults

In considering course and prognosis, it is worthwhile to consider the available adult studies because there are more data. Considering the dearth of data on outcome and course in children and adolescents, and assuming that the disorder is basically the same in children and adults, then qualified but heuristic extrapolations may be made. Comparisons may be made with adult studies when data allow, to indicate what the developmental differences in the disorder are. Findings from adult studies will be described at the beginning of each of the following sections.

Selection of studies

Because of the diagnostic confusion prior to the appearance of DSM-III and ICD-9, only studies published in English since 1980 and which use criteria comparable with DSM-III/IV ICD9/10 criteria (e.g., hallucinations, bizarre delusions or other first rank symptoms, duration at least 2–4 weeks) will be included in this review. Reference will also be made to Eisenberg (1957), who reviewed all studies up to that date. His conclusions will be compared with those of more modern studies. Although the problems of diagnostic criteria and other methodological issues such as clear outcome criteria are even more of an issue in these old studies, the use of adult criteria in diagnosis means that there is some means for comparison, and the fact they were done earlier in the century means that some historical perspective can be gained by considering them. In interpreting the findings, it is important to take into account the shortcomings of these early studies. Some studies used only institutionalized subjects which, of course, would bias outcome toward severity. Also, modern treatment methods, notably antipsychotic medication, were not available then, and this could adversely affect conclusions about outcome.

In limiting the review in this way, the resultant attrition is not great, since, as Werry (1992) points out, there have been very few studies on outcome between Eisenberg's (1957) review and the appearance of DSM-III, and those that there are, are hard to interpret because subjects included those with autism and other pervasive developmental disorders as well as schizophrenia. Some, though reported earlier (e.g., Eggers, 1978), have been encompassed within later studies of the same subjects. Some studies which have appeared since 1980 have had to be rejected because of methodological shortcomings. For example, the widely quoted study by Kydd and Werry (1982) was found in later studies to have consisted mostly of subjects with bipolar or schizoaffective disorder (Werry et. al., 1991).

Studies selected are summarized in Table 10.1. There are seven studies, interestingly, unusually diverse geographically (Germany, Sweden, United States, Canada, Great Britain and New Zealand), though all from developed western countries. The total number of subjects is 380. Most of the studies are of mixed child and (usually predominantly) adolescent onset. Length of follow-up varies within and across studies from 1 to 40+ years with most under 10 years. This is unfortunate since it is held that adult schizophrenia often "burns out" after about 10 years (Westermeyer & Harrow, 1988). Some of the studies do not address schizophrenia specifically, but follow-up adolescent psychosis (Gillberg, Carina et al., 1993; Cawthron et al., 1994) or schizophrenia spectrum disorder (Asarnow & Ben-Meir, 1988), although the latter researchers have more recently reported specifically on a group with schizophrenia (Asarnow et al., 1994). Some data on schizophrenia can be obtained from these studies, where it is reported separately, but in other instances it is impossible to differentiate specific information from that on the wider group, e.g., information on predictors of outcome in the Gillberg study. Attrition of subjects is not a major problem, with only the studies by Cawthron et al. (1994) and the US component of the Werry et al., (1994) study having high levels. A number of studies use comparison groups, mostly with diagnoses of mood disorder.

Organization of the review

As noted in the introduction, data will be organized within four main descriptive concepts: (i) premorbid adjustment; (ii) onset; (iii) course; and (iv) outcome. Within these four broad chronological categories, variables affecting course and outcome will be delineated and results of studies examined within these parameters. Data on adults will be compared with that available for children and adolescents.

Table 10.1. Outcome studies

Author	Number of patients	Age range at onset in years (mean)	Duration of follow-up in years (mean)	Number followed up	Diagnosis	Comparison group	Outcome
Werry et al. (1991)	30[a]	7–17	1–16(5)	30	DSM-III-R Schizophrenia	Mood disorder Schizoaffective disorder	20% recovered 27% suboptimal 53% impaired
Gillberg et al. (1993)	23	13–19	11–17	55/57 with psychosis[b] (96%)	DSM-III Schizophrenic disorder	Other psychotic disorders Community controls	13% possibly good 9% intermediate 78% extremely poor
Cawthorn et al. (1994)	19	12–17	2–13 (7.7)	9/19 (47%)	ICD-9 Schizophrenia	Other psychotic disorders	22% good outcome 87% poor social outcome 78% poor subjective outcome
Asarnow et al. (1994)	21	7–14	2–7	18/21 (86%)	DSM-III Schizophrenia	Major depressive disorder	28% good outcome 28% moderate improvement 28% minimal improvement 17% deteriorating course
Werry et al. (1994)	57	11–17 (13.9)	1–15 (4)		DSM-III-R Schizophrenia		4–13% recovered

Study	N	Age range (mean)			Diagnostic criteria	Outcome
Schmidt et al. (1995)	118	11–16 (16)	Mean 7.4	(82.2%)	ICD-9 Schizophrenia and schizoaffective	Educational 24% no impairment 32% mild impairment 22% moderate impairment 16.5% severe impairment 5% complete impairment Social 20% no impairment 21% mild impairment 25% moderate impairment 29% severe impairment 2% complete impairment
Maziade et al. (1996a,b)	41	5–17 (14)	14.8	40	DSM-III-R	5% total recovery 21% moderate outcome 34% poor outcome 40% very poor outcome
Eggers & Bunk (1997)	71	7–14	42	44/71 (62%)	PSE Schizophrenia	25% complete remission 25% partial remission 50% poor remission

[a] A "few" refused entry to study, the exact number was not reported.
[b] Specific numbers for those with schizophrenia were not given.

Premorbid adjustment

Premorbid adjustment has been defined as the individual's psychological functioning before the onset of the schizophrenic illness (Cannon-Spoor et al., 1982). The period varies according to how onset of illness is defined and is shorter when onset is considered to have occurred at the start of *any* psychopathological symptoms, compared with the start of psychotic symptoms. Larsen et al. (1996) have pointed out that the term prodrome can be misleading in that it includes an expectation of normal functioning, while longstanding non-specific disturbances in function have long been described and may herald the onset of overt psychosis much later in life. A subtype of schizophrenia (formerly called simple schizophrenia) has been described, where only a gradual deterioration may be the earliest manifestation of the psychotic process. Studies of the premorbid period have been necessarily retrospective. Many studies restrict the period they consider to a year or two before onset of overt psychosis, and so are likely to miss any initial deterioration. The development of instruments such as the Premorbid Adjustment Scale (Cannon-Spoor et al., 1982), which rates information throughout childhood, has led to improved description of premorbid adjustment. Adult studies have been done where information is collected at time of first episode to enhance reliability of recall (e.g., Haas & Sweeney, 1992). These studies indicate that around a fifth of the patients with first episode schizophrenia show a pattern of premorbid deterioration, and those that do are more often males with a trend towards more negative symptoms and a long-term history of psychotic symptoms before hospitalization. Other studies such as the current US NIMH (National Institute of Mental Health) on child onset schizophrenia document a high rate of childhood developmental delays, particularly in language and speech, and difficulties in social adjustment (Jacobsen & Rapoport, 1998).

In children and adolescents, a higher degree of difficulty in the premorbid period is reported. Only a quarter of the patients in Werry et al.'s (1991) study had no difficulty premorbidly, with the majority showing more abnormal personalities of the "odd" type and/or brain dysfunction. This is in contrast to children with mood disorder where half had no difficulty. Premorbid problems were also indicated by lower scores on the General Adaptive Functioning Scale over the previous year, with those with schizophrenia having an average score of 53 compared with 71 for those with mood disorder. Eggers (1989) compared the premorbid development of subjects with schizophrenia and those with schizo-affective disorder. Fifty-nine percent of the group of 41 patients with schizophrenia showed poor adjustment premorbidly with "schizothymic personalities," while a third of the group of 16 with schizo-affective disorder were described as shy, inhibited, quiet, insecure and introverted. Nevertheless, it is worth noting that 41% of the group with schizophrenia showed no difficulty in the premorbid period. Green et al. (1992) report a number of non-specific symptoms before the onset of psychotic symptoms in a number of their subjects, while Schmidt et al. (1995) report that 21% of their sample had had former episodes of psychiatric treatment for various diagnoses, mostly neurotic and emotional disorders on ICD-9. Forty percent of the 41 subjects reported by Maziade et al. (1996a) had premorbid developmental abnormalities, and 55% had non-psychotic behavioral disturbance severe enough to warrant consultation. These difficulties are confirmed by other studies where early onset schizophrenia is shown to be associated with higher risk of premorbid social, motor and language impairments (Hollis, 1995; Watkins et al., 1988) and the NIMH study of childhood onset schizophrenia, where 60% of cases had previous developmental disorders and 34% had transient symptoms of pervasive developmental disorder (Alaghband-Rad et al., 1995).

In summary, it appears that premorbid adjustment is variable, with some children exhibiting early signs of non-specific personality and/or neurodevelopmental difficulties and others showing an unremarkable development. Generally, there seems to be a greater degree of poor premorbid adjustment compared with adult studies, with higher rates of developmental delays, and reports of symptoms of pervasive developmental disorder not seen in adults.

Onset

Timing of onset may be determined in a number of ways. Most writers differentiate between age at which:

(i)   Any psychological difficulty (i.e., onset of prodromal symptoms) is first seen which can be defined as "illness onset" (Larsen et al., 1996).

(ii)   Psychotic symptoms first become manifest, i.e., "episode onset" with the suggestion that this be further differentiated into (a) onset of psychosis, positive symptoms, (b) onset of psychosis, negative symptoms, (c) onset of psychotic syndrome (Larsen et al., 1996).

(iii) Clinical care is sought (further complicated by use of first treatment vs. first hospitalization).

Duration of illness before treatment is an important variable. Adult studies indicate that people can suffer from psychosis for considerable periods of time

Table 10.2. Premorbid adjustment and onset of symptoms

Author	Premorbid adjustment	Age at first symptoms	Age at first psychotic symptoms	Prodrome duration (weeks)	Type of onset	Age at first treatment	Age at first hospitalization	Duration of untreated psychosis (weeks)
Eggers (1978)[a]	45.6% normal 54.4% premorbid introversion, difficulties making contact							
Russel et al. (1989)		4.6	6.9	112	Acute 14% Insidious 86%		9.5	135
Werry et al. (1991)	Abnormal personality: None 23% Mild 23% Moderate/severe 54% Abnormal neurological function 23%		13.9		0–2 weeks 31% 3–12 weeks 14% 13+ weeks 55%		14.5	24
Green et al. (1992)		6.4	8.8	116	Acute 21% Insidious 79%		9.6	52
Asarnow et al. (1994)	CGAS mean 59.81 (Normal > 70) PAS Poor peer relationships Poor school adjustment Introverted				Acute (< 1 yr) 5% Insidious 95%			
Maziade et al. (1996a,b)	40% developmental abnormalities	7.2	14.0	354			15.0	52
Eggers & Bunk (1997)		11.8	12.9	56	Acute 75% Insidious 25%		13.4	

[a]Note this group includes subjects with schizo-affective disorder.

before presenting for treatment (Haas & Sweeney, 1992; Beiser et al., 1993). Delay in treatment influences course, since it leads to longer time to remission and lower level of remission (Loebel et al., 1992).

Studies in children also point to a delay in presentation which varied from 6 months (Werry et al., 1991) to nearly 2 years (Green et al., 1992; Russell, 1994). In the latter two studies, the delay is in time to hospitalization, although the authors suggest that this is the time of first diagnosis. Studies which report onset patterns in children and adolescents are summarized in Table 10.2.

Differing onset is described in different studies. In their sample of 44 children and adolescents, Eggers and Bunk (1997) found that 6 (14%) had an acute onset of under a week, slightly over half had a subacute onset, defined as onset under a month and a quarter of their sample (11/44) had an onset of longer than a month. Werry et al. (1991) describe a different pattern with 31% of their 30 cases having a prodrome of less than 2 weeks, and 55% of their sample having a prodrome of 13 or more weeks. This was a longer time of onset than in patients with bipolar disorder where a prodrome of less than 2 weeks occurred in 52% of cases, and only 17% had a prodrome of over 13 weeks. Asarnow et al. (1994) described a much more insidious onset in their group of 7–14-year-olds. They defined "acute" onset as having symptoms for less than a year, and "insidious" or "chronic" onset as over more than 5 years. Ninety-five percent of the children in their group fell into the latter group, and, interestingly, 75% of children presented with major depressive illness. These onset patterns are over longer periods than those reported by other authors, for reasons that are not clear. Green et al. (1992) report an acute onset in 21% of their cases, insidious onset with acute exacerbation in 32% of cases, and an insidious onset in 47% of cases. Unfortunately, their definitions of the above categories are not given. Cawthron et al. (1994) do not differentiate the group of patients with schizophrenia from those with psychosis in their description of onset. They describe an acute presentation (i.e., symptom duration of less than a month) in 20% of their cases.

In summary, onset appears to vary, some cases being relatively acute and others insidious. Some of these differences may, however, be definitional since a significant proportion of subjects in all studies have long-standing personality or other adjustments, which some may call "onset" and others premorbid states. They may also be a function of sample selection since a number of key factors seem to affect onset.

Gender

In adults, males tend to have earlier onset by several years (see Werry, 1992).

Likewise, it has been suggested that, in children and adolescents, boys tend to have an earlier onset of illness than girls and that there is a clear male preponderance in VEOS (e.g., Remschmidt et al., 1994; Maziade et al., 1996a). The study by Eggers and Bunk (1997) failed to confirm this, finding instead that, prior to the age of 15, if anything, there is an excess of girls, but that between the ages of 15 and 24 there is a clear preponderance of boys. The reason for this gender difference may be the protective effect of estrogen, which has an antidopaminergic effect and probably also counteracts the faulty synaptic pruning that is thought to play a part in the expression of schizophrenic symptoms (Eggers & Bunk, 1997). It is postulated that girls who do become psychotic may have lower levels of estrogen, but this has not been investigated to date. As noted above, studies to date have wrongly assumed puberty to occur at specific ages. Those which make explicit links to physical changes indicative of puberty, or indeed measure hormonal levels, have yet to be made.

Age

Older studies (Kolvin, 1971, see also Werry, 1992) state that insidious onset is more common in child onset schizophrenia than in adults, and this has generally been confirmed in most studies and also found to be equally true of child vs. adolescent onset schizophrenia (Eggers & Bunk, 1997; Asarnow & Ben-Meir, 1988; Green et al., 1992; Werry, 1992).

Course

As noted above, course needs to be differentiated from outcome since adult data suggest that the course by which any particular end-stage (good or bad) is reached can be quite variable. There have been a number of studies which have all used different ways of describing and monitoring course with some restricting descriptions to symptoms only, for example, that by M. Bleuler (see Table 10.3), and others incorporating level of functioning as well, for example, that by Huber and colleagues (Marengo, 1994).

An alternative, more simplified description of course is provided by Breier et al., (1991), where schizophrenia is considered to have three phases:

(i)   initial deterioration (over the first 10 years or so of the illness);
(ii)   stabilization (during which symptoms reach a plateau and the illness remains relatively stable over a long period of time);
(iii) improvement (taking place late in the illness).

At this stage, variations in description, of course, are so wide that comparison of studies is difficult, and suggestions for a prototype to be used consistently

Table 10.3. Description of course

Adult schizophrenia (Bleuler, 1978)	Childhood schizophrenia (Eggers, 1978)
Simple	Acute type (74%)
(i) Acute onset, severe chronic end-state (1%)	(i) One acute psychotic episode with full recovery (10%)
(ii) Chronic onset, severe chronic end-state (12%)	(ii) One acute episode, preceded by short transitory (flat) psychotic "waves," with full recovery (9%)
(iii) Acute onset, mild to moderate end-state (2%)	(iii) Frequently recurring psychotic episodes with full recovery (7%)
(iv) Chronic onset, mild to moderate end-state (23%)	(iv) Frequently recurring psychotic episodes leaving a slight schizophrenic defect (relatively good social adaptation) (16%)
Undulating	(v) One acute psychotic episode, leading to a severe defective state (5%)
(i) Undulating with severe end-state (9%)	(vi) Frequently recurring episodes leading to a deep schizophrenic defect (25%)
(ii) Undulating with mild to moderate end-state (27%)	(vii) Acute–recurring onset merging into a sluggish course with continuous deterioration (dementia simplex) (2%)
(iii) Undulating with recovery (22%)	Chronic type (26%)
Atypical (4%)	(i) Chronic–lingering course with amelioration (5%)
	(ii) Chronic–insidious course with slight deterioration (7%)
	(iii) Chronic–insidious course with severe deterioration (9%)
	(iv) Psychotic-like change of behavior for a period of 1 year or longer, leading to a manifest schizophrenic psychosis (5%)

in studies in the future have been made (Marengo, 1994). There is, however, now general agreement that deterioration is an early phenomenon (McGlashan & Johannessen, 1996). This is the reason for the now-accepted need for early and vigorous treatment. A full review of the adult literature with suggestions for future studies can be found in Marengo (1994).

It has been postulated that the course of illness has changed over time, with patterns described early in the century generally of a more severe nature. Some of this may be due to better treatment, some to better referral of milder cases, but some may reflect genuine change in the severity of the illness itself. M. Bleuler described severe unremitting psychosis leading to profound disability or even death. Cases like these are rarely seen today. Similarly, catatonia was seen more often than it is seen now.

In children and adolescents, descriptions of course as detailed as those described in adults, are scant with most details being on outcome. Eggers (1978) provides the most detailed description with the 57 patients in his original sample. These data need to be interpreted, bearing in mind that of his original group, sixteen were deemed to have schizo-affective disorder at follow-up (Eggers, 1989). Despite this, this is the only very detailed description of course available, so is worth including. It is shown in Table 10.3.

Werry et al. (1991) describe a generally chronic course with increasing disability and punctuated by a few psychotic episodes in 90% of patients. These two studies reflected somewhat different epochs with many of Eggers' patients being diagnosed well before the psychopharmacological era which ought to have increased both number of psychotic episodes and disability but appears not to have.

Green et al. (1992) report a relative treatment resistance in their group. None of their children experienced total symptom remission, 60% showed moderate improvement, 20% showed minimal improvement and 17% showed no significant improvement.

Schmidt et al. (1995) found that 73% of their patients experienced at least one further schizophrenic episode, and the mean number of all psychiatric episodes since index admission was 2.5 episodes (SD 3.0; range 0–17). In addition, two of their patients were subsequently diagnosed as having bipolar affective disorder, six as personality disordered, one with a transient organic psychotic condition and one with a disturbance of emotions specific to childhood. A quarter (26.8%) of their patients had no further schizophrenic episodes.

Outcome

There is some difficulty in assessing outcome in both adult and child studies, due to inadequately clear or commonly agreed definitions of outcome and the use of non-specific global terms such as "improved" with differing criteria for judging improvement. Adjustment is a complex function and defining it is not an easy task. DSM's Global Assessment of Function includes, and takes account of, two main components of adjustment: (i) psychopathological symptoms and (ii) social function, probably not very successfully, since, while symptoms and function are correlated, this correlation is not very close and the two domains can behave somewhat independently of each other.

In addition, both in the adult and the child literature, most studies are retrospective. They are carried out over different but often relatively short time periods (1–2 years) and the point at which outcome is reported may not be a true end-state in the disease process.

Overall social and work adjustment

Westermeyer and Harrow (1988) standardized outcome criteria across all studies in adults and found that total or complete remission occurs in 14–30% of patients. However, there are also studies that suggest that this may overestimate recovery. Within a larger study, Vaillant (1978) carried out a 10-year follow-up of a subgroup of 51 schizophrenics who had remitted, and found that 40% eventually relapsed and were repeatedly hospitalized. In addition, those who remained in the community, showed occupational and social impairment. While the other 60% maintained their recovery, this was only 10% of the original sample.

In children, Eisenberg (1957) summarizing studies to that point, found that one-quarter of cases could be expected to attain a "moderately good" social adjustment during adolescence with one-third deteriorating and requiring continuous institutionalization. The remainder had a fluctuating course around a marginal level of adjustment. He thus felt that 50–75% of the total would be expected to do poorly. Despite this, it was felt to be better than the expected prognosis of the 1930s. Later studies of early onset schizophrenia (see Table 10.1), in general, show a similar poor outcome.

Carina Gillberg et al. (1993) followed 55 young people with psychosis, 42% (23) of whom had schizophrenia. They had access to records for social security benefits, names of those on full pension for health-related problems and justice department records. At the age of 30, only 15% were not in prison, hospital, on a pension or social security. Outcome was extremely poor for 18 patients with schizophrenia (78%) and good for only six patients (6%). Only five had married. They report a worse outcome for patients with bipolar disorder, at odds with other studies (e.g., Werry et al., 1991), but the number of bipolar disorder patients is extremely small so that their results have to be interpreted with caution.

A poor outcome is also reported by Werry et al. (1991), with patients with schizophrenia having an average score on DSM-III-R Global Assessment of Functioning Scale (GAF) of 40, compared with 61 for patients with mood disorder. Some of this was accounted for by poor premorbid adjustment with schizophrenia and mood disorders scoring 53 and 71, respectively, on the GAF on function in the year before the illness. At follow-up, only 7% were living independently at an average age of 18 years, compared with 51% of patients with mood disorder, although the latter were a little older with an average age of 20 years. Schmidt et al. (1995) found that a quarter of their sample had no further episodes, but a high number of their patients were still living with their parents, while more than a quarter of the sample were not able to live independently and needed institutional support. Less than a fifth of their sample was financially independent.

Schmidt et al. (1995) compared their sample of patients with schizophrenia beginning before the age of 18 with a group of patients with adult onset from the same area and same clinic, and found that those with earlier onset of schizophrenia had greater social disability on a variety of variables. This may be accounted for by the greater number of patients with insidious onset schizophrenia in the younger age group, as this in turn correlates with poor outcome, or it may be that a schizophrenic illness greatly impedes normal development with greater ensuing disability, or it may indicate that, to have an earlier onset, does indeed indicate a more virulent disease process. Whatever the cause, final social disability appears greater than in adults.

Maziade et al. (1996a) used the outcome categories proposed by Westermeyer and Harrow (1988) and found that only 5% of their sample had total recovery, while 74% fell into the poor or very poor outcome categories. In contrast, adult rates using the same categories are 14–30% and 50%, respectively (Westermeyer & Harrow, 1988).

Education/work

Adult studies indicate that the majority of those with schizophrenia (50–75%) have major deficits in work performance across the lifespan. The percentage of people in the category of "good outcome" declines sharply if full-time employment is used as a measure of recovery. Work capacity is affected more by internal factors such as negative symptoms than it is by factors such as family background. Gender is associated with work performance with women doing better than men.

It is difficult to make statements about work capacity in those with early onset schizophrenia, since many at follow-up are not yet old enough to be at work. However, Werry et al. (1991) included being at school as well as working and found that the figures for being at school were better than for work.

However, as they point out, schools have a legal obligation to take all children, and this is not a particularly good test. Also this study is short term, and the deterioration may not be at an end-state in some of their subjects. Comparative figures for bipolar disorder were significantly better in both respects. Of their sample, only 17% were attending school or working full-time, while a further 35% were doing "some" time at one or the other. In comparison, 48% of patients with bipolar disorder were occupied at school or work full-time. While not reporting specifically on work, Carina Gillberg et al. (1993) report that, at age 30 years, 65% of their patients with schizophrenia were on a full pension so could not have been working. Thus the scarce data available point to considerable educational/vocational deficits for children and adolescents, similar to those seen for adults, though truly long-term data are scarce.

Symptoms

Overall, only 10–25% of adults with schizophrenia are totally symptom free in the long term. Thought disorder is found in the acute phase in 75–80% of patients, with 50% showing signs of thought disorder once out of hospital. Delusions are found more commonly than hallucinations and there seems to be a decline in frequency of these symptoms over time with some improvement after 5 years. Overall, 60–75% of patients with schizophrenia show either equivocal or clear positive psychotic symptoms at any one time in the post-hospital period. Negative symptoms come into prominence later (though it is now thought that they form a substantive part from onset on) and tend to increase with time, with approximately 30% of patients having symptoms early in the course, and 60% later on. Where there is a change in symptoms over the course of the illness, there is a change from more to less organization with time (Westermeyer & Harrow, 1988).

In children and adolescents, there are clear age differences. As with adults, the symptoms are very persistent in the majority of cases with only 4/57 of Egger's original sample being free of symptoms at the initial 27-year follow-up (Eggers, 1978). Carina Gillberg et al. (1993) found that the majority of their group (78%) required ongoing treatment for schizophrenia up to the age of 30. Schmidt et al. (1995) found that 72% of their sample required ongoing care, while a quarter had no further episodes. Werry et al. (1991) report 90% of patients falling into a category they label chronic (more than two episodes following the index episode). Thus continuation of symptoms sufficient to require psychiatric care seems to occur in the vast majority of those with EOS or VEOS. It is not, however, possible to make firm comparisons in this with outcome in adults.

Cognition

It is established that many patients with schizophrenia have cognitive deficits, and twin studies have established that, even where performance is within the normal range, there is often a decline from what would be expected given the performance of the unaffected twin, and compared with tests that measure premorbid functioning. While the deficit is generalized, there appears to be a specific decline in attention (with sustained attention and the ability to attend differentially to different stimuli reduced and ability to process information from stimuli slowed), memory and problem-solving (Gold & Harvey, 1993). These deficits are relatively stable and persist through relapses and remissions. In adults, a clear deterioration between the premorbid period and after the onset of psychosis has been shown (Bilder et al., 1992). Studies of military samples suggest that IQ drops about 10 points with the onset of the illness (Gold & Harvey, 1993).

A recent study has confirmed a similar pattern with children but, unlike with adults, intellectual function continued to decline 24 to 48 months after the onset of psychosis (see Jacobsen & Rapoport 1998).

Hospitalization

It is estimated that 80% of people with schizophrenia are hospitalized at some time, with 40–50% of these rehospitalized within the first year of illness, and 65–85% being rehospitalized eventually. Rehospitalization is frequently used as the sole criterion of outcome, but this is not a good indicator, particularly in comparing studies from different countries and different epochs, since it is greatly influenced by service changes, types and availability .

Studies of early onset schizophrenia have scant information on rehospitalisation with a report that 90% of patients have more than two admissions (Werry et al., 1991) while Maziade et al. (1996a) report that a quarter of their subjects were in a psychiatric institution or in supervised homes at 14-year follow-up.

Suicide

From adult studies, it is well known that about 10% of people suffering from schizophrenia die by suicide (Westermeyer & Harrow, 1988). Where suicide does occur, it is an early phenomenon and the group at greatest risk is that of young, white males. Very few who live past the first 5–10 years will commit suicide subsequently. This rate of suicide is not specific to schizophrenia, but is found in other populations of patients with psychotic illness.

There are little data on this in child and adolescent schizophrenia, and most studies do not extend through the full period of greatest risk. Eggers (1978) points to the high risk of suicide in the prodromal period, with two of the patients in his study attempting suicide and five others expressing suicidal thoughts or intentions. These figures worsened with onset of the illness, and he reports that 65% of his original sample were preoccupied by problems connected with death, 20% attempted suicide and 5% committed suicide. In contrast to adult studies, this was a relatively late phenomenon with the average time between onset of the illness and attempted suicide being 8.5 years, and the three suicides occurring 6, 13 and 14 years after the onset of the disease. The ages at which the suicides occurred is not reported but with the age range at entry into the study at 7–13 years, it may well be that the suicides were committed during the age of greatest risk (17–24 years) and that the difference seen between adults and children in this respect is an interaction between age and disease process, rather than a specific disease-linked phenomenon. Asarnow et al. (1994) also report high rates with suicide attempts in 38% of their sample, and suicidal ideation in a further 38%. At follow-up of up to 7 years, one of their sample had committed suicide at the age of 19. They point out that their sample, having been taken from inpatients, may have had an inflated rate of suicidal ideation, as this is frequently a reason for hospitalization. Other studies report different rates of completed suicide from 2–3% (Schmidt et al., 1995; Maziade et al., 1996a) to 15% (Werry et al., 1991).

In summary, suicide does appear to be a significant outcome in child and adolescents, though attempted suicide seems much more of a risk. It is not possible to make comparisons with adults because most of the studies have not extended long enough nor into periods of independence when presumptively the risk rises.

Factors affecting outcome

While there have been many studies in adults, the ways that outcome has been assessed have varied, and very few have used multivariate methods to assess the power and confounding effects among predictor variables.

In the early onset area, there are very few studies of predictors of outcome, though interestingly two did employ multivariate quantitative methods (Werry & McClellan, 1992; Maziade et al., 1996b). They both found that one of the best predictors of future function was premorbid function. In addition, Werry and McClellan (1992) found older age of onset, delusions, flat affect, length of follow-up, and impairment after first admission, were associated with a poorer outcome. Maziade et al. (1996b) found severity of positive symptoms was the other best predictor of long-term outcome, while age at onset was not related to outcome. In both these studies, because the sample size is small for the number of predictors examined, findings must be regarded as tentative.

Schmidt et al. (1995) examined the correlation of a number of factors with educational/occupational impairment and social disability, and found longer duration of the first episode, lower social competence, more symptoms at discharge and higher number of episodes were all associated with poorer outcome. Age at first admission, symptomatology and social competence at admission, and daily dose of neuroleptics at admission and at discharge, were not correlated with outcome measurements.

Apart from some simple demographic type variables like age and gender, predictors examined have varied. It also goes without saying that, if a variable is not examined (e.g., not recorded initially), its predictive value cannot be assessed, and its absence from the list below does not mean that it is of no interest or importance.

Age

It has been suggested for many years that, in adult schizophrenia, the earlier the age of onset the more malignant the outcome. Weinberger (1987) has suggested that, in many cases, schizophrenia is a congenital developmental disorder. The old idea that there are two types of schizophrenia, one of acute onset and more benign, and the other (formerly known as process or nuclear schizophrenia) of insidious and earlier onset has recently been updated with the suggestion that the latter process schizophrenia is the neurodevelopmental type with a poor prognosis (Murray et al., 1992) . With the tightening of the criteria for schizophrenia over the past 15 years, a poorer prognosis in general now seems apparent, and against such a shifting benchmark it is difficult to make comparisons between adult and early onset schizophrenia.

Nevertheless, in children and adolescents, it has been generally agreed that onset in childhood carries a particularly poor outlook. Kydd and Werry (1982) suggested that the putative poorer outcome in early onset may be due primarily to the high proportion of cases with poor premorbid personality as much as age. Indeed, in the only quantitative analysis of outcome, Werry et al. (1991), and Werry and McClellan (1992) were unable to find any age effect independent of premorbid personality, while Schmidt et al. (1995) and Maziade et al. (1996b) were unable to find any age effect.

Nevertheless, the studies set out in Table 10.1 generally confirm that outcome for child and adolescent schizophrenia is significantly worse than for adult onset. All the studies in Table 10.1 except one (Werry & McClellan, 1992) that have a sufficient age range spread, confirm that child onset carries a worse prognosis. The exception may be due to the fact that the subjects in that study had all been identified as a result of hospitalization, suggesting that this may have biased the sample toward an over- representation of the more malignant type.

Gender

In adults, female gender has a favorable impact on outcome and it has been posited to be a biological (possibly estrogen related) effect, but it may be that, as well as having a later onset of illness with less severe symptoms, the social role of women only makes outcome seem less severe. With women taking a domestic role, unemployment cannot be used as an outcome measure to differentiate those who have a good outcome from those with a poor outcome.

In child onset (VEOS) schizophrenia, there is no discernible gender effect, though the number of females in this group is rather small, and this effect may not be as robust as it seems. However, from adolescence onwards, boys do worse than girls, with a higher proportion ultimately falling into the poor outcome group (Werry & McClellan, 1992; Carina Gillberg et al., 1993; Eggers & Bunk, 1997). The differences between children and adolescents lend weight to the hypothesis of an estrogen-protective effect, though different social roles in females may contribute to these differences.

Premorbid function

Poor premorbid function has been powerfully linked with poor outcome in adult schizophrenia (e.g., Strauss & Carpenter, 1974; Johnstone et al., 1995) and in early onset schizophrenia (Werry et al., 1991; Werry & McClellan, 1992; Gillberg et al., 1993; Maziade et al., 1996b). Werry and McClellan (1992) found that it predicted by far the greatest amount of variance (20%) of any variable. In their contrast group with bipolar disorder, premorbid adjustment explained 8% of the variance while intellectual function was also a powerful predictor (35% of the variance). In these studies the number of subjects was too small to consider the findings anything but tentative; these results are consistent with findings from studies of adult patients.

Pattern of onset

The association of an acute onset and positive symptoms with good prognosis, and insidious onset and predominantly negative symptoms with poor prognosis has been found in several studies (e.g., Werry & McClellan, 1992; Remschmidt et al., 1994). Eggers and Bunk (1997) found that 33% of cases with an acute onset, and none of the cases with chronic onset had complete remission, while 40% of cases with acute onset and 82% of cases with chronic onset had no remissions. Carina Gillberg et al. (1993), by contrast, found early onset possibly associated with better outcome, but this is the only study with this finding.

Intelligence

Eggers (1978) reported that higher level of intelligence was associated with relatively good outcome, whereas less gifted children invariably had a poor outcome. Werry and McClellan (1992) examined low intelligence as a predictor of outcome, but found no association with outcome for patients with schizophrenia, although they did find a strong effect with their patients with bipolar disorder. The picture is thus unclear.

Symptoms

Types of symptoms (Werry and McClellan, 1992), severity of positive symptoms (Maziade et al., 1996b) and duration of first psychotic episode and more symptoms at discharge (Schmidt et al., 1995) have all been shown to have a negative impact on outcome in early onset schizophrenia.

Cultural factors

Adult studies have shown that schizophrenia can be diagnosed reliably in national settings of varying cultures and religion and degree of industrial development. The incidence of core schizophrenic symptoms, characterized by the presence of one or more of Schneider's first rank symptoms is similar across diverse cultural settings. It has been shown in a number of studies that the prognosis of schizophrenia in underdeveloped countries is better than in the western world, regardless of the nature of onset and presenting symptoms. One reason for this may lie in demonstrated greater efficacy of neuroleptics in some cultural groups, although the full effect of this, and the mechanism by which it occurs, remains to be elucidated. A more compelling argument is that this may result from the greater support offered by an extended family network and demonstrable lower rates in the elements of expressed emotion (criticism, hostility and overinvolvement) shown to be correlated with relapse rates (Karno & Jenkins, 1993). Studies looking at course and outcome of childhood schizophrenia in a cross-cultural setting remain to be done.

Interventions

To date, the long-term studies available both in the child and the adult literature, have not been able to look at long-term impact of interventions. In addition, many of those in the studies tend to fall into the poor outcome group, which suggests that interventions are still less than spectacularly successful.

Medication

The changing pattern of illness over the century has led to speculation that medication has reduced the number of people with very severe or catastrophic psychosis as described by Bleuler and others in the past. It remains unclear that medication is the reason for this change, whether it is due to generally improved and better psychiatric services and community supports, or whether it is due to a change in the virulence of the illness. It is now generally held, that with the possible exception of clozapine, medication does not appear to have had an impact on the proportions of people with good or poor outcome, although the ability of medication to reduce the duration and severity of positive symptoms and secondary negative symptoms and the number of relapses is well demonstrated (Lehman et al., 1995). The impact on primary negative symptoms has only been demonstrated for clozapine, while adjunctive pharmacological agents have been shown to augment antipsychotics in the treatment of positive symptoms (lithium) and to be effective in the treatment of ancillary symptoms such as depression and anxiety (Lehman, 1995). Impact of medication on other outcomes has not been demonstrated and definitive studies have yet to be done.

As far as children and adolescents are concerned, comparison between premedication studies (Eisenberg, 1957) and the more recent group listed in Table 10.1, is not possible because of lack of quantitative data in the older studies. However, there is not much evidence that outcome is much better, at least in terms of complete recovery, and supports the view of the effect of medication set out above. Whether or not the newer (atypical) antipsychotics and early intervention programs now in vogue can change this over the next few years, remains to be seen.

Assertive community treatment (ACT) and case management (CM)

There are initial data available on the effectiveness of various community management approaches in ameliorating symptoms and improving function in adult patients with schizophrenia. Programs using ACT require a multidisciplinary team and incorporate assertive engagement, *in situ* delivery of services, continuous responsibility and staff continuity over time, low case load for therapists, and brief but frequent contacts. These have been shown to reduce the rate and duration of psychiatric hospitalization, psychiatric symptoms, and to improve social functioning, promote residential stability and independent living. Moreover, these effects are not maintained if the treatment is with-drawn.

Case management is a far more diverse term that incorporates a variety of approaches but where the fundamental feature is that of an ongoing relation-ship between patient and case manager, designed to enhance continuity and coordination of care. Because of the variability of the case management programs, it is difficult to draw conclusions about effectiveness, although it appears that the more intensive case management programs that approximate closer to ACT are more effective (Scott & Dixon, 1995b). Studies on the effect of either of these strategies on children and adolescents with schizophrenia are still to be done.

Family interventions

There is a consistent and robust finding that family interventions reduce relapse rates in adults with schizophrenia, at least for 2 years, with some evidence that this effect seems to disappear by 2 years unless the intervention is maintained. There is modest evidence that family interventions may improve patients' overall functioning. Much of the research has been done on high expressed emotion families, and more research is needed to see if findings are more generally applicable and whether some subgroups of patients may do better with one approach than another, as is suggested in some preliminary findings (Dixon & Lehman, 1995). Research in this area is needed to see whether the same can be said for child and adolescent onset schizophrenia.

Psychological interventions

Controlled studies in adult patients are few and mostly have serious method-ological problems, but suggest that reality-oriented approaches are superior to insight-oriented psychotherapies, that social skills training can be effective but may or may not generalize to "real life" environments (Scott & Dixon, 1995a). Studies examining effectiveness of cognitive strategies popular in some places are awaited, as are studies in children and adolescents.

Vocational training

In adults, vocational rehabilitation programs have been shown to have a positive influence on work-related activities, but have not shown substantial and enduring impacts on independent competitive employment. They appear, however, to be superior to transitional and sheltered employment programs (Lehman, 1995). Specific studies relevant to children and adolescents, for example, programs to aid education and return to school or college, appear to have not yet been done.

Summary and conclusions

Research into outcome of early onset schizophrenia

Long-term studies of outcome in child and adolescent schizophrenia are few in number, and those that do exist are beset with problems like retrospective design, poorly defined, varying and incomplete outcome variables. For example, there are no good studies of the impact of medication or other major interventions. Time of follow-up varies, and often is less than that required either for the attainment of a plateau (5–10 years) or slow improvement in end-state (> 10 years). The impact of sociodemographic and cultural and ethnic variables also still needs to be studied.

The conclusions which are offered in this review are necessarily tentative, and it requires a major research effort in the next decade to improve the quality of studies, extend the range of variables examined, and lengthen the duration of follow-up to cover the plateau and improvement phases. The long-term impact of the newer interventions is particularly in need of evaluation, while another area worthy of study is that of the impact of puberty, properly defined in biological not chronological terms, on schizophrenia including its long-term outcome.

To improve method, there is need for a change of emphasis from *ad hoc* retrospective to well-planned prospective studies now increasingly figuring in other areas of child and adolescent psychiatry. There is a need to use quantitative methods in analysis of results, particularly in detecting key predictor variables, evaluating the power of their effects, and separating them out from confounding variables. Because of the small number of available subjects, there is a need for multisite studies.

Summary of findings

The onset and course of child and adolescent schizophrenia probably resembles that in adult schizophrenia with a predominance of the classical three phase (deterioration, plateau and slow improvement), though there are little very long-term data to confirm or deny this, and the wide variability of course in children and adolescents needs to be recognized. It is not clear whether the well-demonstrated ability of modern treatments (especially but not confined to medication) to mitigate symptoms, shorten psychotic episodes and delay or prevent relapse in adults is similarly effective in children and adolescents.

Short-term studies detailed elsewhere in this volume suggest that they should, although relative unresponsiveness to medication has been suggested (though not demonstrated) in children and adolescents (Green et al., 1992).

In general, child and adolescent onset schizophrenia has a worse outcome than in adults, though this appears to be more in the degree of disability than in the rate of recovery. The earlier the onset, the greater the disability. Whether this is due to the effect of a devastating illness on the immature organism disrupting and impeding development in all areas remains to be seen. Certainly, the level of premorbid function is an important determinant. Females have a somewhat better outlook, both because they seem to be less vulnerable to early onset than males and less affected by the illness, though it is not clear that their chance of full recovery is any better. Mortality rates are currently unknown, but there is evidence that suicide is a risk as in adults.

The effect of socioeconomic, cultural and ethnic variables is unstudied and requires attention. There are also no good data on the long-term effect of modern treatment and, though outcome is poor, it may be that some of the modalities known to be effective in the short term are not used widely enough or over a long enough period to make an impact on outcome to date. It is to be hoped that some of the more promising approaches to treatment which have an impact in the short term may be found to improve outcome over a long period. This is not to denigrate, in any way, the known and clear effects on course (as opposed to outcome) – acute psychotic symptoms, distress, and support to families.

Conclusions

Though infrequent in childhood, schizophrenia is a major psychiatric disorder of adolescence. In general, course and outcome studies confirm the hypothesis that the disorder is the same one(s) that affects adults, though the impact is more severe. There is also evidence to support the idea that schizophrenia can be a lifelong insidiously developing or even congenital disorder marked at first by personality and neurodevelopmental abnormalities, and that psychosis occurs usually much later in the illness.

The most striking fact, however, is the paucity of good research and the need to remedy this as soon as possible.

REFERENCES

Alaghband-Rad, J., McKenna, K., Gordon, C.T., Albus, K.E., Hamburger, S.D., Rumsey J.M., Frazier J.A., Lenane, M.C., & Rapoport, J.L. (1995). Childhood-onset schizophrenia: the severity of premorbid course. *Journal of the American Academy of Child and Adolescent Psychiatry*, **34**, 1273–83.

Asarnow, J.R. (1994). Annotation: childhood-onset schizophrenia. *Journal of Child Psychology and Psychiatry*, **35**, 1345–71.

Asarnow, J. R. & Ben-Meir, S. (1988). Children with schizophrenia spectrum and depressive disorders: a comparative study of premorbid adjustment, onset pattern and severity of impairment. *Journal of Child Psychology and Psychiatry*, **29**, 477–88.

Asarnow, J.R., Tompson, M.C., & Goldstein, M.J. (1994). Childhood-onset schizophrenia: a follow-up study. *Schizophrenia Bulletin*, **20**, 599–617.

Beiser, M., Erickson, D., Fleming, J.A.E., & Iacono, W.G. (1993). Establishing the onset of psychotic illness. *American Journal of Psychiatry*, **150**, 1349–1534.

Bilder, R.M., Lipschutz-Broch, L., Reiter, G., Geisler, S.H., Mayeroff, D.L., & Lieberman, J.A. (1992). Intellectual deficits in first-episode schizophrenia: evidence for progressive deterioration. *Schizophrenia Bulletin*, **18**, 437–48.

Bleuler, M. (1978). *The Schizophrenic Disorders: Long-Term Patient and Family Studies*. (Translated by S.M. Clemens). New Haven: Yale University Press.

Breier, A., Schreiber, J.L., Dyer, J., & Pickar, D. (1991). National Institute for Mental Health longitudinal study of chronic schizophrenia: prognosis and predictors of outcome. *Archives of General Psychiatry*, **48**, 239–47.

Cannon-Spoor, H.E., Potkin, S.G., & Wyatt, R.J. (1982). Measurement of premorbid adjustment in chronic schizophrenia. *Schizophrenia Bulletin*, **8**, 470–84.

Caplan, R. (1994). Communication deficits in childhood schizophrenia spectrum disorders. *Schizophrenia Bulletin*, **20**, 671–83.

Cawthron, P., James, A., Dell, J., & Seagroatt, V. (1994). Adolescent onset psychosis. A clinical and outcome study. *Journal of Child Pychology and Psychiatry*, **35**, 1321–32.

Dixon, L.B. & Lehman, A.F. (1995). Family interventions for schizophrenia. *Schizophrenia Bulletin*, **21**, 631–43.

Eggers, C. (1978). Course and prognosis of childhood schizophrenia. *Journal of Autism and Childhood Schizophrenia*, **8**, 21–36.

Eggers, C. (1989). Schizo-affective psychoses in childhood: a follow-up study. *Journal of Autism and Developmental Disorders*, **19**, 327–42.

Eggers, C. & Bunk, D. (1997). The long-term course of early-onset schizophrenia. *Schizophrenia Bulletin*, **23**, 105–18.

Eisenberg, L. (1957). The course of childhood schizophrenia. *AMA Archives of Neurology and Psychiatry*, **78**, 69–83.

Gillberg, Carina., Hellgren, L., & Gillberg, Christopher (1993). Psychotic disorders diagnosed in adolescence. Outcome at age 30 years. *Journal of Child Psychology and Psychiatry*, **34**, 1173–85.

Gold, J.M. & Harvey, P.D. (1993). Cognitive deficits in schizophrenia. *Psychiatric Clinics of North America*, **16**, 295–312.

Green, W H., Padron-Gayol, M., Hardesty, A.S., & Bassiri, M. (1992). Schizophrenia with childhood onset: a phenomenological study of 38 cases. *Journal of the American Academy of Child and Adolescent Psychiatry*, **31**, 968–76.

Haas, G.L. & Sweeney, J.A. (1992). Premorbid and onset features of first episode schizophrenia. *Schizophrenia Bulletin*, **18**, 373–86.

Hollis, C. (1995). Child and adolescent (juvenile onset) schizophrenia: a case control study of premorbid developmental impairments. *British Journal Of Psychiatry*, **166**, 489–95.

Jacobsen, L.K. & Rapoport, J.L. (1998). Childhood onset schizophrenia: implications of clinical and neurobiological research. *Journal of Child Psychology and Psychiatry*, **39**(1), 101–13.

Johnstone, E.C., Frith, C.D., Lang, F.H., & Owens, D.G.C. (1995). Determinants of the extremes of outcome in schizophrenia. *British Journal of Psychiatry*, **167**, 604–9.

Karno, M. & Jenkins, J.H. (1993). Cross-cultural issues in the course and treatment of schizophrenia. *Psychiatric Clinics of North America*, **16**, 339–50.

Kolvin, I. (1971). Studies in the childhood psychoses. I. Diagnostic criteria and classification. *British Journal of Psychiatry*, **118**, 381–4.

Kydd, R.R. & Werry, J.S. (1982). Schizophrenia in children under 16 years. *Journal of Autism and Developmental Disorders*, **12**, 343–57.

Larsen, T.K., McGlashan, T.H., & Moe, L.C. (1996). First-episode schizophrenia: I. Early course parameters. *Schizophrenia Bulletin*, **22**, 241–56.

Lehman, A.F. (1995). Vocational rehabilitation in schizophrenia. *Schizophrenia Bulletin*, **21**, 645–56.

Lehman, A.F., Carpenter, W.T., Goldman, H.H., & Steinwachs, D.M. (1995). Treatment outcomes in schizophrenia: implications for practice, policy and research. *Schizophrenia Bulletin*, **21**, 669–75.

Loebel, A.D., Lieberman, J.A., Alvir, J.M., Mayeroff, D.I., Geisler, S.H., & Szymanski, S.R. (1992). Duration of psychosis and outcome in first-episode schizophrenia. *American Journal of Psychiatry*, **149**, 1183–8.

McGlashan, T.H. & Johannessen (1996). Early detection and intervention with schizophrenia: rationale. *Schizophrenia Bulletin*, **22**, 201–22.

Marengo, J. (1994). Classifying the courses of schizophrenia. *Schizophrenia Bulletin*, **20**, 519–36.

Maziade, M., Gingras, N., Rodrigue, C., Bouchard, S., Cardinal, A., Gauthier, B., Tremblay, G., Cote, S., Fournier, C., Boutin, P., Hamel, M., Roy, M., Martinez, M., & Merette, C. (1996a). Long-term stability of diagnosis and symptom dimensions in a systematic sample of patients with onset of schizophrenia in childhood and early adolescence. 1: Nosology, sex and age of onset. *British Journal of Psychiatry*, **169**, 361–70.

Maziade, M., Bouchard, S., Gingras, N., Charron, L., Cardinal, A., Roy, M., Gauthier, B., Tremblay, G., Cote, S., Fournier, C., Boutin, P., Hamel, M., Merette, C., & Martinez, M. (1996b). Long-term stability of diagnosis and symptom dimensions in a systematic sample of patients with onset of schizophrenia in childhood and early adolescence. 11: Positive/negative distinction and childhood predictors of adult outcome. *British Journal of Psychiatry*, **169**, 371–8.

Murray, R.M., O'Callaghan, E., Castle, D.J., & Lewis SW. (1992). A neurodevelopmental approach to the classification of schizophrenia. *Schizophrenia Bulletin*, **18**, 319–32.

Remschmidt, H., Schulz, E., Martin, M., Warnke, A., & Trott, G. E. (1994). Childhood-onset schizophrenia: history of the concept and recent studies. *Schizophrenia Bulletin*, **20**, 727–45.

Russell, A. T. (1994). The clinical presentation of childhood-onset schizophrenia. *Schizophrenia*

Bulletin, **20**, 631–46.

Russell, A.T., Bott, L., & Sammons, C. (1989). The phenomenology of schizophrenia occurring in childhood. *Journal of American Academy of Child and Adolescent Psychiatry*, **28**, 399–407.

Schmidt, M., Blanz, B., Dippe, A., Koppe, T., & Lay, B. (1995). Course of patients diagnosed as having schizophrenia during first episode occurring under age 18 years. *European Archives of Psychiatry and Clinical Neurosciences*, **245**, 93–100.

Scott, J.E. & Dixon, L.B. (1995a). Psychological interventions for schizophrenia. *Schizophrenia Bulletin*, **21**, 621–30.

Scott, J.E. & Dixon, L.B. (1995b). Assertive community treatment and case management for schizophrenia. *Schizophrenia Bulletin*, **21**, 657–68.

Strandberg, R.J., Marsh, J.T., Brown, W.S., Asarnow, R.F., & Guthrie, D. (1994). Information processing deficits across childhood- and adult-onset schizophrenia. *Schizophrenia Bulletin*, **20**, 685–95.

Strauss, J.S. & Carpenter, W.T. (1974). The prediction of outcome in schizophrenia: 11. Relationships between predictor and outcome variables. *Archives of General Psychiatry*, **31**, 37–42.

Vaillant, G.E. (1978). A 10-year follow-up of remitting schizophrenics. *Schizophrenia Bulletin*, **4**, 78–85.

Watkins, J.M., Asarnow, R.F., & Tanguay, P.E. (1988). Symptom development in childhood onset schizophrenia. *Journal of Child Psychology and Psychiatry*, **29**, 865–78.

Weinberger, D.R. (1987). Implications of normal brain development for the pathogenesis of schizophrenia. *Archives of General Psychiatry*, **44**, 660–9.

Werry, J.S. (1992). Child and adolescent (early onset) schizophrenia: a review in light of DSM-III-R. *Journal of Autism and Developmental Disorders*, **22**, 601–24.

Werry, J.S., McClellan, J.M., & Chard, L. (1991). Childhood and adolescent schizophrenic, bipolar, and schizoaffective disorders: a clinical and outcome study. *Journal of the American Academy of Child and Adolescent Psychiatry*, **30**, 457–65.

Werry, J.S. & McClellan, J.M. (1992). Predicting outcome in child and adolescent (early onset) schizophrenia and bipolar disorder. *Journal of the American Academy of Child and Adolscent Psychiatry*, **31**, 147–50.

Werry, J.S., McClellan, J.M., Andrews, L.K., & Ham, M. (1994). Clinical features and outcome of child and adolescent schizophrenia. *Schizophrenia Bulletin*, **20**, 619–30.

Westermeyer, J.F. & Harrow, M. (1988). Course and outcome in schizophrenia. In: *Handbook of Schizophrenia: Nosology, Epidemiology and Genetics*, Vol. 3, (ed. M.T. Tsuang & J.S. Simpson), pp. 205–44. Amsterdam: Elsevier.

Index